Cesarean Section

Cesarean Section

An American History of Risk, Technology, and Consequence

Jacqueline H. Wolf

Johns Hopkins University Press
Baltimore

Printed in the United States of America on acid-free paper

Johns Hopkins Paperback edition, 2020
9 8 7 6 5 4 3 2 1

Johns Hopkins University Press
2715 North Charles Street
Baltimore, Maryland 21218-4363
www.press.jhu.edu

The Library of Congress has cataloged the hardcover edition of this book as follows:

Names: Wolf, Jacqueline H., author.
Title: Cesarean section : an American history of risk, technology, and consequence / Jacqueline H. Wolf.
Description: Baltimore : Johns Hopkins University Press, 2018. | Includes bibliographical references and index.
Identifiers: LCCN 2017039404 | ISBN 9781421425528 (hardcover : alk. paper) | ISBN 1421425521 (hardcover : alk. paper) | ISBN 9781421425535 (electronic) | ISBN 142142553X (electronic)
Subjects: | MESH: Cesarean Section—history | Risk Assessment | History, 19th Century | History, 20th Century | United States
Classification: LCC RG761 | NLM WQ 11 AA1 | DDC 618.8/6—dc23
LC record available at https://lccn.loc.gov/2017039404

A catalog record for this book is available from the British Library.

ISBN-13: 978-1-4214-3811-5
ISBN-10: 1-4214-3811-9

Special discounts are available for bulk purchases of this book. For more information, please contact Special Sales at specialsales@press.jhu.edu.

Johns Hopkins University Press uses environmentally friendly book materials, including recycled text paper that is composed of at least 30 percent post-consumer waste, whenever possible.

To Cora for the family she has always been to me
and
To Chris for the family he will be to me
and
To the family they will make together

Contents

Cesarean Section

Introduction

From Risk to Remedy

During the 1960 US presidential campaign, the wife of the Democratic candidate was pregnant. Shortly after John F. Kennedy won the election, Jackie Kennedy gave birth to their first son by emergency cesarean section. While the emergency was unexpected, the surgery had long been planned. At the time, the dictum "once a cesarean, always a cesarean" prevailed in American medicine. As someone who had given birth by cesarean previously—to a stillborn daughter in 1956, followed a year later by the now-3-year-old Caroline—Kennedy was subject to that guideline. Thus, from the moment he learned of her latest pregnancy, her obstetrician, John Walsh, had anticipated a third surgery. Originally, Walsh scheduled the surgery for mid-December. When Kennedy began to hemorrhage on November 25, he moved up his plans.[1]

Birth by cesarean section was rare in the United States in 1960, representing fewer than 4 percent of births overall. Doctors performed cesareans so infrequently that a significant number of Americans did not even know the meaning of the term. In the aftermath of John Jr.'s birth, however, few escaped the torrent of information about the surgery. Newspapers and magazines provided explanations of how and why physicians performed cesareans. The birth of John-John, as the president's toddler son quickly came to be known by a smitten citizenry, was one of the first public signs of the normalization of cesarean birth.[2]

Two years after John Jr.'s birth, Jackie Kennedy was pregnant again, and her obstetrician planned another cesarean. For a second time, the press used one of her pregnancies to demystify and destigmatize the surgery. *Time* magazine likened the operation to a wholesome athletic event, assuring Americans that having multiple cesarean sections was "hardly more dangerous" than the president's well-publicized 50-mile hikes. Another article informed women that the drugs doctors routinely administered during labor to ease pain posed a greater threat to maternal and infant health than cesarean surgery. Cesarean section was to be neither dreaded nor feared. If the first lady of the United States needed one, anyone might.[3]

The newfound acceptance of the surgery was short-lived, however. On August 7, 1963, the Kennedys' second son, Patrick, was born via emergency cesarean almost six weeks before his due date. Weighing only 4 pounds 10½ ounces, and suffering from hyaline membrane disease, Patrick lived less than two days. Every detail of her baby's brief life and death was so widely reported that Jackie Kennedy complained that the press had turned her family's personal tragedy into "a theatrical production."[4]

While the birth of John F. Kennedy, Jr., sparked greater public and medical acceptance of cesarean surgery, the death of his younger brother seemed to highlight its dangers. *Newsweek* noted that while Patrick Kennedy's death had been traumatic for the entire nation, "it will have a special trepidation for the 200,000 American women who each year are delivered of babies by Caesarean section." Indeed, the Kennedy baby's death had such a profound effect on such a vast audience that it spurred scientists to discover the cause of, and develop a cure for, hyaline membrane disease. Patrick Kennedy has since been credited for saving more lives than any other child in history, a claim that perhaps mitigated Jackie Kennedy's understandably distraught reaction to the relentless publicity surrounding his death.[5]

The starkly opposing views of cesarean surgery engendered by the very different outcomes of the Kennedy sons' births reflected the two traditional, contradictory perceptions of cesareans in US history. Throughout the nineteenth century, and into the early decades of the twentieth, the vast majority of American doctors termed cesarean surgery death-dealing; only a slim minority viewed it as potentially life-saving. Patrick's birth harkened back to the old fear and discomfort, while John's birth represented the relaxed attitude toward the surgery that would prevail 20 years after his birth. The two births thus became a fault line between the trepidation, even horror, that was common before World War II if physicians faced the possibility of cesarean surgery and the surgery's post-1980 normalization, when doctors were often relieved to be able to perform a cesarean section and avoid what they, and increasingly their patients, perceived as the discomfiting vagaries of vaginal birth. While before the 1970s doctors and their patients almost always saw the risk as being inherent in the surgery itself, in the 1980s and after, the risk seemed to be in not performing the surgery.[6]

The change in attitude and practice—although long in the making, as this book will demonstrate—seemed to occur rapidly. Between 1965 and 1987, the cesarean section rate in the United States rose 455 percent—from 4.5 percent to 25 percent of births. Today, the rate is considerably higher—almost one in three births is by cesarean. Once among the most vilified and scrupulously avoided surgeries, by the early twenty-first century, cesarean section, at almost 1.4 million in 2010, had become the most commonly performed surgical procedure in the country. This book, a study of the medical, historical, cultural, social, political, and economic factors that reframed the meaning of risk in relation to both cesarean birth and vaginal birth, is an examination of how and why that happened.[7]

A cesarean birth, particularly today when effective means of ensuring surgical safety are a given in industrialized countries, is at times appropriate and necessary. In cases of cord prolapse, placenta previa, placental abruption, and persistent transverse lie of the fetus, the procedure can be life-saving. These life-threatening conditions are rare, however. Each occurs in considerably fewer than 1 percent of births. In contrast, there are abundant reasons to anticipate that a birth is likely to go well: 99 percent of the time there is only one fetus in the womb, 97 percent of infants deliver headfirst, and 97 percent of fetuses have no major structural or genetic abnormalities. Thus, today, cesareans seem to be occurring far more often than is medically necessary. The World Health Organization (WHO) has for many years contended that the optimal cesarean rate is between 10 and 15 percent of births, that new studies reveal cesarean rates higher than 10 percent are not associated with reductions in maternal and neonatal mortality at the population level, and that any rate above 15 percent is more likely to do harm than good given the maternal and neonatal side effects long associated with the surgery.[8]

As the WHO asserts, medical records across time indicate that, on average, only about 5 percent of human births run into trouble when labor begins spontaneously. A midwife with a large practice in the late eighteenth century classified 5.6 percent of the births that she attended as "difficult." Joseph DeLee, a Chicago obstetrician now often referred to as "the father of modern obstetrics," estimated that, left to its own devices, childbirth "would be natural, would be spontaneous" in all but 5 percent of cases. A study of maternal mortality in New York City published by the New York Academy of Medicine in 1933 made the identical claim;

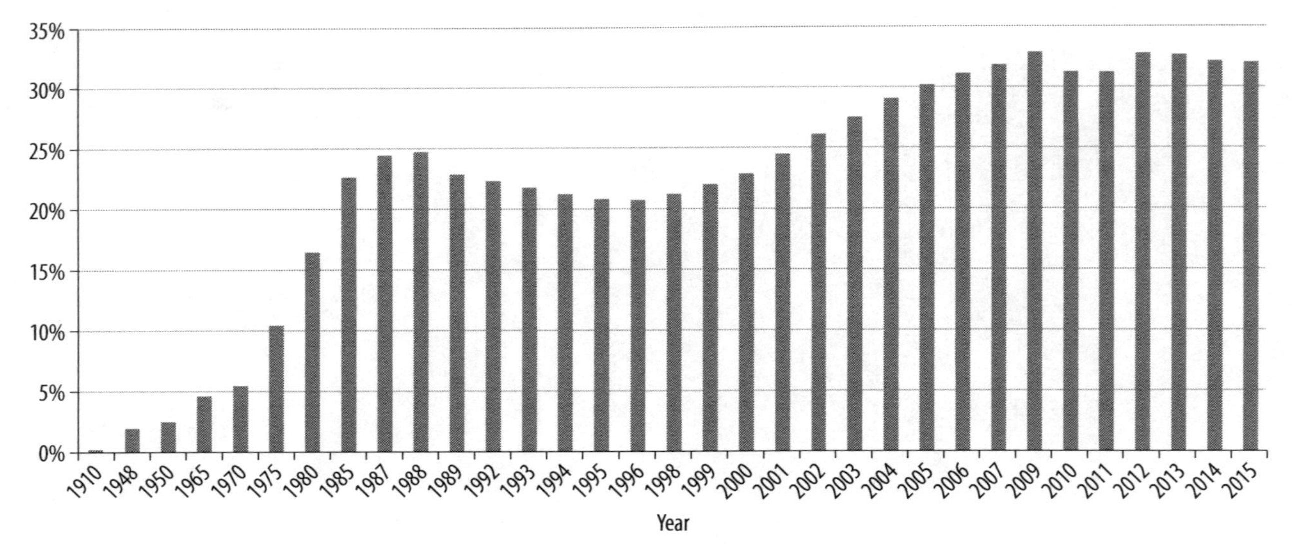

Cesarean section rates in the United States, 1910–2015. The rates rose 455 percent between 1965 and 1987. The rate reached its high point, 32.9 percent, in 2009. The most recently available data are for 2015, when 31.9 percent of births were by cesarean.

Sources: See note 7 of the introduction for several contemporary sources and note 1 of chapter 3 for assorted sources for the first half of the twentieth century. Other figures collected from the ACOG Resource Center, for 1970 to 1985: MMWR 42(15), table 1; 1995: MVSR 45(11 Supp), table 39; 1996: MVSR 46(11 Supp), table 39; 1998: NVSR 48(3), table 39; 1999: NVSR 49(1), table 39; 2000: NVSR 50(5), table 39; 2001: NVSR 51(2), table 39; 2002: NVSR 52(10), table 39; 2003: NVSR 54(2), table 39; 2004: NVSR 54(8), table E. All years after 2004 are CDC data.

the optimum rate of "operative interference"—a reference most often in that era, when the cesarean rate was barely 1 percent, to the use of forceps—was generally accepted to be about 5 percent. In other words, according to both the contemporary WHO appraisal and historical evidence, in the early 1950s, after antibiotics and blood transfusions became available to the public, obstetricians probably kept the cesarean section rate—then about 2.5 percent—too low. Consensus among physicians' professional organizations today is that the 32 percent rate in the United States is too high.[9]

Even as physicians began to resort more often to the surgery beginning in the 1920s, skilled obstetricians continued to take pride in their ability to avoid a cesarean, even in the face of imminent need. Obstetricians described the expertise that allowed them to circumvent invasive treatments as "conservative obstetrics"; the phrase signified high praise. As J. Whitridge Williams, head of the Department of Obstetrics at Johns Hopkins University, admonished his students in 1926: "any one with two hands and a few instruments can do a cesarean section, but . . . it frequently requires great intelligence not to do it."[10]

Today, conservative obstetricians do the opposite: They perform a cesarean in the face of even niggling doubt about a birth's outcome. One typical obstetrician, who graduated from medical school in 1991, explained why she always errs on the side of cesarean birth. Just as doctors once feared performing a cesarean, she fears not performing one "and have it be a bad outcome because then everybody loses on that one. Right?" While doctors once viewed cesarean section as the riskiest of obstetric procedures, today vaginal birth represents the risk. The physician's query—"everybody loses on that one. Right?"—implies that a cesarean is more likely to result in a good outcome than a vaginal birth, even if the vaginal birth in question poses only minor difficulties.[11]

Patients have changed their attitude toward cesarean section alongside doctors. While women who gave birth by cesarean section in the 1970s tended to be unprepared for, and long resentful of, their experience, beginning in the mid-1980s women who gave birth by cesarean more often expressed the belief that their cesarean, as a methodical surgical procedure, assured a better outcome. One woman, who gave birth to her first child in 1996 by a planned cesarean due to what her doctor told her were "very small pelvic bones," was typical in that she was grateful to her doctor for scheduling what she perceived to be a prophylactic surgery. She is certain that a century earlier, when she would have had little choice but to give birth vaginally, she would have been "one of those women who . . . died in childbirth." The interconnected messages that there are risks inherent in vaginal birth and that cesarean section provides an assuredly safe avenue no matter the circumstance have served to normalize the surgery.[12]

Perceived risk, however, is not risk. A high cesarean rate not only fails to mitigate risk at the population level, it is risky in and of itself. Full-term infants delivered by cesarean despite no medical need have a death rate almost three times their vaginally born counterparts. Their morbidity rates are higher too. One of the many ways that vaginal birth benefits the neonate is by removing amniotic fluid from the lungs; the slow, tight squeeze through the birth canal is of value to the neonatal pulmonary bed. In contrast, infants surgically removed from the uterus are at an immediate disadvantage. They are born with lungs full of amniotic fluid. Wet lung at birth can have lifelong effect—children born by cesarean section have higher rates of asthma. Infants born by cesarean also are deprived of exposure to their mothers' vaginal flora, which in a vaginal birth colonizes the neonatal gut, crowding out harmful bacteria in the first months of life. After a cesarean birth, on the other hand, the aberrant colonization of the neonatal gut persists for up to six months; researchers have connected the lack of exposure to mothers' vaginal microbiome to a higher incidence of allergic disorders throughout life. A high cesarean rate has nationwide economic costs too: a cesarean surgery with no complications costs twice as much as a vaginal birth.[13]

Mothers' health is also affected detrimentally. The risk of postpartum infection after a cesarean is nearly fivefold that of vaginal birth. Even when all goes well, births by cesarean section result in longer recovery times and greater and lengthier postpartum discomfort. Worst are the downstream effects. In subsequent pregnancies, the likelihood of stillbirth, placental anomalies, and uterine rupture increases with each cesarean. Thus, a cesarean, so often described as a life-saving measure during one birth, increases the chances of serious, even life-threatening, conditions in later births. Of particular concern to obstetricians today is the increase in the United States of placenta accreta—a condition in which the placenta grows into the uterine wall and will not release after birth, often because it has grown into the scar from a previous cesarean. In the 1950s, accretas occurred in fewer than 1 in 30,000 births; by 1980 the rate was 1 in 2,500. Today, 1 in 533 births sees an accreta—a 55-fold increase in 60 years. The life-threatening condition portends massive maternal blood loss. To staunch the hemorrhage, doctors almost always remove the uterus. Worse, maternal mortality in the face of an accreta is as high as 7 percent. One obstetrician, in connecting a cesarean section today "to the complications [of] tomorrow," described a mother who had recently given birth at his hospital and died shortly after due to postpartum hemorrhage caused by placenta accreta: "72 units of blood, the entire hospital stopped."[14]

If more births by cesarean have not resulted in improved maternal and neonatal outcomes, then what factors prompted (and over time sustained) the relatively recent surge in the cesarean rate? Physiological and demographic change (such as the increase in the incidence of maternal obesity, more mothers giving birth to multiples due to fertility treatments, and the higher incidence of women over 30 giving birth for the first time) account for only a small portion of the rise. I argue that the increase has been driven less by medical need and more by change in American society and American medical culture in the last quarter of the twentieth century, changes that created the perception that vaginal birth is risky and that cesarean section serves as its infallible guardrail. Salient influences in the medical culture have included new diagnostic tools that redefined "normal" labor and birth, the vagaries of American healthcare financing, a series of medical malpractice "crisis points," changes in the training of obstetric residents, and the enormous increase in female obstetricians. In the culture at large, faith in medical technology, the American penchant for scheduling and time-keeping, and the sweeping change in women's lives beginning in the 1970s converged with the changes in medical culture to normalize cesarean section and pathologize vaginal birth.

The Ever-Changing Meaning of Risk

Tying together these disparate influences is the concept of risk—actual risk, perceived risk, fear of risk, the desire to control risk, the use of risk to persuade patients, and the ever-changing meaning of risk. The paradox today is that despite living in a sanitized society and enjoying unprecedentedly long and comparatively healthy lives, Americans perceive risk as looming large in everyday life. The unrelenting media focus on the Ebola outbreak in West Africa in 2014 and its "threat" to the United States is one example. Although doctors treated only 11 cases of Ebola in the United States between August 2014 and March 2015—and only 2 of those 11 cases were contracted within the country—coverage of Ebola was close to nonstop on 24-hour news stations throughout the fall, prompting one comedian to observe wryly, "Fortunately, folks, for every medical professional out there reassuring us, there's a TV professional re-scaring us." The specter of risk is so easily conjured today that, no matter how inflated or improbable a health risk might be, many Americans are willing to accept measures that can include expensive monitoring, testing, or prophylactic treatment, all with potential side effects, to ward off the insignificant threat.[15]

Alleviating risk has become a particularly pronounced focus of contemporary medicine. Indeed, some of the medical treatments prescribed most often in the United States today are not designed to ease symptoms but to reduce risk. Treating high cholesterol with powerful drugs that are prescribed for life is one example. Since the notion of "modifiable risk" has become mainstream, and medication has made cholesterol levels modifiable, high cholesterol has come to be viewed as a greater de facto threat than the side effects of cholesterol-lowering drugs. Now that physicians have come to define an unhealthy state according to how much a level of something—cholesterol, serotonin, or Vitamin D, for example—deviates from a predetermined norm, asymptomatic individuals become perpetual patients.[16]

Childbirth has not been impervious to the modern-day medical propensity to measure bodily functions against a standard and offer treatment when the patient deviates from the standard. As just one example, since the 1950s, if any segment of labor takes much longer than the Friedman curve indicates it should, then an obstetrician diagnoses dystocia; today the treatment for dystocia is often cesarean section. This contrasts sharply with the early part of the twentieth century, when dystocia was a rare, life-threatening condition. Physicians defined it as blocked labor, often caused by a sizeable tumor in the uterus or birth canal. After Emanuel Friedman formulated his graphic curve indicating how long a "normal" labor should last, however, "dystocia" came to have a broader meaning—a labor that had strayed outside the temporal parameters of the Friedman curve. Given its new meaning, labor dystocia became such a frequent diagnosis that today it is the number-one indication for a primary cesarean section. Yet critics of the high cesarean rate dismiss the diagnosis as largely meaningless—"vague," "non-diagnostic," and "catch-all."[17]

Of all the normal physiological conditions to be treated medically in the last seven decades, pregnancy and childbirth have arguably prompted the creation and use of the most diagnostic tools leading to treatment; the Friedman curve is only one of many. In his examination of American obstetricians' unremitting focus on risk during prenatal care visits, one physician criticized this tendency to overdiagnose and overtreat. In a book, cleverly titled *Expecting Trouble*, he observed that, in the United States, pregnant women are instructed to see their obstetricians for prenatal exams an average of 13 to 14 times, as opposed to mothers in Switzerland (5 times), France (6 times), and Denmark (8 times), where infant and maternal mortality rates are far lower than in the United States despite the comparatively lax surveillance of pregnancies. Overtreatment becomes even more conspicuous during childbirth—the cesarean section rate in the United States is only one example. One group of academics (a mix of obstetricians, ethicists, sociologists, and anthropologists) recently argued that during childbirth in the United States, medical interventions are so frequent, and so seldom questioned, that they continue to be used even when studies show they do not work. They cite two oppositional historical themes as the source of this tendency—"purity in pregnancy," when drugs tend to be avoided even at the risk of maternal health, and "control in birth," when medical interventions are used "unreflectively" to deflect "*any* risk to the fetus, however small or theoretical." Both proclivities, these researchers contend, "can lead to reasoning about risk that is oriented more by magical thinking than evidence."[18]

While the consequences of ignoring a bona fide health threat are usually obvious, the ramifications of exaggerating threats are less so. Yet medical overtreatment—defined as a medication, diagnostic scan, or procedure that does more harm than good—has become increasingly common in our risk-averse society. As just one admittedly contentious example of overtreatment, the US Preventive Services Task Force (USPSTF) has warned since 2009 that low-risk women should not have a mammogram before age 50, and after that only biannually. The USPSTF explains that an annual mammogram, particularly beginning at 40, encourages false positives that lead to unnecessary biopsies and the treatment of conditions—such as intraductal carcinoma in situ—that are highly unlikely to become invasive cancers. Some of the treatments for intraductal carcinoma in situ, such as tamoxifen, can themselves increase the risk of cancer.[19]

Yet today medical and lay thinking in the United States lean toward the aphorism, the more medicine, the better the outcome. And in the case of childbirth, popular and medical thought seem to suggest, contrary to the facts, that the higher the cesarean rate, the better off infants and mothers will be. It is a difficult notion to shake. The medical model of birth requires obstetricians to assign a risk category to all pregnant women, ensuring that even the most robust women will view themselves as trouble-prone. After all, the most desirable pregnancy category, "low-risk," still implies the potential for problems rather than the overwhelming likelihood of smooth sailing.[20]

The concept of risk as currently understood in English is relatively new. Derived from the French word *risqué*, the word first appeared in its Anglicized form in the early nineteenth century to describe a gamble made after considering all potential gains and losses. Thus, in its original sense, "risk" implied neutrality—the likely outcome in a given situation. Today, the term has an unambiguously negative connotation—the likelihood of an undesirable result in light of a potential threat. One sociologist has argued that this change in emphasis ensures a "mixed-up perception of risk" that permeates American culture. Magnifying the danger of an exceedingly rare event, such as the chance of being sickened by Ebola while going through the motions of daily living in an American city or town, exemplifies this muddled view.[21]

Another sociologist contends that the public's perception of risk has been similarly inflated by the forensic use of risk. When authorities employ risk retrospectively to explain a calamity, those experts mean to invoke risk in a reassuring way—to predict the likelihood of disaster if the scenario is ever repeated. Yet in alerting the public to danger in order to diminish the sense of danger, pundits unintentionally magnify minor threats. With constant attention being drawn to risk, Americans feel perpetually vulnerable, even in a largely safe society.[22]

Whether individuals are in control of a situation also influences their perception of risk. When participating in voluntary activities, such as smoking or eating fast food, people tend to dismiss even significant threats. Involuntary circumstances, however, such as polluted air or loose bricks tumbling from buildings, draw ire. In the words of Chauncey Starr, a physicist and expert in risk analysis, "we are loath to let others do unto us what we happily do to ourselves." Other scholars have argued that individuals are especially likely to accept any risk associated with medical procedures—such as a diagnostic scan, prescription drug, or surgery—because medicine is intended to benefit us, in theory if not always in reality.[23]

Cesarean section, then, is subject to a double whammy—both the illusion that it confers a measure of control to the individual and the fact that it is a medical procedure make the surgery uniquely vulnerable to "mixed-up perception of risk." Since the 1990s, obstetricians have increasingly framed cesarean section as a voluntary activity (because, some argue, the patient should have the right to choose a cesarean birth—CDMR, cesarean delivery upon maternal request, has become a recognized medical acronym) and also as a beneficial treatment (because the implicit message is that agreeing to the surgery ensures a good outcome, while refusing the surgery courts disaster). As lay and medical publications increasingly portray vaginal birth as a dangerously unpredictable avenue into the world, cesarean section has become the antidote—a presumably methodical, controlled, and controllable path to an assuredly healthy mother and baby.[24]

Location, Location, Location

Initially, the increase in cesarean birth that began in the United States in the late 1960s was unique in the world, and that singularity persisted for almost two decades. In the mid-1980s, the *New England Journal of Medicine* reported that, among 19 industrialized countries, the US had a rate 50 to 200 percent higher than any other country except Canada and Australia. Since then, other countries have also seen significant increases. In fact, a few developing countries have surpassed the US rate; in the mid-1980s, Brazil's c-section rate was the first to outstrip the US rate, which, at 22.7 percent, was considered inordinately high at the time.[25]

As a sizeable segment of any healthcare system, maternity care is impacted by economic and political pressures. And because obstetrics, more than any other medical specialty except plastic surgery, is consumer-driven, birth practices also can be a bellwether for the changing role of women in society, attitudes toward medical technology, public and medical perceptions of health and illness, and the value a culture accords women and children. Separately and together, these factors help shape the definition of "normal" birth. The effect of this array of forces becomes especially clear through a cursory examination of the cesarean rates in countries other than the United States—namely, the Netherlands, Brazil, China, and the United Kingdom.

Largely because birth outcomes have been so much better in the Netherlands than in the United States, the Dutch experience provides a particularly compelling example of the role of perceived risk in increasing cesarean rates. Today, the Dutch infant mortality rate is half the American rate; at less than one-quarter the American rate, maternal mortality is even more impressive. Due to its strikingly good outcomes, the Dutch midwifery system has become the model that American midwives and some childbirth educators point to when making a case for the normalcy and safety of vaginal birth. Yet even in the Netherlands, the cesarean section rate has risen. In 1986, at 6.6 percent, the Netherlands had one of the lowest rates in the world. The rate has been increasing ever since—to 8.2 percent in 1992 and 13.5 percent in 2002. Today, the rate is 17 percent.[26]

Although the Dutch rate is still only slightly more than half the American rate, this steady upward trend in the Netherlands belies the country's prevailing obstetric philosophy and practice. Dutch midwives, not obstetricians, are the medical gatekeepers for all pregnant women; midwives send their patients to an obstetrician only if a medical condition warrants a referral. Birth is considered such a nonthreatening event that midwife-attended home births are common—midwives attend 70 percent of births in the Netherlands, and 60 percent of the births they attend take place in the home. Nevertheless, even in the Netherlands the association between perceived risk and vaginal birth (and by implication cesarean section and safety) seems to be making an inroad.[27]

Birth in Brazil exemplifies another cultural phenomenon—that a woman's class shapes lay and medical notions of appropriate obstetric care and "normal" and "necessary" medical interventions. The overall cesarean section rate in Brazil today, at 54 percent, is among the highest in the world but is far higher at private, as opposed to public, hospitals: 84 versus 40 percent. Indeed, the rate is so high in Brazil's private hospitals—institutions frequented by the affluent—that vaginal birth is effectively unknown in those facilities. If a woman giving birth in a private hospital wants a vaginal birth, she must doggedly seek and retain a *parteiro*—the rare obstetrician who supports and promotes vaginal birth. Roughly translated as "male midwife," *parteiro* implies low professional status. Desire for midwives is a rarity in Brazil today, and use of this pejorative maintains the status quo.[28]

Even as the culture denigrates vaginal birth, the Brazilian lay and medical communities literally celebrate cesarean births. Middle- and upper-class women begin early in their pregnancies to plan for a cesarean as if for a wedding, choreographing the components of their birth as they plan for the requisite birth video. The Brazilian cesarean video has become so essential an element of childbirth that private hospitals devote an entire wing of their maternity wards to a film department. Rather than the impromptu, homemade affairs common in the United States, the Brazilian birth video is months in the making and correspondingly costly.[29]

During their pregnancies, women consult with the secretary of their hospital's film department to select the music, fonts, backgrounds, colors, captions, voiceovers, and animated characters (a stork is a favorite) to frequent the film. Women also preselect the video's before- and after-birth shots. The hospital exterior is one of several popular before-birth shots. The baby sleeping peacefully in the nursery and the grinning father are the two most common finales. Because their cesareans are filmed for posterity, women prepare for the surgery as they would any important social event—getting their hair and nails done and their bodies waxed before checking into the hospital. In describing her birth from start to finish, one Brazilian woman began by describing her visit to the salon. "I had to look good for the film, right?" she explained. "I had to be beautiful to receive a beautiful baby." Brazil's experience with cesarean section seems to indicate that once a certain threshold has been reached, both doctors and their patients normalize cesarean birth so fully that exalted cultural rituals and high social status become associated with the surgery, further marginalizing vaginal birth.[30]

China offers a different lesson—that economic and regional pressures shape medical treatment. Between 1988 and 2008, the cesarean section rate increased in China even more dramatically than it did in the United States between 1965 and 1987. China's overall rate went from 3.4 percent in 1988 to 39.3 percent in 2008; in urban areas, at 64.1 percent, the rate rivaled Brazil's.[31]

The initial increase coincided with the second of four incarnations of the Chinese healthcare system after the Chinese civil war ended in 1949. After 35 years of experimentation with government-owned and -operated health facilities, China's conversion to a market economy in 1984 encompassed the healthcare sector. Government funds allocated to hospitals decreased, and most healthcare organizations became for-profit institutions. But to ensure all citizens retained access to basic care, the Chinese government set limits on the prices doctors and nurses could charge for their services. The government was far more generous, however, with the pricing of drugs and technical services; doctors responded to their salary loss by increasing prescriptions, laboratory tests, and medical procedures, including cesarean sections. Although by 2008, the Chinese government recognized the shortcomings of the market-driven healthcare system and instituted government-subsidized health insurance, some effects of the short-lived, market-driven experiment lingered, including a high cesarean section rate.[32]

Regional differences have also influenced the cesarean rate in China—unsurprising in a country of more than 1.3 billion people occupying a diverse landmass. Indeed, in China, a factor more potent than social class, ability to pay, or educational level in determining the odds of giving birth by cesarean is place of residence. The urban/rural divide is most predictive—urban women, even with a low level of education, have a much higher cesarean rate than their rural counterparts. As in Brazil and the United States, the Chinese experience also seems to indicate that the more cesareans doctors perform, the likelier patients are to anticipate cesarean birth as routine. The geographic angle, too, holds a lesson for the US, where the cesarean rate varies dramatically on a macro level, from region to region, and on the micro level, from hospital to hospital within the same region.[33]

Controversy over the cesarean rate in the United Kingdom demonstrates another propensity in medicine: that in a conflict between health economics and cultural preferences, cultural preferences generally prevail. As the cesarean section rate rose in the UK, the National Health Service (NHS) ruled that only medically necessary cesareans would be permitted in NHS hospitals. This did not sit well with some women, who responded with an orchestrated, well-publicized protest against the guideline, accusing NHS administrators of infringing on their right to choose how they would give birth. Newspapers and magazines satirized the controversy by describing protestors as "too posh to push." In reaction to the kerfuffle, the NHS withdrew its mandate in 2011 and granted women the right to give birth by cesarean section even in the absence of medical need. Today, between 25 and 30 percent of the 700,000 annual births in the United Kingdom are by cesarean. The NHS estimated that obstetricians performed one-third of those cesareans due to maternal request, at an estimated excess cost of £1,000 each.[34]

The controversy in the United Kingdom has continued. The National Institute for Health and Care Excellence (NICE) issued guidelines, updated in 2016, urging low-risk pregnant women to consider giving birth either at home or in a "midwifery-led unit" because rates of medical intervention were lower in those locales and saw outcomes similar to hospitals'. What that advisory will mean for the cesarean section rate is unclear, however. But as the experiences of all these countries indicate, cultural, economic, political, and geographic trends shape cesarean birth practices at least as much as, and often more than, medical need.[35]

Looking only at the numbers, the rise in the cesarean section rate in the United States appears to have begun in earnest in the late 1960s. Yet the forces driving the dramatic change in the experience of childbirth coalesced long before that. The complex trajectory of the story began in 1827, when the first description of a cesarean performed by a physician in the United States appeared in a medical journal, and is likely far from over. Today, with childbirth the leading cause of hospital admission in the United States and the costliest component of health-care spending, the story is especially relevant. A history of cesarean section contributes to our understanding of how physicians formulate diagnoses, why some medical treatments come to the fore as others retreat, and how the public comes to view treatments, even major surgical procedures that were once marginal practices, as both standard and beneficial.[36]

I organize the book chronologically, with chapters overlapping somewhat in time. Each chapter centers on the medical and public perception of childbirth-related risks during the era under examination, the social and medical forces shaping those perceptions, and the effect of those perceptions on the use of cesarean surgery. The book begins in the early nineteenth century and ends with descriptions of the cultural forces buffeting obstetricians' contemporary use of cesareans (chapter 6) and women's experience of and attitudes toward cesarean section since the 1970s (chapter 7). Chapter 2 describes physicians' struggle in the early twentieth century to determine appropriate indications for cesareans. Chapter 3 examines the public's growing understanding of cesarean section, as magazines and newspapers began to run articles on the surgery—some macabre, others sensationalist, still others strictly educational—beginning in the 1930s. Chapters 4 and 5 describe the effect of assorted diagnostic tools, developed in the 1950s and 1960s, on mothers' and obstetricians' perceptions of the risks of childbirth in general and cesarean section in particular. Chapter 5 also describes women's orchestrated reaction, picking up speed in the early 1970s, to obstetric treatments that they argued had become mechanized and inhumane. So as not to disrupt the narrative flow, I do not define medical terms as I use them. Instead, a comprehensive glossary appears at the end of the book.

Since 1996, I have conducted dozens of oral history interviews with physicians who performed cesarean sections and with mothers who had them. These mothers and doctors represent several generations; the doctors interviewed were trained anywhere between the late 1930s and the 2010s, the mothers gave birth by cesarean between the early 1970s and the 2010s. Some of the interviewees reside in a major urban area—Chicago—and others in a rural area—southern Ohio. Their tales enliven this book and substantiate archival evidence. If I use names for any of the mothers and physicians—and I name mothers far more often than I do physicians because mothers' stories tend to be longer and more involved—the names are pseudonyms due to Ohio University Institutional Review Board requirements. Reflecting the American cultural deference to doctors and the power differential between physicians and their patients, I refer to mothers using a first name and physicians using a last name.

Readers will discover that physicians' voices and stories are far more pervasive than mothers' in the first four chapters. Historians can do no more than unearth and examine the evidence. Although there are many records in diaries and letters of women's personal experiences of vaginal birth from earlier eras, cesarean surgery was so rare before the 1970s that, even if women did undergo the surgery, there are neither archival nor published sources describing the experience from their point of view. Consequently, I could only extrapolate women's experiences before the late 1960s from physicians' reports. Beginning in the early 1970s, however, as the cesarean rate increased precipitously, the voices of women who experienced the surgery become plentiful and strong.

While the factors contributing to today's cesarean rate are numerous and complex, it is obvious why physicians made a concerted effort to keep the rate low before World War II. They had no way of adequately treating the most common side effects of cesarean surgery, infection and hemorrhage. Without antibiotics and the ability to store and transfuse blood, a cesarean was customarily riskier than whatever condition prompted a physician to contemplate performing one. After those treatments became available, the average nationwide cesarean rate rose slightly—to 2.5 percent of births. In other words, the rate increased—from negligible to measurable—in the immediate aftermath of World War II for medically justifiable reasons. What is less clear is why the surgery became, by the first decade of the twenty-first century, the most commonly performed surgery in the United States. That the dramatic increase did not occur until 30 years after cesareans had become dramatically safer suggests that today's high rate is attributable to something other than medical need. This exploration of the historical emergence of cesarean section as a routine medical intervention is an examination of the factors that undermined what is customarily a prerequisite for any medical treatment, especially a treatment with as many side effects as cesarean section: an evidence-based foundation for its frequency. As readers will discover, the story is riddled with ironies—unsurprising when the tale being told is how the most dreaded and denounced of all surgeries in one era became the most commonly performed surgery in another.[37]

Chapter One

The Epitome of Risk

Cesarean Sections in the Nineteenth Century

In 1827 John L. Richmond performed a cesarean section in a tiny town in the southwest corner of Ohio. His harrowing account of the surgery—the first published account of a cesarean section performed by a physician in the United States—appeared in the *Western Journal of the Medical and Physical Sciences* three years later. While Richmond's experience typified doctors' encounters with the surgery later in the century in many respects, the case veered from the nineteenth-century norm in three crucial ways. The operation occurred in the northern, not the southern, United States; the patient was white; and she survived.[1]

Other than those anomalies, over the next seven decades, cesarean surgeries were strikingly like the one documented by Richmond. The setting for the surgery was far from ideal—Richmond arrived at the laboring woman's house during a violent storm, just as night fell. He noted that the woman's bleak home, with its dirt floor and gaping crevices in the logs that constituted walls, would likely compound the daunting task before him. He immediately exhibited impatience with the midwives who had summoned him, complaining that the two women were unable to provide useful answers to his questions. The paltry information they did supply—that the patient "had fits and the pains did no good"—provided nothing useful to help Richmond establish a diagnosis and formulate a treatment.[2]

During his initial examination, Richmond was unable to find any sign of cervical dilation. The discovery baffled him. The patient seemed to be in the throes of a shockingly strenuous labor. Each contraction culminated in three- to five-minute "general convulsions" followed by "alarming faintings" lasting 10 to 20 minutes. To tame the convulsions, Richmond administered laudanum and sulphuric ether and applied "flannel wet with hot spirits" to the patient's feet. While the treatments eased the convulsions, they increased the fainting spells.[3]

After four hours of futile attempts to trigger productive labor, Richmond still had not pinpointed the source of the problem. Unconsciously mimicking the action of the midwives he had ridiculed hours earlier, he sent for additional help. The help never arrived. The fierce storm prevented his colleagues from making their way to the cabin. The patient's obesity compounded the mounting difficulties.[4]

Eventually, Richmond decided the woman's life was likely lost. Only a cesarean section offered a slim hope for survival. He shared his conclusion with everyone present: the exhausted, semiconscious patient, the midwives, and the friends and family members who had convened at the patient's bedside. Everyone agreed to the plan. As the storm continued unabated, "feeling a deep and solemn sense of my responsibility, with only a case of common pocket instruments," Richmond commenced the operation with "an incision through the integuments, down to the *linea alba* from the umbilicus, to within an inch and a half of the pubis." The woman's friends helped by holding blankets in front of candles to prevent the howling wind from leaving the surgical scene in total darkness.[5]

Richmond was momentarily heartened when the patient's convulsions ceased during the surgery. Then he encountered another problem. The infant was so "uncommonly large" that no amount of force permitted extraction. In a final attempt to remove the child intact through the uterine incision, he passed his hand around the baby's body to grab the feet. The mother begged him to stop. She could not endure the pain. Reminding himself that "a childless mother [is] better [off] than a motherless child," Richmond altered course and proceeded to remove the fetus in pieces from the wound in the mother's abdomen.[6]

As Richmond's account attests, his patient suffered during the surgery; the discovery of anesthesia was still two decades away. Although there is no record of the ordeal from the patient's perspective, a letter written by another surgical patient, who underwent not a cesarean but an oophorectomy in 1844, suggests how a woman undergoing surgery without anesthesia, and surviving, might recall the experience. Forty-nine years after the removal of her ovaries, Catharine E. Reitzel wrote a letter to the son of her surgeon, John L. Atlee. She praised Atlee as "the happy instrument in the hands of the Almighty" and expressed gratitude for the surgery and Atlee's skill: "Had I never fallen into his hands I would long since have passed to that . . . whence no traveller returns . . . . I am glad that I submitted to the dangerous and painful ordeal . . . . Your father's invaluable services can never be erased from the tablet of my memory while memory lasts."[7]

According to Richmond, his patient was similarly stoic after her surgery. During the "whole course of the cure," she never complained. Richmond visited her regularly, draining and cleaning her wound, and periodically infusing saline into her rectum to induce bowel movements. Twenty-four days after the surgery, she returned to work. Two weeks after returning to work, she took a lengthy walk. After she healed, Richmond examined her thoroughly and discovered an abnormally shallow vagina with no discernable cervical opening. He ended his account wondering how she had conceived a child in the first place.[8]

A Lengthy Process Demanding Patience

Richmond's report did not garner significant notice. Few physicians exhibited interest in cesarean surgery, other than as a curiosity, largely because it ran counter to medical ethos. Early-nineteenth-century obstetric texts counseled physicians to refrain from interfering with the birth process, warning that medical intervention heightened risk rather than mitigated it. Birth was a lengthy process demanding patience, and doctors' forbearance was generally rewarded with a living mother and a living child. Medical meddling, on the other hand, often saw deadly results.[9]

Because of poor or nonexistent training, few physicians attended births anyway, leaving the normally mundane process to midwives. Medical educators considered childbirth so routine that the vast majority of medical schools did not offer even rudimentary education in that area. Thus, the average doctor did not know what to do at an uneventful birth, let alone a difficult one. Before 1831, the medical school affiliated with the University of Pennsylvania specifically stipulated that it was unnecessary to amass knowledge of childbirth before graduation. As late as 1910, most medical schools adhered to that philosophy. One typical late-nineteenth-century physician confessed to such complete ignorance of birth that, when he examined his first laboring patient, he mistook the baby for a massive tumor blocking the birth canal. Horrified, he prepared himself for the woman's death. He did not know what else to do. Not until the baby arrived quite safely, without his assistance, did he recognize his blunder.[10]

Doctors called to a birth tended to rely on the guidance provided by obstetric textbooks. In the event of a prolonged labor—defined as the active portion of first-stage labor lasting more than 24 hours—these manuals suggested rousing a woman's "uterine energies" by employing benign measures: giving a mother a warm drink, for example, or encouraging her to change position. The customary care tendered by Charles D. Meigs, who practiced obstetrics in Philadelphia for 44 years beginning in 1817, and who was widely recognized during much of his career as the leading obstetrician in the United States, reflected this advice. While he believed that a medical expert capable of rendering "prompt scientific aid" was essential at all births, he also cautioned that "*meddlesome midwifery* is bad" and urged shunning all "impertinent interferences." Meigs observed that, under most circumstances, nothing more was needed from midwives and physicians than "receiv[ing] and protect[ing] the child."[11]

As the overarching medical advice implied, births tended to go well in the eighteenth and nineteenth centuries. The experience of Martha Ballard, a midwife who practiced in Maine between 1785 and 1812, is considered typical of the era. She classified only 46, or 5.6 percent, of the 814 births that she attended as "difficult." None of Ballard's mothers died during labor or delivery; five died within two weeks of giving birth. Although one maternal death for every 198 births (just under 0.5 percent of births) is exceedingly high by today's standards (when 0.028 percent of births in the United States end in a mother's death), the maternal death rate in Ballard's practice was 33.3 percent lower than in 1930, when the principal site of birth began the move from home to hospital. The death rate spiked at that time because hospitals failed to institute basic precautions for maternity care—institutions only rarely separated healthy, laboring women from the general patient population. In the preantibiotic age this proved disastrous; hospital-acquired postpartum infections were numerous and deadly. Childbirth was thus safer for American mothers in 1800 than in 1930.[12]

Thanks to the generally good birth outcomes, coupled with the medical philosophy of noninterference, cesarean births were exceedingly rare in the nineteenth century. Even after a lifetime of practicing medicine, only a tiny minority of physicians ever witnessed a cesarean. Fewer still performed one. Even when encountering an especially troubling condition, such as severe placenta previa, doctors seldom considered the surgery. Francis Ramsbotham, a second-generation obstetrician who in 1853 became the first doctor to be appointed physician and lecturer in obstetrics at the London Hospital, so detested cesareans that he suggested that anyone "called upon to perform this dreadful operation" sever the fallopian tubes afterward to prevent the patient from ever conceiving another child.[13]

Customarily, laboring women relied on midwives. A midwife, in turn, summoned a physician only when she needed help. Her call for assistance often meant forceps were required to culminate the birth; midwives were not permitted to apply forceps and they certainly were not permitted to perform surgery. Yet even during births at charity hospitals catering exclusively to impoverished populations, where doctors were always present, the need for forceps was rare. At Sloane Maternity Hospital in New York City, doctors treated patients in "bad condition . . . owing to neglect or unskillful treatment." Yet only 8.3 percent of that high-risk population needed the aid of forceps.[14]

Given the rare use of forceps, it is unsurprising that cesarean section, the most extreme obstetric intervention, was virtually unheard of. An 1833 obstetric text translated from French into English and published in New York dismissed the surgery as "more or less detrimental to the mother and child." In his lengthy *Treatise on Obstetrics*, first published in 1849, Charles Meigs did not even mention the surgery. At Sloane Maternity Hospital, between January 1, 1888, and October 1, 1890, when the hospital's first 1,000 births occurred, doctors did not perform a single cesarean. And despite the poverty and poor physical condition of most of the mothers giving birth at Sloane, only 6 of the first 1,000 mothers giving birth there died.[15]

All but Helpless at the Bedside

When a birth did go badly in the nineteenth century, however, it often went nightmarishly badly. Infection or hemorrhage caused the clear majority of maternal deaths, and not until antibiotics and blood transfusions became widely available to the public after World War II were effective treatments available for either condition. Even today, laboring women are uniquely vulnerable to hemorrhage. The uterus and ovaries are highly vascularized organs; the ovarian artery arises from the aorta. Thus, any one of several medical conditions during or immediately after birth—uterine rupture, failure of the uterus to contract, or an incompletely expelled placenta—can produce profuse bleeding. In the nineteenth century, hemorrhage was such an upsetting complication of childbirth that, as one prominent obstetrician noted at the time, laypeople bearing witness to the horror aptly dubbed the condition "flooding."[16]

Doctors' descriptions of postpartum hemorrhage confirm that the colloquialism was no exaggeration. One physician, summoned to a laboring woman's home by a desperate midwife in 1888, arrived to find the woman bleeding so copiously that blood oozed from the soaked mattress onto the floor. Postpartum hemorrhages in hospitals were equally alarming. Doctors described the consequences of a case of placenta previa at the Philadelphia Lying-In Charity Hospital in 1899: "profuse hemorrhage prior to admission, awakened (in hospital) by another hemorrhage and continuous streams of blood flowed from the vagina." Both mother and baby died.[17]

Professional and lay witnesses described postpartum infection in equally grisly terms. "Childbed fever," as it was commonly known, sparked "the utmost alarm in the physician." Signs of infection included intense shivering, rapid pulse, high fever, and abdominal pain so excruciating that the weight of even light bedclothes caused a mother to writhe in agony. Just as nineteenth-century physicians were helpless at the bedside when a mother hemorrhaged, in the preantibiotic age there was nothing a doctor could do for a mother with a postpartum infection other than be present at her death. That is why cesarean section was an unsatisfactory remedy for a difficult labor: extreme blood loss and postpartum infection were frequent side effects of the surgery. In other words, a cesarean section was likely to produce diseases and conditions even worse than the condition the surgery sought to alleviate.[18]

Rationales for the Rare Intervention

Thus, owing to many factors—the paltry number of births attended by physicians, their lack of training in obstetrics, the gruesome side effects of surgery—cesarean sections were so rare in the nineteenth century that only a physical anomaly as extraordinary as no discernable cervical opening would prompt a doctor to even contemplate such a drastic course of action. At Philadelphia Lying-In, the only cesarean performed in the 121 births occurring there between October 1895 and March 1896 was for an abdominal pregnancy. The black, married patient had been suffering "with constant pain somewhat colicky localized at the umbilicus" when, during the latter part of her pregnancy, doctors felt the umbilical cord pulsating through her skin. Shocked, they administered ether and tried to forcibly dilate the woman's cervix. With "no presenting part detected" in the uterus, physicians initiated abdominal surgery only to find the amniotic sac adhered to the peritoneum. With "placental tissue protruded into the incision," they delivered a dead fetus. The mother died 90 minutes later. This surgery was typical of nineteenth-century cesareans in several ways: performed on a black patient, for a highly unusual reason, with a bad outcome.[19]

Indeed, the surgery at the Philadelphia Lying-In Charity Hospital was anomalous only due to its locale; the Ohio outback or a southern plantation were more characteristic locations for nineteenth-century cesareans than a New England hospital. Even with a hospital or lying-in charity nearby, physicians deemed women's homes the safest place for any birth, including birth by cesarean section.

In an era when even the sick avoided hospitals, those institutions were particularly abhorrent to laboring women. One doctor observed in 1880 that cesareans performed by even the most renowned practitioner "in the putrid atmosphere of an infected hospital" would prove fatal far more often than cesareans performed in "healthy rural localities." As he explained, only "the most unpromising and hopeless class of cases"—indigent women, single women, and women deserted by their families—labored and birthed in hospitals.[20]

No matter how meager their worldly goods or how low their class status, the vast majority of women gave birth in their homes. As the first published account of a cesarean performed in the United States indicated, midwives and/or laboring women's friends gathered in homes to assist at a birth as a matter of course. In the unlikely event they had to summon a physician, he almost always implied that the incompetence of the original birth attendants had prompted the unfolding calamity. Yet an unusual physical condition, rather than the ineptitude of a midwife, customarily proved to be the source of the problem. If the physician eventually decided to perform a cesarean, or offer any treatment for that matter, he sought consensus from everyone present, including the patient, before proceeding.

Journal articles written by physicians about the cesareans they performed in women's homes consistently confirm that doctors did not perform an operation without the consensus of everyone present. In 1868, after a woman had labored for more than five days, Dr. D. Warren Brickell of New Orleans arrived at the patient's bedside to assist two other doctors and a midwife. After a lengthy physical examination, Brickell suggested a cesarean, "but some great fears of Caesarean section being expressed," he tried forceps first, followed by a craniotomy, both to no avail. Only then was it "unanimously agreed that Caesarean section should be resorted to, and the patient and her friends readily assented." In an 1881 case, a woman with a misshapen pelvis suffered a stillbirth, followed by two miscarriages. When she became pregnant for the fourth time, a doctor suggested cesarean surgery but "the patient, taking advice of some female friends at this juncture, declared her unwillingness to have any interference. We could do nothing but wait." Eventually, she did agree to the surgery and gave birth to her first living child.[21]

As Francis H. Ramsbotham, the premiere obstetrician in London in the mid-nineteenth century, explained, "no operation in what is called *pure surgery*, is undertaken without the concurrence of the patient, and I do not know why we should place the obstetric branch of the science on a different footing." Walter Channing, the most famed obstetrician in Boston in his day, agreed. No matter how beneficial he believed a treatment might be, he never administered it without the express permission of the patient. During a particularly difficult labor in 1857, Channing proposed culminating the birth by applying forceps, a procedure referred to in that era as an "operative delivery." He explained why he believed the use of forceps was imperative: "The labor was proceeding slowly. Suddenly contractions ceased. There was slight haemorrhage. Sinking rapidly followed." Yet the patient rejected his proposal. "She said she was perfectly easy and would sooner die than submit to any operation. . . . She died in a few hours."[22]

Consultation with the patient in the face of a difficult birth was typical only in the case of white patients, however. When the patient was black and a slave—and before the Civil War most, if not all, black women who underwent cesarean surgery were slaves—the physician consulted with the slave owner, not the patient. In one case in Arkansas in 1863, immediately after one woman's second birth by cesarean because of a deformed pelvis, her owner instructed the physician to remove her ovaries to prevent another pregnancy. The child survived the birth; the mother died 10 days later of peritonitis. One doctor attributed the deadly infection not to the cesarean but to the procedure ordered by the mother's owner "to render her barren."[23]

Most of what is known about cesarean births in the nineteenth-century United States is due to one man's obsession with the surgery. Robert P. Harris, a Philadelphia physician originally trained as an ophthalmologist, received his medical degree from the University of Pennsylvania in 1844. After postgraduate training in the United States and Europe, he abandoned ophthalmology for medical research, gaining renown as a medical statistician. Although he gathered data on assorted treatments and conditions, he was particularly interested in cesarean surgeries, boasting that save for his efforts, many cesareans "would soon have been lost beyond the possibility of being ever recovered by the medical world." His claim was not hyperbole; descriptions of 35 of the first 85 cesareans performed by doctors in the United States before 1872 were never published. Only Harris's keen interest, and neatly inscribed journal, saved them for posterity.[24]

Harris appealed to a vast network of informants to amass his data. His records ultimately included descriptions of cesareans performed in 22 states and territories between the very early nineteenth century (exact dates for the first two surgeries are not known) through 1871. His accounts appear to be inviolable. After receiving the initial description of a surgery, he followed up by contacting witnesses and the patient, if she had survived, for corroboration. His data represented, in his words, descriptions of "genuine Gastro-hysterotomies, these being

1. 15

Case 1.
Year. Early in present century.
Locality. Near Donaldsonville - Louisiana
Operator. Dr. François Prevost. D.M.P.
Color. Black.
Result to woman. Recovered.
" " child. Lived.
1. Case communicated by Dr. Thomas Cottman, of New York, formerly of Donaldsonville, and successor in practice to Dr. Prevost, March 26th 1878.

Dr. Prevost was born at Pont-de-Cé, in the south of France, about 1764, and went to Louisiana about 1803. He was a graduate of the School of Paris; went to San Domingo, from which he escaped during the insurrection under Toussaint L'Ouverture. Nearly one half of the Caesarean operations of the State, were performed in this section, in St James, and Ascension Parishes.

65

Case. 42. Dwarf No. 8.
Year. 1855. October 17th.
Locality. Corning. New York.
Operator. Dr. Joshua B. Graves.
Age. 26.
Color. White. Mrs B——. primipara.
Height. Body of medium length, legs like those of a girl of ten years old. Was exhibited about the country as a curiosity.
Cause of difficulty - Deformed Pelvis.
Conj. diam. 1 inch.
Condition of woman at time of operation. } Much exhausted.
Length of labor. Four days.
Result to woman. Died in six days - the rectum had been perforated in three places, by Smellie's scissors in the hands of a young accoucheur, who mistook the sacral promontory for the fœtal head.
Result to child. Lived - was alive in 1869.
27. There case is reported. Philad^a Med. & Surg. Reporter. 1869. Decr. page 375.

Two of the 85 cases described in Dr. Robert Harris's handwritten log, *The Caesarean Operations of the United States*. Thirty-five of the cases described by Harris in this journal were unpublished. "Case 1" describes a cesarean, exact date unknown, performed by François Prevost, the physician who performed more cesareans recorded by Harris than any other physician. "Case 42" describes a cesarean performed on a woman Harris labels "Dwarf No. 8."

Source: Robert P. Harris, *Caesarean Operations of the United States* (1879), 15, 65, Robert Harris Collection, courtesy of the Wangensteen Historical Library of Biology and Medicine, University of Minnesota, Minneapolis.

alone recognized by the writer as 'Caesarean.'" He accumulated so much knowledge about the surgery that, even though his training was in ophthalmology, he was tapped to be one of the founders of the Philadelphia Obstetrical Society.[25]

Doctors performed the majority of the 85 cesareans documented by Harris on women of color: 46 of the operations were on women described as black, mulatto, quadroon, or creole; 38 on women described as white; and one on a woman described as Mexican. Race appeared to be a significant factor when doctors decided to perform the surgery; while a preponderance of the women undergoing cesareans were black, blacks constituted only between 12.6 and 14.6 percent of the population during the first three-quarters of the nineteenth century. Disability was a likely consideration as well; Harris found that doctors performed 20 percent of cesarean surgeries on women he described as "dwarfs," most of whom had severe pelvic malformations. In short, what is referred to today as "othering"—a dismissive attitude toward marginalized groups—probably factored into white, male, able-bodied physicians' decisions to perform the surgery, although records of doctors' explicit thinking are rare.[26]

Harris used location to justify the racial disparity. More than half of the 85 cesareans he documented occurred in the South; 15 of the 85, including 6 of the first 9, occurred on Louisiana plantations. Harris attributed the geographic concentration to the unusual number of cesareans performed on "both white and black subjects" in the French West Indies in the eighteenth and early nineteenth centuries. He surmised that doctors there shared their knowledge and experience with "French surgeons in the colony of 'Louisianne,'" where rachitic deformities were common among the slave women." Harris lauded Louisiana physicians for their "greatest proportion of successful results," naming one doctor in particular, François Prevost, who performed 4 of the first 85 cesareans—more cesareans than any other American doctor in Harris's records.[27]

Slavery and pervasive racism, however, clearly steered doctors toward some patients and away from others. While doctors favored the life of a white mother over the life of her newborn, and thus largely avoided performing cesarean surgery on white women because of the high maternal death rate connected with the procedure, physicians evaluated the lives of pregnant slaves according to the interests of the slave owner, who might value a surviving infant more than a mother exhibiting poor health. And unlike white women, slaves had no choice in the matter—their owners made all medical decisions for them. Physicians were also more willing to experiment on black women, deeming them hardier than white women and thus more likely to survive the surgery. Although Harris disagreed with the latter supposition, he confirmed the belief was widespread among his colleagues: "It has been argued from the success in Louisiana, that the black race, like the Chinese, is less subject than the white, to the inflammatory sequellae of surgery, and hence that the slave has more frequently recovered than the white woman." Harris, however, once again invoking geography, deemed locale a better predictor of outcome than race: "whites in the West Indies and Southern States have done equally well; and blacks in our Northern States have not escaped any more frequently than the whites."[28]

Doctors customarily avoided performing cesareans no matter the locale or patient's characteristics. Drastic circumstances were always required to tip the scales. Before undergoing her first cesarean, one woman, a slave in Louisiana, had four miscarriages followed by a delivery of a full-term stillborn baby via forceps. Only after she labored for 12 hours during her sixth pregnancy in 1846 did someone summon a physician; he discovered a bony tumor blocking the birth canal. The information was relayed to the woman's owner who, "after some delay," consented to cesarean surgery. The doctor, who had no surgical instruments with him, improvised with the household tools at his disposal. The baby died shortly after birth. Three years later, the same woman survived a second cesarean birth, as did her first living child. As this story of seven pregnancies resulting in only one live birth attests, the surgery was a last resort no matter the patient. Indeed, cesareans were so unusual that, for some, the operation became part of their lifelong identity. The daughter of one of the slaves operated on by Prevost was christened "Cesarinne" as a permanent testament to the mode of her birth. The surgery, coupled with the fact that both mother and baby survived, was so extraordinary that the owner of the mother celebrated by freeing Cesarinne.[29]

Class played at least as significant a role as race in shaping doctors' attitudes toward cesarean surgery. Harris observed that women undergoing cesareans were "very largely derived from the lower classes" in every country he studied. Yet, just as he credited geography for the unusual number of black women giving birth by cesarean, he attributed the class differential to necessity rather than bias, contending that undesirable habits innate to working-class and indigent women—poor diet, heavy drinking, slovenly habits—made the greater incidence of cesareans among them inevitable.[30]

Harris similarly deemed the pregnant women he described as "dwarfs"—between three feet four and four feet eight inches tall—to be at inherent risk for cesarean surgery. In his ledger recounting the details of all known cesarean births in the United States through 1871, "dwarf" was the only characteristic he highlighted, penning the word in red ink in the upper right corner of relevant cases. For the vast majority of these cases, he listed "pelvic deformity" as the "cause of difficulty" prompting the surgery. One of those surgeries, the first cesarean birth in New York City, was performed in 1838 on a 42-year-old woman who was four feet tall. Five physicians were in attendance; one initially favored an embryotomy over a cesarean. A colleague disagreed, insisting that mutilation and removal of the fetus was more likely to kill the mother than a cesarean—the patient's unique pelvic deformity made damage to her bladder or rectum likely during an

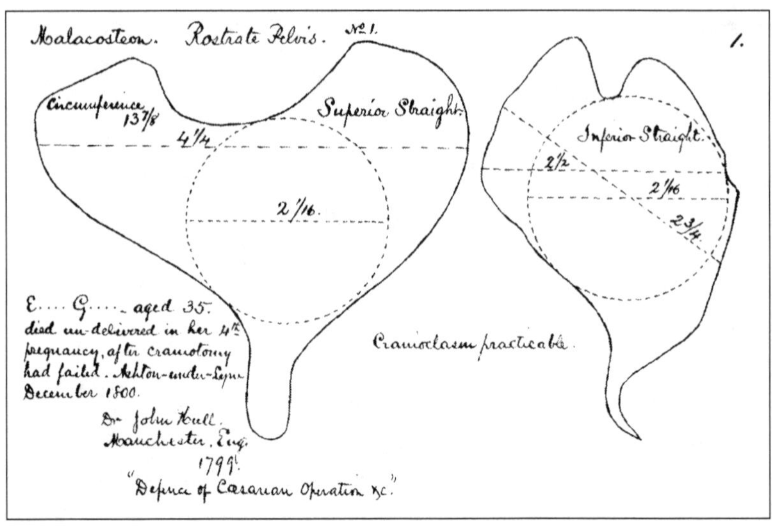

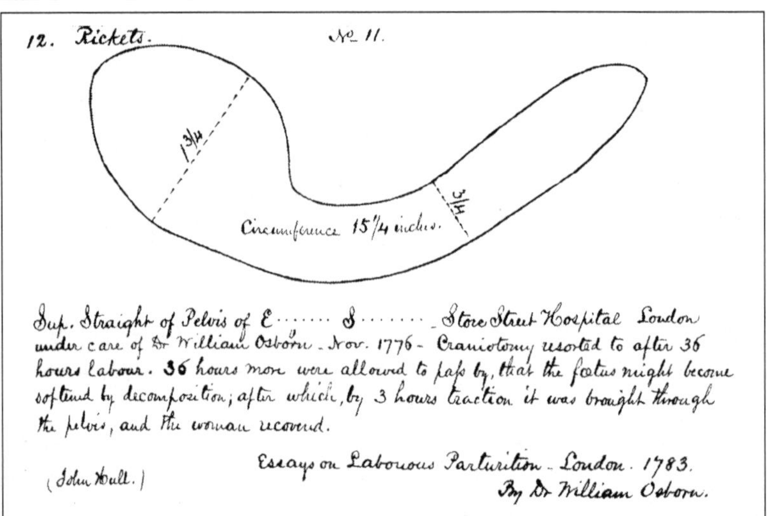

Dr. Robert Harris, a medical statistician with an enduring interest in cesarean sections, collected and documented pelvic deformities that required cesarean sections in the eighteenth and nineteenth centuries. Both drawings above illustrate the consequences of what would likely be classified today as rickets. *Top*: "Malacosteon," or osteomalacia, is a softening of the bones equivalent to rickets. A "rostrate pelvis" is a pelvic deformity common to the condition. *Bottom*: Rickets is a softening of the bones caused by severe vitamin D deficiency.

Source: Robert Harris Collection, courtesy of the Wangensteen Historical Library of Biology and Medicine, University of Minnesota, Minneapolis.

embryotomy. Only after much discussion did the five doctors agree a cesarean was the safest route. The mother survived the surgery; the baby, who doctors described as "deformed in the lower extremities," died shortly after birth.[31]

While the majority of cesareans documented by Harris ended in a mother's death, mothers he designated "dwarf" were even less likely to survive. Not only did the vast majority of the 16 women of unusually small stature listed in Harris's records die shortly after the surgery, usually of peritonitis, but the cesarean birth was often a miserable end to a difficult life. One of the women described in Harris's chronicles as being three feet six inches tall had never walked without crutches due to a rachitic pelvis. She died 20 hours after giving birth in 1869, with an unsutured, festering wound. Another woman, "exhibited about the country as a curiosity" for most of her life, died six days after giving birth by cesarean in 1855. She suffered enormously in the hours preceding her death—"a young accoucheur, who mistook the sacral promontory for the foetal head" had perforated her rectum in three places. Her child survived.[32]

The Obstetrician's Dread

Maternal death was so common after a cesarean that one physician dismissed the surgery as "sacrificial midwifery." Among Harris's 85 cases, 44 women died—a death rate of almost 52 percent. European statistics were far grimmer. Francis Ramsbotham reported in 1841 that 90 percent of the cesareans performed in the British Isles had ended in a mother's death.[33]

Harris made what was perhaps the most chillingly persuasive case for the surgery's dangers. Because his interest in cesareans encompassed every manner of abdominal birth, in addition to gathering data on conventional cesarean surgery he sought accounts of "laparo-hysterotic rips"—the medical records of pregnant women who had been gored by cattle and forced to deliver their babies through the gaping wound. These "rips" did occur from time to time in what was then a largely rural United States, where even urban families kept livestock in proximity to their homes. Of the nine abdominal gorings by cattle of pregnant women documented by Harris, five women and five children survived. He called this an admirable record, considering that only two women and three children had survived the 11 documented cesarean sections performed in New York before the late 1880s. Cesarean surgery was so deadly, he observed, there is "a far better showing for the cow-horn than the knife."[34]

Knowing more about the nature of the surgery and its outcome than any other physician in the country, Harris identified, and sought to mitigate, its risks. In studying his 85 accounts, he concluded that women were most likely to die from a cesarean after laboring for days, as opposed to hours. Although this was not always true—women giving birth by cesarean who labored more than two days sometimes lived, and women who had short labors sometimes died—Harris nevertheless theorized that extreme fatigue due to prolonged labor created optimal conditions for peritonitis and septicemia. Fewer pregnant women had died after being gored by cattle, he reasoned, because the fetus had been removed from the womb before labor began and exhaustion could set in. Delay, he argued, was the underlying cause of the operation's significant mortality.[35]

According to Harris, while fewer than 50 percent of women survived cesarean sections in the United States, 70 to 75 percent of them survived "timely operations." Consequently, he riddled his otherwise objective descriptions of cesarean sections in his handwritten journal with criticisms of "delay." One woman, for example, "exhausted by futile attempts at delivery, and delay in giving consent to the use of the knife," died five or six days later of peritonitis. Another woman underwent the surgery after a 50-hour labor, 24 of them spent in "useless delay." She died of exhaustion four hours after the surgery. Another, "almost hopeless from long delay . . . under the care of a midwife" before her cesarean, died of peritonitis three days after the surgery. While Harris recognized the dangers of cesarean sections, he was so certain that swift action made the surgery safer that he characterized most medical interventions performed in the hope of avoiding a cesarean (applying forceps being the most common) as "postponement and futile meddling" that rendered "the work of the surgeon of no avail."[36]

Harris promoted his protocol even when faced with evidence contradicting its alleged benefits. Although English doctors, unlike their American counterparts, did perform cesareans early in labor exactly as Harris advised, they saw significantly higher mortality than in the United States. Yet Harris theorized that the flawed character of the British women who seemed to need cesareans in the highest numbers, namely "the peasantry" prone to "beer-drinking habits," was responsible for their demise. Why else, he observed, "should skill and promptness be so entirely thrown away in the great majority of cases in which they have been exercised?"[37]

The call for timely performance of the surgery was as much an attempt to quell his colleagues' fear of the operation as it was a studied recommendation. Doctors deemed the surgery so risky that, if they performed it at all, they did so only after attempting every other maneuver and eventually deciding the mother's life was likely lost anyway. Harris lamented in 1879, "About three fourths of our caesarean operations are too late in their performance, and we are growing worse instead of better in this respect, hence the greatly increased mortality of the last ten years over any previous decade." Although he did not impose a strict timeline, he suggested that if a doctor harbored any suspicion that a cesarean might be necessary, he not allow a woman to labor more than five to 10 hours. Directly countering the supposition that black women weathered cesareans better than white women, he argued, "No race or color can by natural immunity, compare in the measure of security with that which is given to the patient by a timely resort to the knife, while the membranes are unbroken, the uterine tissues normal, and strength not exhausted." He declared prompt performance of the surgery especially crucial in the case of "dwarfs . . . whose strength must be readily wasted," even during a short labor. In 1878, Harris observed that in his native Philadelphia, with a population of over 800,000, only one cesarean had been performed in the previous 40 years. He admonished, "Will anyone pretend to say that this was the only woman who required it?" He clearly believed that the Philadelphia mothers who had died undelivered and in agony might have survived if his advice had been followed.[38]

While Harris's view of cesarean section was aggressive compared to his compatriots', he could be circumspect about the surgery as well. He roundly condemned several of the physicians whose surgeries he had documented, one for being a "quack-surgeon" and "bold bungler," others for being "reckless" and exhibiting "lamentable ignorance." He deemed several of the operations he documented "uncalled for." A woman who had previously undergone two cesareans in quick succession, one in 1833 and the other in 1834, went into labor with her third child without anyone nearby to assist her. By the time a physician arrived, she "had already delivered herself of 'healthy, vigorous twins.'" Harris concluded that if she could give birth to twins vaginally, without assistance no less, her cesareans must have been unnecessary. Although according to the medical record both cesareans had been due to an arm presentation likely caused by transverse lie of the fetus, Harris nevertheless condemned the physician as "a better surgeon than obstetrician." Ultimately, the consequence of the mother's two cesareans was dire. She bled to death during her fourth labor in 1838, after her uterus ruptured along the scar left by the two surgeries.[39]

No matter the incompetence of some physicians, doctors were more likely to blame the actions of the patient or her other birth attendants for any untoward effects of a cesarean. Physicians often cited "indiscretions in diet" as the proximate cause of a death. One mother, who seemed to be doing well, "dined on animal food, with cider" just before she died. Harris insisted another patient would have survived "but for her own folly in eating, an indiscretion begotten of ignorance, which has proved fatal several times, after the Caesarean operation." Doctors blamed another woman for her own death because she consumed dumplings. Another mother was doing fine three days after surgery until "her husband came home intoxicated and got into a quarrel with his wife's mother. The patient jumped out of bed to protect her [mother], and died in consequence in 12 hours."[40]

Doctors so dreaded the surgery's high death rate that some favored procedures that were likely to render a woman severely disabled, essentially choosing permanent physical damage over the likelihood of death. Some physicians, for example, chose symphysiotomy—cutting through the cartilage between the ends of the two pubic bones—rather than cesarean section when confronted with a hopelessly blocked birth. Symphysiotomy allowed the bones to separate about one and a half inches—often, but not always, permitting passage of the fetal head. Yet even when the treatment worked, the bones did not always reunite, and the patient never walked again. J. Whitridge Williams, the obstetrician-in-chief at Johns Hopkins Hospital, said of the sole symphysiotomy at his hospital, "the death of the only patient upon whom it was performed did not serve to increase our enthusiasm."[41]

Physicians intervened so seldom during birth that they hesitated to employ even forceps—the most benign of the so-called operative obstetric techniques—for fear of doing damage. Obstetric texts described the "operative" birth procedures in ascending order, according to risk to the mother: first how to select and apply forceps, then how to execute a craniotomy (a procedure that was obviously fatal to the infant but safer for the mother than a cesarean), and finally how to perform assorted surgeries, including cesarean section. While doctors wielded forceps or performed a craniotomy specifically to save a mother's life, they viewed a cesarean quite differently—as more desperate than deliberate. One typical physician admitted, "there is nothing in surgery, about which the surgeon is so timid, as the Caesarean operation; and nothing in obstetrics, of which this obstetrician stands so much in dread."[42]

Applying Forceps, Avoiding Cesareans

Having learned through experience of the potentially disastrous effects of medical intervention, most doctors shrank from any interference, including the use of forceps. Although forceps generally had fewer deadly and debilitating effects for mothers than cesarean section and symphysiotomy, one Chicago physician observed that even under ideal conditions "the most skillful forceps operation is but a clumsy imitation of natural labor." Knowing this, another doctor refused to interfere during labor for any reason. He told Walter Channing, Boston's leading obstetrician for a good portion of the nineteenth century, "I wait . . . hours and days, nourish, stimulate, encourage, and at length in three or four days, the labor finishes itself. I never give aid; I never will."[43]

Physicians tended to characterize forceps as the least objectionable operative intervention, even though a pair of forceps had always been a difficult tool to master. Without the benefit of sight, doctors must place the instrument precisely, not only within the birth canal but also upon the infant's head, so as not to damage either vaginal tissue or the infant's skull and face. After the instrument is properly placed, the work is no less daunting. The "operator" must apply exactly the right amount of tension, taking into account the position of the infant and its location in the birth canal. Then the physician must intuit the amount of force needed and at what angle to pull, even as the angle changes multiple times, depending on the strength of uterine contractions, condition of the mother, and position of the fetus. As one early-nineteenth-century obstetrician declared in an understatement, forceps demanded "the union of much dexterity and intelligence."[44]

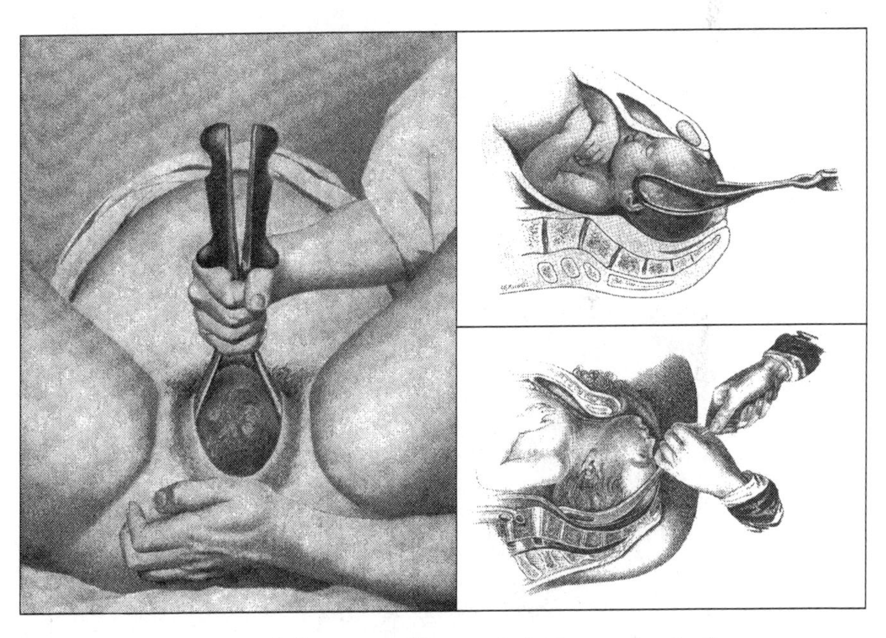

Each drawing illustrates a different use of forceps. Left: the use of outlet forceps, described in the text as "protecting the pelvic floor." *Top right*: The use of forceps when the infant presents in the occiput posterior position ("sunny side up" in contemporary lay vernacular). *Bottom right*: The use of forceps during a face and brow presentation. Sources: E. Davis, *Operative Obstetrics*, figures 111 and 101; Ramsbotham, *The Principles and Practice of Obstetric Medicine*, figure 102.

The most dangerous and least-used category of forceps was the "high" type—designed to dislodge an infant stuck at the top of the birth canal or still in the uterus long after the cervix had fully dilated. High forceps could do so much damage that in 1879 one Boston doctor, who compared 125 births ending in cesarean section with 119 terminated with high forceps, noted that cesarean section, despite its appalling death rate, had better outcomes. High forceps challenged even the most adept obstetrician. During a birth in 1898, the instrument "bruised" a baby's eye. A pair of high forceps was the source of another child's permanent facial paralysis and another's "markedly wounded" head. There were also times high forceps failed utterly ("1 p.m. high forceps applied but head couldn't be made to engage even with extreme traction"), in which case the birth often ended in a cesarean—the very surgery doctors had hoped to avoid when they applied high forceps. Just as Harris warned, this compounded the dangers of the cesarean; when a cesarean occurred after a failed high forceps procedure, the odds that a woman would die from postpartum infection increased significantly.[45]

A particularly difficult case in 1892 at New York's Sloane Maternity Hospital illustrates the intricate skill needed to wield the instrument successfully. A mother's labor with her second child started well enough—she went into labor at 8:45 p.m. and was fully dilated and ready to push seven hours later. After five and a half hours of pushing, however, the fetal head had not descended into the birth canal. At 8:58 a.m., a physician applied high forceps through the cervical opening and into the uterus, placing one blade over the infant's face and the other over the occiput portion of the head. After four minutes of fruitless maneuvers, the doctor was unable to bring the head into the pelvis. He removed the forceps and reapplied the instrument, grasping the sides of the skull and "pushing up a very little and rotating with some force." Eventually, the experienced doctor succeeded in moving the baby into the birth canal. After removing the forceps, he massaged the mother's perineum in anticipation of the birth. The final sentence of the medical record reads: "Skin broke long before head was well down but slow delivery prevented deep laceration." As this case intimated, while the correct use of forceps in the hands of a skilled physician could be lifesaving, one careless maneuver could irreparably mangle, even kill, mother, child, or both.[46]

Thus, doctors applied high forceps judiciously, although more often than they performed a cesarean section. From 1891 to 1901, in 2,800 births at Philadelphia Lying-In Charity Hospital, obstetricians used high forceps during 19 births. They employed the most common and least dangerous type—low or outlet forceps to remove a baby stuck at, or near, the vaginal opening—in 119 births. When added to the nine births ending in cesarean section and the two ending in craniotomy, Philadelphia Lying-In saw, during that 10-year period, operative interventions in 5.3 percent of births—a rate essentially identical to the 5.6 percent of births that Martha Ballard deemed "difficult" in her eighteenth-century midwifery practice.[47]

The obstetricians who wrote obstetric manuals acknowledged the skill needed to apply forceps by devoting a great deal of space to use of the device. In Charles Meigs's 1856 textbook, how to choose the correct pair, apply the instrument to the fetal skull, and maneuver it adeptly through the birth canal consumed 40 illustrated pages. Well into the twentieth century, obstetric texts devoted far more space to forceps than to cesarean surgical technique. Even the most fundamental aspect of decision-making—which type of forceps to use in which situations—entailed lengthy discussion. There were dozens to choose from, each composed of a different material and molded into a different shape and size. Smellie's wooden forceps sported chunky handles and smooth, curved blades; Smellie's straight forceps showcased leather covers. Others included Burton's lobster claw forceps, Hamilton's forceps with a hinged handle, and Chapman's forceps featuring inward-facing hooked handles and paddle-shaped loops for wrapping around the fetal skull. Even the Chamberlens—the family that spawned multiple generations of obstetricians and whose patriarch, William, who died in 1596, invented the first forceps—redesigned their prized instrument many times before stopping with great-great-grandson Chamberlen Walker's early-eighteenth-century design.[48]

Doctors disagreed bitterly about the efficacy and risks of each type. One physician who preferred curved forceps charged that colleagues opting for the straight version harbored "a prejudice fatal to life and fatal to all scientific progress." Another doctor dubbed a pair of short forceps—characterized by wide, flat-edged blades—"a murderous weapon." Choosing the appropriate instrument and using that tool judiciously and deftly was indeed a matter of life and death, hence the tense debates.[49]

Yet forceps, despite the difficulties the instrument posed, were the main reason nineteenth-century doctors were able to avoid cesareans almost completely, and with impunity. Without the instrument, doctors were as helpless at a "stuck" birth as they were when facing hemorrhage or postpartum infection. With forceps in hand, a practiced physician could ensure, far more often than not, that he would leave behind in the birthing chamber the living mother of a living child, despite a difficult birth.[50]

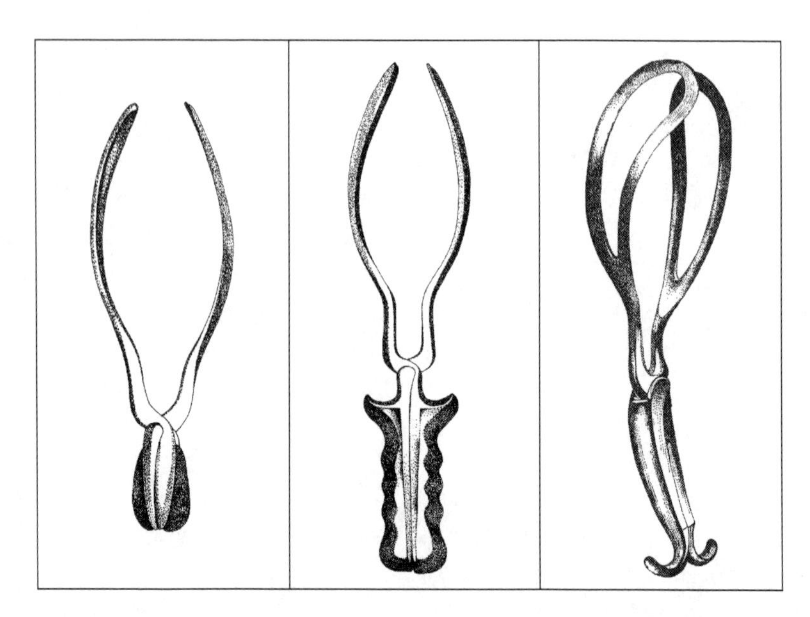

Forceps came in a constantly changing array of shapes, sizes, and materials. *Left*: James Young Simpson's short forceps. Simpson, an obstetrician practicing in Edinburgh, Scotland, beginning in the 1830s, gained renown for championing obstetric anesthesia. *Middle*: Simpson's long (14.75 inches) forceps, 4.5 inches longer than his short forceps. *Right*: Sawyer's forceps with David Davis's blades, dated 1896. David Davis was the author of *The Principles and Practice of Obstetric Medicine* (London: Taylor and Walton, 1836). Illustrations by Maryam Khaleghi Yazdi, adapted from illustrations in Hibbard, *The Obstetrician's Armamentarium*, 93, 103.

A Grisly Task

If forceps failed to remove the infant from the birth canal, a doctor's next course of action was usually craniotomy—collapsing the fetal head by draining a large portion of the brain. Doctors employed a variety of instruments to perform this grisly task, but often the tool was as simple and ubiquitous as a crochet hook. Although disturbing to all involved, the procedure was less lethal to a mother than a cesarean, and so, just as doctors reached for forceps first during a difficult birth, they opted for craniotomy far more often than cesarean surgery. Faced with a decision between craniotomy, ending in the certain death of the fetus, versus cesarean section, ending in the likely death of the mother, doctors invariably chose craniotomy.[51]

A chapter title in an 1836 obstetric text reflected the unequivocal importance of maternal life over survival of the fetus: "Of Obstetric Operations Calculated to

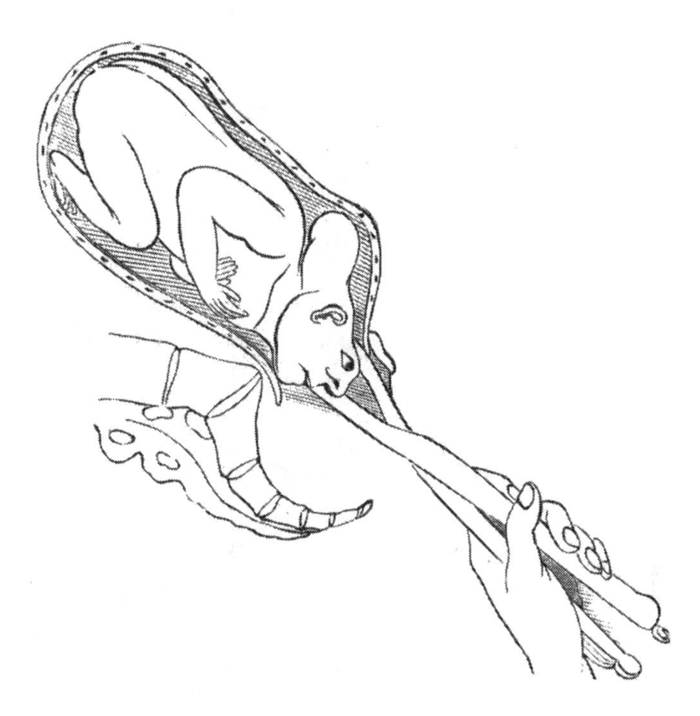

Seizing the base of skull with craniotomy forceps after removal of the cranium.
Source: Herman, *Difficult Labour*, 393.

Ensure the Preservation of the More Important Life of the Mother." One Boston physician explained that his medical education had been clear: a woman, "a member of society and the potential mother of many children," was always to be favored over her "unborn fetus." When summoned to a difficult labor, doctors thus took care to place craniotomy instruments in their satchels alongside forceps. While mothers would survive a newborn's death, a newborn was not likely to survive its mother's death. In an era before refrigeration, pasteurization, and pure food laws, motherless babies were doomed to short, miserable lives for want of mothers' milk if a wet nurse could not be found.[52]

Performing a craniotomy was not necessarily any more straightforward than applying forceps, however. After a mother labored fruitlessly for four days, Boston obstetrician Walter Channing executed a particularly prolonged, gruesome procedure in the mid-nineteenth century. Following his ineffectual use of forceps, "the perforator & crochet were next used, & such was the difficulty after removing the brain that it was necessary to take away most of the vault of the cranium before the head descended." The experience of a 24-year-old Irish woman at Sloane Maternity Hospital in New York City in 1892 similarly demonstrated how difficult craniotomies could be for women to endure and physicians to perform. For five and a half hours during second-stage labor, physicians tried in vain to use low forceps to deliver the woman's baby. For almost two addi-

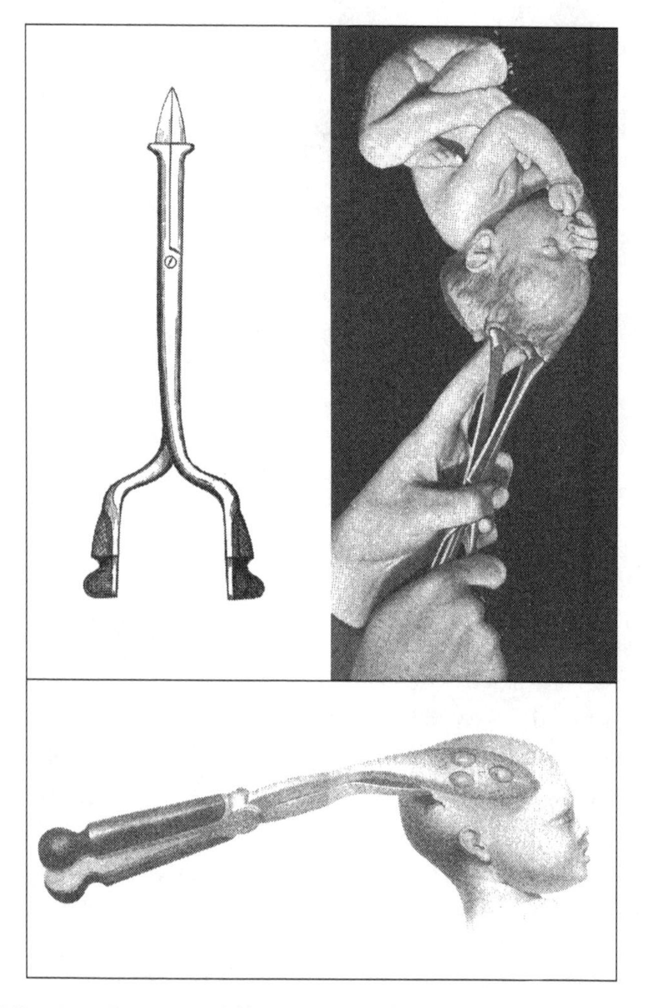

Top left: Oldham's perforator, used for piercing the fetal skull to remove brain matter and effect delivery without resorting to a cesarean. This design allowed operators to open the blades by squeezing the handle of the instrument. *Top right*: Using the perforator. *Bottom*: Piercing and grasping the fetal skull.
Sources: Herman, *Difficult Labour*, 387; E. Davis, *Operative Obstetrics*, figure 150; D. Davis, *The Principles and Practice of Obstetric Medicine*, 1158.

tional hours, they applied median forceps—again to no avail. Finally, doctors decided to perform a craniotomy. With median forceps still in place, one physician perforated the fetal head with a trefine and then drained brain matter. Yet even after applying strong traction, the dead fetus remained in place. The doctor removed the forceps and inserted a cephalotribe in the birth canal to crush the fetal head. The fetus remained firmly in place. Only after using a smaller cephalotribe to remove still more brain matter did the physician succeed in removing the mutilated fetus from the mother's body.[53]

If craniotomy proved insufficient to permit passage of what was now a dead fetus, a few doctors went on to perform a cesarean in a final attempt to save the mother. Although craniotomy followed by cesarean was among the rarest of rare scenarios, the combination did occur in 6 of the 85 cesareans documented by Harris. Half of those six mothers survived, a slightly better ratio than the overall maternal death rate after a cesarean alone, although the small number of women in the cohort hardly constituted a definitive test. In an even rarer scenario, during a birth in Louisiana in 1849, doctors executed all three of the major "operative" procedures. When forceps proved insufficient ("was unable to effect delivery in consequence of the monstrous size of the child's head"), another doctor in attendance punctured the infant's brain and removed its parietal bones. When that, too, proved unhelpful due to the unusual structure of the mother's pelvis, doctors agreed that "to take the child away by pieces" would be more dangerous to the mother than removing the dead infant through an abdominal incision. The woman survived the cesarean surgery.[54]

Developing Cesarean Surgical Techniques

Because doctors performed cesareans so rarely—the Philadelphia Lying-In Charity Hospital saw a 0.3 percent rate during its first 10 years—even the few physicians who performed the surgery disagreed on the most basic aspects of its protocol. When in the course of a pregnancy or labor was the best time for the operation? What step-by-step actions should the surgery entail? What surgical instruments should be employed? Did uterine sutures cause peritonitis or prevent it? What was the best anesthesia to administer? At least one British physician insisted it was opium. There were no uniform answers to even the most fundamental questions.[55]

Professional jealousy was likely a significant reason for obstetricians' inability to agree on fundamental practices. The type of professional rivalry that prevented any consensus was on display in the animated correspondence between

Max Sänger, a gynecologist from Leipzig, Germany, and Robert Harris, the American medical statistician who collected data on cesarean sections. In one letter to Harris in 1887, written in Sänger's imperfect English, Sänger criticized a colleague—German obstetrician Christian Gerhard Leopold. Sänger said of Leopold's first cesarean section: "Not a single step of this first operation . . . is originally to him, except that he cutted off the muscular flap not as proposed by myself from the serous surface to the decidua, but in opposite direction!" When Sänger wrote that letter, both he and Leopold had already gained a measure of professional renown. Sänger was well known in both the United States and Europe because, after performing his first cesarean on August 22, 1880, he did something unprecedented—he sutured the uterine wound. Before Sänger, doctors sutured only the abdomen, leaving the uterus to heal unaided. Leopold was a well-respected teacher of midwifery at Leipzig University and director of the Royal Gynecological Infirmary in Dresden. Today, Leopold is still remembered for what came to be known as the "Leopold maneuvers"—a means of manually ascertaining the position of the fetus in the uterus.[56]

Sänger's harangue against Leopold continued in the letter to Harris: "Notwithstanding in his latest paper . . . he has not quoted me and, perhaps, he imaginates now to have done more for the improved caesarean operation as myself. . . . You don't know the arrogant, self-glorious and intriguant character of this man, who is indebted for his carriere only to his father-in-law Prof. Crede." Carl Siegmund Franz Credé, Leopold's mentor, was, at the time Sänger wrote the letter to Harris, better known in obstetric circles than either Sänger or Leopold. In the letter, Sänger claimed that Credé said of his son-in-law, "After having performed several times a new operation of another he imaginates always to be the inventor."[57]

Sänger described his difficulties with Leopold to explain to Harris why he was unable to answer a question Harris had posed to him in an earlier letter: How many cesarean sections had been performed at the Dresden maternity hospital? "Now you will understand," he told Harris, "why Dr. Leopold not communicates to me . . . so I don't know how many operations there has been performed at the Dresden Maternity till the present time." Sänger attributed his inability to communicate with Leopold entirely to Leopold's piracy of Sänger's surgical method: "And now he also imaginates to have improved my own technique and don't find it necessary to quote my name before the students at the same clinic, which saw the first triumph of the reconciliated caesarean section! He does not inform me, when he operates he does not communicate me the result after having operated." That two such influential and talented obstetricians refused to either acknowledge or communicate with each other probably stymied many attempts by the obstetric community to achieve professional consensus.[58]

Professional jealousies aside, the paucity of information about the operation available to the average physician likewise stifled the ability of obstetricians and surgeons to agree on a safe set of surgical techniques. In the 1840s, if an obstetric text offered any information about cesarean surgery, it did so only cryptically: "The Caesarean Operation consists in dividing the abdominal parietes, cutting into the cavity of the uterus, and extracting the child, placenta, and foetal membranes, through the incision thus made." Thirty years later, descriptions of the surgery remained equally terse, although the latter-day explanations often dwelled more on what to avoid doing than on what to do: "The assistants support the abdominal wall on either side, looking out to prevent the escape of intestine. The *uterine incision* is made in the middle line, sparing the fundus and lower segment as much as possible, as these parts are not well adapted to close by contraction."[59]

Not until the late 1870s, when the work of Italian obstetrician Edorado Porro garnered attention, was there significant effort to ascertain the most efficacious protocol. Porro culminated every cesarean he performed with amputation of the uterus and ovaries in order to prevent post-operative hemorrhage and infection—or, as obstetricians explained in recalling this practice in the 1950s, "to remove the septic focus." After acceptance of Porro's innovation, doctors began to refer to the traditional cesarean section, leaving the unsutured uterus to fester, as "gastro-hysterotomy" and Porro's cesarean as "gastro-hysterectomy." Porro's contribution to cesarean surgery was so significant that Harris, who had taken over editorship of W. S. Playfair's classic text *Midwifery* in 1878, highlighted the Porro operation in the first sentence of the 1889 edition of the book by lauding the recent "revolution" in obstetric surgery, particularly the enhanced safety provided by the "Porro-Cæsarean operation."[60]

Yet obstetricians and surgeons did not immediately embrace Porro's work. Even Harris was unimpressed initially. In a speech before colleagues at a meeting of the Obstetrical Society of Philadelphia, he at first denounced Porro as a fraud, noting that James Blundell of London had performed the identical operation in 1828, as had Horatio Storer in Boston in 1869. Harris asked sarcastically, "Shall we introduce this unsexing operation into the United States?" And while Harris eventually reversed his judgment, professional jealousy likely prevented Sänger from ever being impressed with Porro. He wrote to Harris in 1891, "Myself, I am the owner of a little private hospital of 24 beds, where I promote science to the utmost of one's power. Porro, who takes out the womb, is Senator of the Italian

Kingdom, myself, who conserves it, is neither knight nor baronet, but I am content with my fate."[61]

Porro first performed the surgery that would bear his name in 1876. The 25-year-old woman he experimented on was a first-time mother of very short stature; Harris would have labeled her "dwarf." She had suffered rickets as a child—a case so severe that for much of her childhood she could not stand without assistance. Upon arrival at the woman's bedside, Porro immediately determined a cesarean was necessary and proposed removing the woman's uterus immediately after the birth to prevent a life-threatening hemorrhage. After Porro extracted a healthy female infant, a hemorrhage did ensue. Porro recalled, "It was providential that we had made all the preparations necessary for hysterectomy; otherwise the patient would surely have died." After the surgery, Porro was so pleased with the result that he recommended, in a widely circulated, 63-page report, that doctors perform "utero-ovarian amputation" immediately after every cesarean. For a time, the Porro cesarean became standard in many maternity centers in Europe and the United States. By 1890, doctors around the world had performed more than 300 Porros.[62]

Porro's influence on the development of cesarean surgical technique was ultimately indirect, however. When Max Sänger died at age 50 in 1903, his obituary

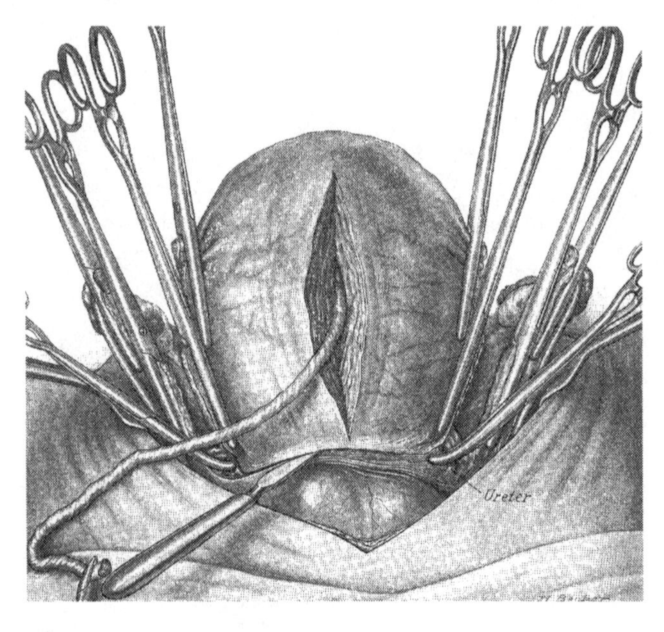

A Porro cesarean, with uterus in position to be amputated immediately after delivery.
Source: DeLee, *The Principles and Practice of Obstetrics* (1918), 1027.

noted that Porro's operation had "roused to fresh efforts the obstetric surgeons of a quarter century ago." Peter Müller, a Swiss obstetrician, was one. He modified the Porro by lifting the uterus from the abdominal cavity before removing the newborn. Max Sänger, who retained the uterus and sutured it, was another. Professional rivalry had its pluses as well as minuses.[63]

As the first physician to write a lengthy tome devoted solely to cesarean surgery, Sänger ultimately exerted the greatest influence on the development of the modern operation. Porro's fleetingly favored technique to remove the organ entirely to avoid infection was useful only until physicians accepted Sänger's suturing of the uterus. Professor Paul Zweifel, a noted Swiss gynecologist, explained the meaning of Sänger's innovation: before Sänger, "it was like a death warrant for a woman to undergo a caesarean operation." After Sänger, postsurgical maternal mortality dropped dramatically—he was able to boast of a personal 5.8 percent maternal death rate after a cesarean, plus "all children living before the operation . . . born living."[64]

Doctors eventually dubbed Porro's technique the "radical cesarean." Sänger's form of the surgery was given one of two monikers—either the "conservative cesarean," because it conserved the uterus, or, more commonly, the "classic cesarean," because suturing the uterus soon became standard practice. Sänger's achievement was so significant that his 1903 obituary ended with this high praise: "whatever minor services to science and to humanity may shrink into insignificance, or perhaps be forgotten, one great achievement will stand out in all future histories of obstetrics and gynecology by the association of the name of Max Sänger with the Conservative Caesarean Section."[65]

Until the antibiotic era, however, postpartum infection remained a significant risk of the surgery despite Sänger's innovation. Thus, even after Sänger's protocol triumphed, disagreement remained. While most obstetricians came to prefer the classic cesarean, others stuck to Porro's radical version of the surgery. In 1921, obstetrician J. Whitridge Williams of Johns Hopkins University continued to defend the occasional use of the Porro operation because in "infected or exhausted patients" removal of the uterus saved lives. Others were less certain: "it is a frightful price for a young primipara to pay on the chance that she may develop a serious infection." Well into the twentieth century, conflict remained a hallmark of obstetrics.[66]

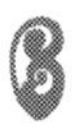

Physicians viewed cesarean section as inherently risky in the nineteenth century because they deemed mothers' lives paramount. On that there was no disagreement. Doctors preferred the grisly task of craniotomy over cesarean surgery because destroying a fetus often ensured the mother would survive. In contrast, a cesarean section performed to save a fetus often ended in the mother's death. Hence, cesareans were to be avoided. Only at the end of the century were there signs of that conviction softening. In 1894, Chicago obstetrician Junius Hoag assured a group of colleagues that when confronted with a difficult birth, cesarean section had become a viable option. With the operation now performed "according to modern methods"—anesthesia, asepsis, timely performance, and changes in surgical technique that included suturing the uterus—the maternal recovery rate had risen to 69 percent, as opposed to below 50 percent just a few years earlier. He cited specific instances where outcomes were even better than the average: 6 recoveries out of 8 operations in Ohio, 14 of 19 in Louisiana. Although Hoag doubted the surgery would ever be performed to the extent it was in Europe, where conditions associated with poverty, such as rickets and osteomalacia, were more prevalent than in the United States, he lauded his European counterparts for their "proper appreciation of the diameters of the parturient canal." In issuing that praise, he indirectly criticized his American colleagues for assuming that virtually every woman was capable of giving birth vaginally.[67]

The controversy surrounding cesareans was far from over, however. Immediately after Hoag issued his assertion, a doctor in the audience rose to disagree, noting that during his career he had witnessed only one cesarean and he was loath to ever witness another. The infant died soon after birth; the mother died two days later of postpartum infection. He was aware that cesareans had become the subject of "a great deal of talk," even "in little country towns." He suspected, however, that the surgery's death rate was far higher than the optimistic numbers supplied by Hoag. He called for decreasing, rather than increasing, the incidence of the surgery.[68]

Yet enhanced surgical safety, as Hoag's pitch intimated, was about to lead to a half-century-long discussion of the benefits of broadening indications for cesareans. Medical advances were indeed making cesarean sections safer. Antiseptics in particular had decreased postsurgical mortality across the board—with improvement in outcomes after a cesarean the most striking, likely because physicians had traditionally performed the operation under uniquely difficult circumstances. So why not perform more cesareans? The early-twentieth-century debate would resolve little, however. While some physicians supported performing more cesareans, others fought the proposal with equal vigor—citing the identical concern their progenitors had. The surgical risks were simply too great.[69]

Chapter Two

Still Too Risky?

1900–1930s

By the end of the nineteenth century, medical developments allowed physicians to view cesarean surgery as a rational, although still rare, option rather than a desperate, last-ditch effort. The introduction of ether in 1846, followed by the discovery of the anesthetic properties of chloroform in 1847, allowed surgeons to discard the makeshift measures they had used traditionally to ease their patients' agony during surgical procedures. Even more far-reaching, affecting every corner of medical practice, was acceptance of the germ theory of disease.[1]

The cause of postsurgical infection had always mystified doctors. They mulled many possibilities over the years—predisposition of the individual, seasonal change, environmental miasmas, overcrowding, and exposure to sewer gas, to name only a few. Not until 1857, when Louis Pasteur's investigation of a catastrophe befalling the French wine industry led him to connect bacteria with pathological change in organic matter, did anyone suggest that invisible organisms caused illness in people.[2]

Even then, physicians did not link Pasteur's discovery to surgical practice until 1865, when Joseph Lister became one of the first physicians to adopt aseptic techniques. Lister, an English surgeon who worked variously in Glasgow, Edinburgh, and London, theorized that just one microscopic germ might prompt sepsis. He explained, "Upon this principle, I have based a practice." Lister's success was soon manifest. Using carbolic acid as an antiseptic during amputations, he saw mortality in his surgical practice drop 67 percent—from 46 to 15 percent of cases.

Although many in the medical community remained skeptical of the germ theory, attentive surgeons on both sides of the Atlantic began to adopt the practices that came to be known collectively as "Listerism." Institutional acceptance was slower in coming; the first sterile surgical room in the United States did not open until 1889, when surgeons at Johns Hopkins Hospital inaugurated it. The establishment of that lone room, however, signaled a sea change. By the end of the nineteenth century, routinely disinfecting surgical instruments, donning sterile gowns, and dressing wounds postsurgically with an antiseptic were universal practices.[3]

Before anesthesia and asepsis, surgeons performed operations quickly, hoping to minimize patients' suffering and reduce their chance of infection. By quelling pain and diminishing postoperative sepsis, the life-saving combination of anesthesia and Listerism afforded surgeons an opportunity to work methodically as opposed to frantically. For mothers undergoing cesareans, this meant fewer postpartum infections, nicked intestines, and wounded offspring. Indeed, women undergoing cesarean surgery probably profited from the increase in surgical safety more than the average surgical patient; not wasted by disease, their odds of recovery were greater than the majority of patients who underwent abdominal surgery due to a ravaging illness. As one physician observed, cesarean surgery had finally been "shorn of its terrors."[4]

Although still rare, cesarean births rose accordingly. At the New York Nursery and Child's Hospital, cesareans increased from 2 in 1,000 deliveries in 1910 to 25 in 1,000 in 1927; at the Chicago Lying-In Hospital, while 6 in 1,000 births were by cesarean in 1915–1916, 30 in 1,000 were by cesarean in 1928 and 1929. Similarly, at Johns Hopkins Hospital in Baltimore, from 1899 to 1921 doctors performed 183 cesareans in about 20,000 deliveries, a rate of 0.9 percent. Then, from 1921 to 1926, doctors performed 180 cesareans in 8,000 births—a 146 percent increase. The Manhattan Maternity and Dispensary saw comparable statistics. From 1905 through 1919, Dispensary physicians attended 6,212 births that included 103 by cesarean—a 1.66 percent rate. In the following decade, from 1920 through 1932, the Dispensary saw a 73 percent increase—342 cesareans in 11,896 births.[5]

Ongoing Caution

All urban hospitals seemed to be seeing at least some upsurge in the surgery. The increases, however, even among institutions in the same city, varied enormously. In 1929, Boston Lying-In Hospital was at one end of the spectrum, with 1 in 12 births a cesarean. At the other end was New York Lying-In, with 1 in

585 births a cesarean. In between the outliers were San Francisco Hospital (1 in 40 births), Cook County Hospital in Chicago (1 in 88), Long Island College (1 in 125), and Detroit Hospital (1 in 217).[6]

The variations could be attributed to three factors: patient population, the experience of each institution's physicians, and the basic philosophies of those physicians. At some hospitals, difficult births were the norm; in an era when the majority of births still took place in the home, the few hospitals providing maternity care catered to the most desperate women, many of whom were single and homeless, essentially shunned by their families and consequently the most likely mothers to experience difficult births. The best of those institutions also employed the most skilled obstetricians. The obstetrician-in-chief at Johns Hopkins Hospital, for example, was the famed J. Whitridge Williams. The equally renowned Joseph B. DeLee helped found the Chicago Lying-In Hospital. Some gifted obstetricians tended to perform more cesareans simply because they were confident of their ability to ensure good outcomes. Other, equally talented physicians exhibited the opposite tendency: they performed fewer cesareans because they were capable of managing difficult births without resorting to surgery. Still others had learned that the likelihood of a poor outcome did not justify the risks of surgery. Marked inexperience elicited the same contradictory behaviors. Some doctors acknowledged their lack of skill by avoiding cesareans; ignorance allowed others to plunge headlong into performing them.

The most experienced obstetricians condemned overly confident, novice colleagues. One obstetrician working at both Massachusetts General and Boston Lying-In Hospitals explained that one of the many dangers of cesarean section was the operation's simplicity—it was easier to perform than any obstetric maneuver "except perhaps an easy low forceps." And that, he lamented, was the reason some inexperienced doctors chose cesareans "in improper cases." A New Orleans physician similarly cautioned: "The mortality of the average operator and the average mortality of all operators are much truer indices of the value of a given procedure than are the brilliant results of a single skilful [*sic*] surgeon or a single well organized clinic."[7]

Thus, despite an uptick in the surgery at some urban hospitals, obstetricians worked so hard to avoid cesareans that they touted an early form of labor induction as a preventive measure. In the 1924 fourth edition of his classic text, *Principles and Practice of Obstetrics*, DeLee listed contracted pelvis as the primary reason for induction. To spare those women the "frightful mortality" of cesarean surgery, he theorized that they would have little difficulty giving birth to their smaller (albeit premature) babies if doctors forced them, via induction, to give birth several weeks early. Although induction as a means of avoiding a cesarean was slower to catch on in the United States than in England (the first 1,000 births, occurring between 1888 and 1890, at Sloane Maternity Hospital in New York City saw only a dozen inductions), the lofty goal of sparing a mother a cesarean lent an air of prudence to the otherwise radical procedure. The most common induction techniques in the early twentieth century included rupturing the amniotic sac, inserting a bougie into the uterus, and forcibly dilating the cervix using successively larger bags injected with liquid.[8]

J. Whitridge Williams was one of the many obstetricians who deplored the early-twentieth-century rise in cesareans. Despite his extraordinary skill, and the skill of the doctors who worked with him, he feared that any increase in the surgery would erode the talent that allowed physicians to facilitate difficult vaginal births. A doctor who worked at the Preston Retreat, a medical charity in Philadelphia serving "indigent married women of good character," likewise urged colleagues to avoid "the more brilliant and oftentimes spectacular Caesarean section." He adhered to his own advice, mustering his skill, for example, to position a laboring woman "with rachitic lordosis and ankyloses of the left hip" to effect a vaginal delivery. He wrote of the birth, "This happy termination of a case promising serious obstruction saved the Retreat's record of 2,000 consecutive deliveries without a Cæsarean section and with but one craniotomy and that upon a dead infant."[9]

Reasons for performing the surgery had not changed markedly between 1875 and the first decade of the twentieth century. In both eras, physicians most often listed "profuse hemorrhage," "generally contracted pelvis," or "flat pelvis" in obstetric records as justifications. And just as in the first published account of a cesarean in the United States, when the physician could find no cervical opening, doctors also described the infrequent extraordinary circumstance. In 1905 at the Manhattan Maternity and Dispensary, for example, "united twins" posed a series of problems. The first child presented in the breech position. Unable to extract the infant, "the lower extremity of the presenting child was then amputated above the pelvis." Fearing uterine rupture if labor continued, doctors decided to deliver the remaining baby "& amputated head" by cesarean. In short, unspeakable difficulties still triggered most cesareans, and lack of operative interference remained the salient characteristic of obstetric practice.[10]

Nevertheless, a few obstetricians were beginning to argue that the new surgical safety measures offered unprecedented promise to women facing exceptionally serious threats. Those doctors urged widening the indications for cesareans beyond the standard severely contracted pelvis, insisting that the severest cases of placenta previa and eclampsia, for example, now posed greater risk to mothers than cesarean section. Anything approaching consensus on such a radical proposal remained elusive, however. Still wary of the surgical risks, most doctors resisted these suggestions, continuing to insist that severe pelvic deformity—an immutable, lifelong condition—remain the only legitimate reason to perform a cesarean.[11]

Williams was particularly adamant in this regard. He cautioned that any broadening of indications invited "considerable margin for abuse." He was not alone. In 1929, a New Orleans doctor ridiculed the physicians pressing for more surgeries by publishing a list of "Miscellaneous Indications [for cesareans] Quoted Verbatim" that included children born in rapid succession, "arthritis ankle," varicose veins, and "low grade mentality." A California doctor compiled a similarly frivolous inventory almost a decade later: "wish of the family doctor," "economic reasons," "to preserve a normal pelvic outlet," "repeated attacks of false labor," and "premature rupture of the membranes without labor pains although the pelvis is not contracted or abnormal."[12]

These physicians likely resorted to mockery because the advocates for more cesareans were making some headway, at least in the literature. By the end of the second decade of the twentieth century, obstetric texts had begun to classify the indications for a cesarean as either "absolute" or "relative." In the event of an absolute indication, a baby could not be born in any other way. Relative indications relied on physicians' subjective judgment. While the child had a chance of being delivered vaginally without incident, a cesarean might afford the mother and child better odds than "delivery from below"—physicians' slang for vaginal birth.

Assorted editions of Joseph DeLee's *The Principles and Practice of Obstetrics* demonstrate how the conditions prompting a cesarean changed over the first half of the twentieth century. The 1918 third edition of DeLee's tome listed only one absolute indication for the surgery—a "parturient canal" so narrow that the infant, "even reduced by mutilating operations," could only be removed by cesarean surgery. He dismissed relative indications as "largely subjective," lamenting the surgery "is being done too often and for insufficient indication."[13] Ten years later, in the 1928 fifth edition of his text, DeLee displayed both greater flexibility and ongoing ambivalence. Although he listed more relative indications than he had previously (cord prolapse, death of the fetus in or just before labor in previous births, placental abruption in several previous pregnancies, abnormal presentation, eclampsia, fibroids, and heart disease, to name only a few), he bemoaned the "wide field for the play of individual preference, the influence of isolated experience, and the clash of contending statistics" afforded by the additional indications. He continued to characterize cesarean surgery as "much abused . . . even by men whose intentions are honest."[14]

Not until the mid-twentieth century did obstetricians exhibit a shift in sensibility. In the 1951 edition of DeLee's text, now authored by J. P. Greenhill (DeLee died in 1942), "absolute" and "relative" categories had disappeared altogether. All indications, now numbering 17, rested on a level playing field and included "definite disproportion between the baby's head and the pelvic inlet," "extreme narrowing of the pelvic outlet," a previous cesarean, preeclampsia, total placenta previa, severe cases of placental abruption, and breech presentations in first-time mothers older than 40. The limitations placed on most indications appearing on the expanded list were telling, however; constraints implied obstetricians' ongoing reluctance to perform the surgery. Except for "a previous cesarean" and "preeclampsia," Greenhill qualified every indication according to the extremity of the condition. Conditions mandating cesarean surgery had to be "definite," "extreme," "total," "severe," or "in first-time mothers older than 40."[15]

During the first half of the twentieth century, the most vocal opponents of more cesareans contended that the surgery's growing safety was largely illusory. In 1921, Franklin Newell, professor of clinical obstetrics at Harvard University, devoted an entire book to discussion of cesarean surgery "in the hope that it may have some influence in diminishing the prevalent abuse of one of the most valuable obstetric procedures." While cesarean surgery may have been seeing better outcomes in large urban hospitals employing highly skilled obstetricians, Newell contended it was a different matter for "local operators in small communities," where cesarean section remained "one of the most fatal of surgical operations." Another physician declared "the wonder" was not the lower maternal death rate thanks to improvement in surgical techniques but that anybody ever survived the surgery. He urged "letting mothers and babies take their chances by natural channels alone."[16]

Williams credited only the recent innovation of "elective cesareans" for the improvement in the postsurgical maternal death rate. The phrase referred to a planned operation prompted by a compelling medical indication, a starkly different meaning than the elective cesareans of today. Physicians theorized that scheduled cesareans ensured that skilled obstetricians would be present, limited the surgery to "uninfected and unexhausted women," and helped to reduce the number of operations that were little more than a dangerously impromptu response to a birth exhibiting a seemingly endless cascade of difficulties. Williams argued that if the so-called elective episodes were eliminated from the data pool, the maternal death rate after a cesarean remained as "murderous" in 1922 as half a century earlier.[17]

Infant Deaths Decrease, Maternal Deaths Increase

The early-twentieth-century elective cesarean became an acceptable option because, for the first time, doctors were factoring into their decision-making the value of not only maternal but also fetal life. As one physician observed in 1912, "the living foetus should always be a part of the obstetric problem, and a considerable part at that." His observation ran so counter to what had been longstanding medical priority that he immediately tempered his remark by adding, "provided the life of the mother is not too greatly jeopardized thereby." The thrust of his statement was nonetheless clear. Now that cesarean surgery was safer for mothers, doctors should consider employing it not only to save an otherwise doomed woman but also to save an otherwise doomed fetus. While, traditionally, risk during childbirth had been defined strictly in maternal terms, risk to the fetus was now a consideration as well. Within two decades, cesarean surgery had become so clearly linked to saving the fetus that, in 1930, the chief of the Gynecology and Obstetrics Department at the University of Kansas warned medical students not to perform a cesarean if the fetus had died "in as much as Caesarean section is essentially an operation in the interest of the baby."[18]

Given the increased focus on the fetus, physicians' aversion to craniotomy grew, and both the proponents and the critics of the increase in cesarean surgeries exploited that abhorrence to make their case. If destroying "a living child" was obscene, one doctor argued, "so should an abdominal operation be that demands such a heavy toll" on women. Advocates for the surgery countered by insisting that a cesarean was more humane than a craniotomy. Franklin Newell touted cesarean surgery as benefiting the two patients equally—terming it "one of the most valuable operations yet devised . . . as a life and health saving procedure for both mother and child."[19]

Not only doctors discussed maternal, infant, and child health. Those concerns were one impetus for the social activism that characterized the Progressive Era, from roughly the 1890s through World War I. Progressivism subsumed many causes—women's suffrage, abolition of child labor, prison reform, tenement reform, control of infectious disease, prohibition, and access to contraception, to name a few. The disparate movements shared one purpose: to mitigate the effects of rapid urbanization and industrialization. As crucial drivers of Progressivism, women demanded action on their special concerns, most notably preventing the premature deaths of the nation's most vulnerable citizens—infants. "Save the Babies" became a national rallying cry, leading to well-funded, intensively publicized efforts, for example, to bottle and pasteurize cows' milk. Dramatically fewer infant and child deaths from diarrhea were the result.[20]

Obstetricians' concern for infants became even more pronounced after World War I. During the war, almost 30 percent of draftees had been declared unfit for military service due to defects traceable to poor care and disease in childhood. Inspired by these findings, pronatalism—concerted governmental efforts to encourage women to have more children and to provide women with the means to better care for them—became national policy. One concrete manifestation of pronatalism was the Sheppard-Towner Act, passed by the US Congress in 1921, which funded pre- and postnatal education for mothers that included visits from public health nurses during pregnancy and immediately after birth.[21]

Cesareans remained a thorny issue in this era. While a cesarean might save an infant's life, the surgery also posed a threat to a mother's ability to bear more children. Since life-threatening maternal complications increased with each cesarean, most obstetricians, even into the 1970s, advised that a woman's uterus be removed immediately after her third cesarean. Yet truncating a woman's reproductive years ran counter to the government-sponsored pronatalism of the 1910s and 1920s.[22]

The stubbornly high maternal mortality rate in the United States remained the primary reason for the ongoing cesarean debates. Even as Progressive Era activists saw success in lowering infant mortality, maternal mortality increased. Between 1900 and 1920, as infant mortality plunged 42 percent, maternal mortality rose 27 percent. In 1926, the United States placed nineteenth among the 20 countries then compiling maternal death data, ahead of only Chile. The disgraceful ranking prodded the New York Academy of Medicine (NYAM) to launch an investigation into every maternal death in New York City from 1930 through 1932. The resulting report concluded that 64 percent of the deaths had been avoidable. NYAM blamed physician "incompetence," singling out cesarean sections as a particular hazard: "the proportion of living mothers and infants obtained by caesarean operation fails to justify its use . . . average mortality figures show plainly that caesarean is a dangerous measure."[23]

The rise in maternal deaths during the first three decades of the twentieth century was due largely to the principal site of birth moving from home to hospital.

Maternal outcomes in New York City, where the death rate from postpartum infection was 47 percent less in home as opposed to hospital births in the early 1930s, exemplified the problem. Chicago obstetrician Henry Benaron explained that laboring women, "probably immune to their own bugs in their own homes," were better off giving birth there. A microbiologist agreed, characterizing hospitals as "a sort of armed camp of streptococci"—no place for healthy women undergoing a physiological process. DeLee heeded the call "to isolate mothers from death" by helping to open the Chicago Lying-In Hospital, an institution devoted solely to childbirth.[24]

As late as the 1930s, 15,000 women died annually in the United States as a direct result of childbirth; the "fight for life," as one American microbiologist with a special interest in maternal health put it in 1938, was ongoing. The claim of some physicians that cesarean surgery remained too dangerous to justify, and the counterclaim of others that mothers would benefit if there were more cesarean surgeries, were part of a broader discussion about how best to mitigate high maternal mortality in general.[25]

This is not to say that the maternal death rate following a cesarean had not seen improvement since the turn of the twentieth century, or that cesareans were singularly responsible for high maternal mortality. By the second decade of the twentieth century, deaths after a cesarean birth had plummeted to an average 8.1 percent (from greater than 50 percent for most of the nineteenth century), with cesareans at the country's best hospitals seeing a 2 to 4 percent death rate. Yet the most difficult cases—a cesarean performed after a prolonged labor, preceded by multiple attempts to terminate the labor with forceps—saw mortality as high as 34 percent.[26]

The physicians who championed more cesareans attributed bad outcomes to poorly selected cases. They claimed that in "clean cases," cesareans performed on mothers uncompromised by either exhaustion or medical meddling, "mortality is almost nil." While the surgery had long been a panicked, last-minute, most likely deadly effort, it had become far safer as physicians began to adhere to certain provisos. The operation was "almost universally successful" when performed just before or immediately after the onset of labor, on a well-rested patient in good condition, in an appropriate locale, with expert assistance at the ready. And the best obstetricians at the most elite institutions observed those rules, avoiding patients whose membranes had ruptured or who had been given an internal vaginal exam. By not performing the surgery on those patients, doctors hoped to circumvent the invariably fatal sequence of events seen too often in the nineteenth century—a mother exhausted by an inordinate number of hours in labor, multiple failed attempts to employ forceps accompanied by trauma to soft tissue, the introduction of pathogenic bacteria, then the surgery resulting in hemorrhage and/or infection and death. As cesarean births began to see a maternal mortality ranging from less than 1 to, at most, 5 percent in the best hospitals with an accompanying neonatal mortality close to zero, cesareans began to replace high forceps, which saw a maternal death rate of 4 percent and fetal demise between 40 and 80 percent.[27]

Only the best obstetricians and the most renowned urban hospitals could boast of these statistics, however. For the vast majority of physicians and hospitals, the numbers remained grim. Seven percent of the 900 women who gave birth by cesarean in largely rural Iowa in the late 1930s died; the overall maternal death rate in the state at the time was only 0.07 percent. Other states and cities fared even worse during the same time period: Texas, Cincinnati, New Orleans, and Indiana saw post-cesarean maternal mortality of 14.4, 16, 16.1, and 17.3 percent, respectively. One physician argued that any other surgery seeing such a high death rate would "never be performed except for the most compelling indications." With high maternal mortality as the backdrop, medical opinion over cesareans remained divided.[28]

Measuring Pelvises

Through the nineteenth century, pelvic abnormality had been the number-one reason for performing a cesarean, and the prevalence of this diagnosis persisted well into the twentieth century. From 1894 to 1909, severe pelvic deformity was the reason given for 96 of the first 100 cesareans performed at Boston Lying-In Hospital. Of the 112 cesareans performed through 1913 at the Sloane Hospital for Women in New York City, 78 percent were for a gravely contracted pelvis. Similarly, 79 percent of the 183 cesareans performed at Johns Hopkins Hospital between 1899 and 1920 were, in Williams's words, "done on account of disproportion between the size of the child and the pelvis, and I believe that great conservatism was observed in the indications for its performance." Yet pelvic anomalies were not always obvious to the naked eye, hence enthusiasm for what obstetricians dubbed "pelvimetry."[29]

Pelvimetry was the intricate art of taking pelvic measurements in relation to the presumed dimensions of a full-term fetus. Obstetricians deemed the art to be so vital that when the Obstetrics Department at Johns Hopkins opened in 1896, "carefully and accurately" measuring patients' pelvises was top priority. For at least the next three decades, either the chief of obstetrics, his surrogate, or the resident obstetrician (with three or more years' experience) was responsible for ensuring the accuracy of those measurements and dutifully recording them. The calculations were so painstaking, physicians figured them to the half-centimeter. Indeed, a half-centimeter could dictate the difference between a vaginal birth and an elective cesarean. Franklin Newell put so much stock in pelvic measurements that in 1921, after noting "the excellent results of cesarean section . . . under modern conditions," he called for liberalizing the definition of pelvic contraction from "a true conjugate diameter of less than 7.5 centimeters" to a pelvic diameter up to and including 7.5 centimeters.[30]

Pelvimetry yielded many diagnoses, each subtly different. They included the "uniformly contracted pelvis," the "obliquely contracted pelvis," the "flat non-rhachitic pelvis," the "simple flat rhachitic pelvis," the "rhachitic dwarf pelvis," the "spondylolisthetic pelvis," and the "transversely contracted pelvis." Each diagnosis, depending on its severity, was then classified as either absolute or relative. Like other indications for cesarean section, absolute abnormalities demanded a cesarean birth. Relative pelvic abnormalities, on the other hand, could be confounding—the identical condition might lead to a cesarean birth for one woman and a vaginal birth for another.[31]

Diagnoses, and whether they were a relative or an absolute indication for a cesarean, stymied even the most seasoned obstetricians. Edwin Cragin, professor of obstetrics and gynecology at the Columbia University College of Physicians and Surgeons, would declare a pelvis normal according to pelvimetric analysis, only to find during labor that an abnormal pelvic angle created an "impassable

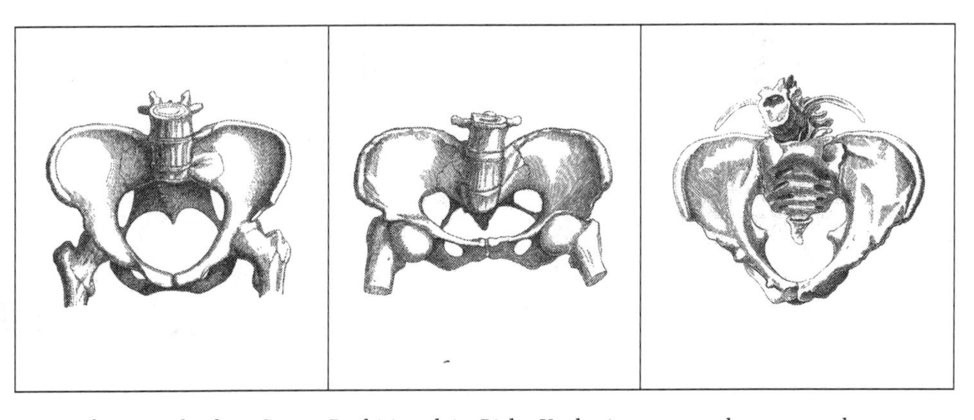

Left: Normal pelvis. *Center*: Rachitic pelvis. *Right*: Kyphotic transversely contracted pelvis.
Source: Barnes, *Lectures on Obstetric Operations*, figures 98, 99, and 100.

dystocia" requiring a cesarean. The opposite occurred as well: measurements that indicated the need for a cesarean delivery in one pregnancy would be refuted in the next as the same woman, unable to get to the hospital in time, would give birth to a subsequent baby at home, vaginally, without medical supervision and without difficulty. Even more perplexing, the baby born vaginally was often larger than the infant born by cesarean. Thus, even as some physicians swore by the "science of pelvimetry," others condemned any "arbitrary standard" dictating the need for cesarean surgery.[32]

Despite the doubts, pelvimetry long remained a valued obstetric tool. One obstetrician recalled that in the 1960s, he and his colleagues took a diagnosis of fetal-pelvic disproportion so seriously that they mulled over multiple factors when trying to predict the size of a full-term fetus. "We looked at things like how tall was the patient [and] the husband's hat size." One of his partners conducted a perpetual contest among the obstetric residents: "If you could come within 10 percent of the weight of the baby . . . he would give you a bottle of scotch. If you were wrong, you had to give him a package of cigarettes. And he said he . . . never had to buy cigarettes, and rarely did he have to give up a bottle." The obstetrician's overflowing cigarette stash evidenced a dilemma—the seeming importance of accurately estimating fetal weight and its relationship to maternal pelvic size

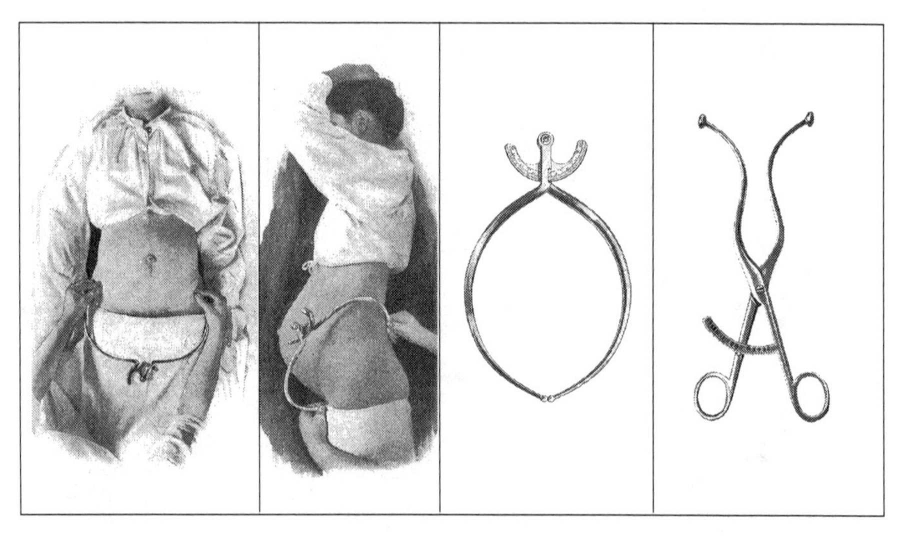

Left and center left: Taking external pelvic measurements. *Center right*: An external pelvimeter. *Right*: An internal pelvimeter.
Source: DeLee, *The Principles and Practice of Obstetrics* (1918), 238, 240, 241.

versus the slim chance of estimating either fetal weight or maternal pelvic size accurately. Yet the measuring ritual persisted, even as late as the 1970s.[33]

In the 1940s, "x-ray pelvimetry" gave pelvimetry new life. X-rays seemed to provide an accuracy no one could argue with. Yet the ambiguous results that plagued hand measurements dogged pelvimetry's more sophisticated descendant. As one doctor noted in 1950 of what had become the routine maternal pelvic x-ray, "A normal pelvis tolerates great discrepancies between fetal head and the pelvis." In other words, both the maternal pelvis and the fetal skull are malleable, rendering the static measurements taken during pregnancy useless. The reliance on pelvic measurements, whether by hand or x-ray, commonly steered a physician in the wrong direction—"either [toward] radicalism or sad conservatism." Yet not until the dangers of x-raying pregnant women became universally acknowledged did all obstetricians finally reject pelvimetry as "medical nonsense."[34]

Until then, the best-known obstetric textbooks, particularly in the 1920s, devoted a hundred or more pages to discussion of the size, shape, and degree of distortion of assorted pelvic abnormalities. J. Whitridge Williams devoted seven chapters to the pelvis in the 1923 edition of his text, *Obstetrics*. In the 1925 fourth edition of Joseph DeLee's *Principles and Practice of Obstetrics*, he urged colleagues to hone "as exact a knowledge as possible of the size and shape of the parturient passages," warning that ignoring pelvimetry in favor of a trial of labor was "a blundering method . . . both unscientific and costly in human life."[35]

Although Williams paid even more attention to the pelvis in his text than DeLee did in his, Williams did not suggest that pelvimetry be used to justify cesareans—quite the contrary. He hoped that careful pelvimetric analysis would steer obstetricians away from the surgery. He believed the more precise the diagnosis, the more likely a physician would avoid radical intervention. Of the almost 1,200 pregnant women he had treated who exhibited "the usual types of contracted pelvis," only 1 in 30 of those 1,200 required a cesarean. The skill and sense of the physician, Williams argued, should be the primary determinant of whether a cesarean was necessary, not pelvic measurements.[36]

Despite Williams's homage to obstetricians' skills, physicians' diagnoses, including Williams's, were not necessarily dispassionate. Class, race, and ethnicity were omnipresent subtexts when doctors evaluated pregnant patients. Obstetricians believed that certain women were simply more likely to need a cesarean than others. In the 1910s, a physician at Michael Reese Hospital, an institution built in Chicago in the 1880s with the help of charitable contributions from the city's German Jewish community, could not recall a single cesarean performed on their service despite an average 1,000 births a year there. He ascribed the hospital's record to "pelvic indications being absent among the women coming to us." Although he did not describe the women he referred to, presumably he was alluding to a mainly Jewish group of central European lineage. DeLee, on the other hand, complained of "a large contracted pelvis clientele from the foreign born population, particularly the Italians and Poles." Williams claimed that Johns Hopkins Hospital saw "the largest contracted pelvis material in the country, owing to the fact that one half of . . . patients are negroes." Williams was so wedded to the notion that race and pelvic deformity were linked that he used "the large Negro population of Baltimore, with its unusual incidence of abnormal pelves," to demonstrate "important and fundamental differences" between his white and black patients. Another obstetrician compared the pelvises of Filipina women with "European[s] or American[s]" and found the pelvises of the former to be significantly smaller than the latter. The discovery confounded her because, despite their small pelvic dimensions, Filipina women had far fewer cesareans than white women. She ultimately concluded that the Filipina habit of squatting while working compensated for their small pelvises.[37]

Eugenics, a philosophy calling for improvement of the human gene pool through the separation of races and classes and sterilization of "the unfit," fueled the racist assumptions about pelvic size and shape and a woman's ability to give birth. Influential in the United States from the turn of the twentieth century through World War II, eugenic thought permeated public policy and legislation. The 1927 US Supreme Court decision *Buck v. Bell*, for example, declared constitutional a Virginia law permitting the forced sterilization of "socially inadequate" people. In agreeing that the state of Virginia had a legitimate interest in sterilizing the plaintiff, Carrie Buck, Supreme Court justice Oliver Wendell Holmes, Jr., said of the teenage Buck, her mother, and her "illegitimate" infant daughter, conceived when an older relative raped her: "Three generations of imbeciles are enough."[38]

Politicians, public health officials, and physicians embraced eugenics in many realms, but especially in matters pertaining to human reproduction. During his presidency, Theodore Roosevelt characterized white, Protestant married women without children, or with only a few children, as "criminal against the race." S. Josephine Baker, head of New York's Bureau of Child Hygiene, similarly warned that if native-born American women continued to have children at a rate lower than immigrants, "extermination of the Anglo-Saxon race" was inevitable. Eugenics also shaped doctors' rationales for surgical protocols when performing a cesarean. At Johns Hopkins, one-third of the cesareans performed in the 1920s were Porros—which by definition included removal of the uterus—long after other institutions had switched to Sänger's conservative cesarean. Williams described the Porro technique as essential for his patient population because "a large number of our patients are colored women of relatively low intelligence in whom we have felt that an unlimited number of repeated Caesarean section was not justifiable."[39]

"Once a Cesarean, Always a Cesarean"

Several factors thus ensured an increase in cesarean births during the first two decades of the twentieth century. Surgeries were safer. Pronatalism had become national policy, putting greater emphasis on the fetus. And the mere act of ascertaining and recording pelvic measurements rendered cesarean surgery an omnipresent possibility if not a common occurrence.

The most durable contribution to an increase in cesareans, however, was a pronouncement by obstetrician Edwin Cragin. In a speech before the New York State Medical Society in 1916, and published subsequently in the *New York Medical Journal,* Cragin advised that no matter how carefully a doctor sutured a uterus after a cesarean, the uterus would never again be as sturdy as it had been. The scar would be prone to rupture in subsequent labors—leading to uncontrollable hemorrhage and death. This downstream consequence of just one cesarean birth prompted Cragin to famously recommend to colleagues, "Once a Cæsarean always a Cæsarean," a dictum that would hold sway in the United States for the next 80 years.[40]

Cragin based his edict on a known hazard of the surgical technique employed by American obstetricians. When performing a cesarean, they cut a long vertical incision that began high on the expanded uterus; the resulting scar was notoriously weak and, as Cragin observed, prone to rupture in subsequent labors. Another peculiarity of the cut was that it invited infection. One obstetrician explained in 1929, "the classical operation is never safe late in labor, for no suture line is water-tight, and no amount of packing can lessen the danger of the intraperitoneal spill of uterine contents which, at this stage, are never sterile."[41]

Cragin was by no means the first physician to suggest that after one cesarean a woman not be permitted to give birth in any other way. He has likely been credited with the proviso only because he described it in a memorably pithy manner. Well before his pronouncement, other obstetricians had already adopted the rule. In 1909 at Boston Lying-In Hospital, for example, physicians did not allow any woman who had had a previous cesarean to labor for long; as one physician explained, "our custom [is] never to subject a patient who has had one Caesarean section to the strain of labor on account of the danger, which is always present in such cases, of rupture of the uterus through the old scar."[42]

In addition to ensuring an increase in the surgery, the "once a cesarean, always a cesarean" credo also came to serve as the strongest argument against the surgery. Cesareans were antithetical to pronatalism; just one cesarean put a woman "in a position of reproductive inferiority" by threatening to place irrevocable limits on her family size. For this reason alone, Williams urged restricting the indications for a cesarean to "the narrowest possible limits." Only if a woman had previously given birth to multiple children before facing her first cesarean was Williams more amenable to considering the surgery. As he explained, "the patient has already done her duty to the State, and the possibility of further childbearing may be regarded as a matter of relative indifference." Cragin agreed, advising against cesareans in "all borderline cases" to prevent women from experiencing "a great dread, which otherwise would shadow each pregnancy."[43]

In the United States, the problem persisted despite a solution developed in Europe. In 1906 a German obstetrician had devised a safer surgical technique—a cut placed low on the uterus in a horizontal line that was less prone to uterine rupture in subsequent labors than the classic cut. Yet American obstetricians were slow to embrace the innovation. In the 1930s, the chief of the Department of Gynecology and Obstetrics at the University of Kansas explained to medical students and residents that American obstetricians and surgeons preferred the classical form of cesarean surgery. Even in the late 1950s, American obstetricians continued to doubt the benefits of the low transverse incision. The authors of one obstetric text published in New York in 1956 assured colleagues, "neither type of incision is clearly superior to the other." Not until the 1970s did American obstetricians definitively agree with their European counterparts that the low transverse incision had unparalleled advantages: it was easier to suture, resulted in less blood loss, and left a scar that was less likely to rupture in subsequent pregnancies and labors.[44]

The reluctance of American obstetricians to adopt the safer European technique was likely due to nationalism, a prejudice often evident in medicine. During World War I, when a handful of American socialites wrote about their experience giving birth in Germany under an anesthetic technique known as "twilight sleep," American physicians voiced their displeasure. One decried the magazines that gave women the false impression that "it is only these Europian [*sic*] masters of the hypodermic needle that have been capable of such wonderful clinical practises in medication." Another doctor admonished, "We

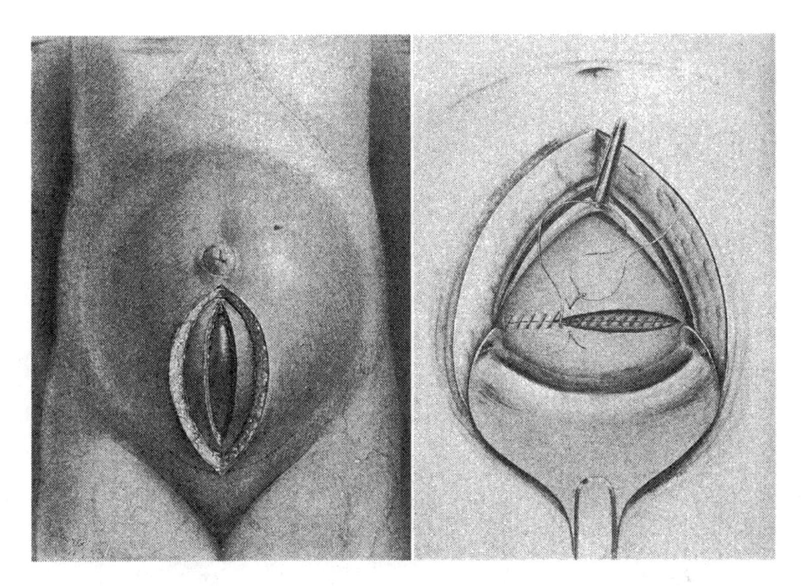

Left: The classic cesarean cut, a long vertical line starting at the umbilicus and ending at the bottom of the uterus. The scar left by the classic cut is weak and prone to rupture in subsequent labors. *Right*: The newer, low transverse cut, performed at the bottom of the uterus in a horizontal line. The scar left by this cut is far less prone to rupture. A European obstetrician invented the low transverse cut in 1906 and American physicians were exceedingly slow to adopt it despite its advantages.
Source: Newell, *Cesarean Section*, 111, 294.

have perhaps more reliable and less dangerous methods *not* 'made in Germany.'" Medical innovations introduced in one country are rarely appreciated quickly by physicians in another country.[45]

The Lowly Obstetrician

As obstetricians debated the merits, dangers, and assorted techniques of cesarean surgery, they also sought respect for their medical specialty, with only marginal success. Mothers had long been content with midwives; in the early twentieth century, few consulted a general practitioner during pregnancy, let alone an obstetrician. S. Josephine Baker observed with dismay that when a midwife was unavailable to attend a birth, most immigrants sought assistance from "the janitor's wife or the woman across the hall" rather than a physician. Joseph DeLee similarly complained that most women thought of childbirth as an activity that was as mundane and automatic as respiration and digestion and thus did not require specialized medical supervision. Most physicians treated obstetrics with similar disregard. Charles Ziegler, professor of obstetrics at the University of Pittsburgh, acknowledged in 1922 that the word "obstetrics" had come from a Latin word meaning "'to stand before' or, as a sneering colleague once observed, 'to stand around.'" As Ziegler's admission implied, the vast majority of doctors agreed with the public that childbirth was a straightforward activity requiring little medical expertise.[46]

Medical school training reflected this conviction. DeLee complained in 1898 of recent medical school graduates who had never examined a pregnant woman or witnessed a labor. Williams lamented similarly in 1917 that "ordinary doctor[s]" were so ignorant of the basic physiology of childbirth that few recognized that cervical dilation occurred spontaneously and slowly over many hours and sometimes days. On multiple occasions, he had been called to aid colleagues who had inflicted damage upon women by attempting to pry open their cervixes "when all that [had been] necessary [was] to give nature a chance." Physicians' educational deficit in obstetrics was so pronounced that in 1910, when Abraham Flexner issued his blistering criticism of the inadequacy of American medical schools that became known as the "Flexner Report," he reserved his harshest condemnation for the absence of training in obstetrics.[47]

Before the improvement in medical education prompted by Flexner, the few doctors who limited their practice to obstetrics took it upon themselves to remedy the omission in medical schools. DeLee was one of the most effective in this regard; in 1895, he opened the Chicago Lying-In Dispensary, a medical charity that dispatched trained physicians to attend home births in the vicinity of Jane Addams's Hull House—one of the most densely populated immigrant neighborhoods in the country. Medical students flocked to the dispensary to serve as apprentices. DeLee touted this as the primary reason for the charity's existence: "It is a fact that midwifery has been and still is the most neglected branch of medical teaching and the mortality records of the Board of Health bring melancholy proof of this fact." Although women's resistance to physician-attended births made it difficult initially for DeLee to attract patients, his medical charity soon became popular not only among impoverished women but also among the city's upper class. Chicago's wealthiest families—including the McCormicks (farm equipment manufacturers) and the Schaffners (men's clothiers)—recognized that physicians trained in obstetrics benefited all women, no matter their social and economic status. Bequests to the charity thus represented self-interest as well as benevolence.[48]

In this setting, surrounded by colleagues who devalued their specialty, obstetricians argued about widening the indications for cesareans. Some obstetricians explicitly linked cesareans with their own marginalization, contending that any increase in the surgery would further degrade their specialty. They characterized cesarean surgery as the recourse of the less skilled. Williams, for example, contended that cesareans required "only a few minutes of time and a modicum of operative experience," as opposed to a difficult vaginal birth that demanded "active mental exertion, many hours of patient observation, and frequently very considerable technical dexterity." He taught his students that "any carpenter with a little training can do a section, but . . . the highest grade of obstetrical intelligence is required to predict in a given case of moderate pelvic contraction that the child can be born spontaneously."[49]

DeLee agreed. He charged his private patients less for a cesarean than for a vaginal birth because, as he explained to a patient's husband, "there is less difficulty and it consumes less time. A normal labor takes from four to twenty hours of my time and a cesarean section is over in an hour and a half." Another obstetrician likewise observed that performing a straightforward surgical procedure was easier than obstetric maneuvers that took years to perfect and "half the night perhaps" to execute.[50]

The Nature of Childbirth and the Nature of Risk

Although obstetricians agreed that they were the best-suited medical professionals to mitigate any risk posed by childbirth, they disagreed about the nature of those risks and how to approach them. The disagreement was so foundational to their professional identity that obstetricians tended to self-identify with one of two informal philosophical camps—"operators" and "nonoperators." Operators argued that risk was omnipresent during childbirth. Nonoperators downplayed risk, contending that obstetricians were necessary at births to deftly handle the rare problem that might materialize. Each camp used its claim about the nature of childbirth to justify and elevate obstetrics as a medical specialty. The writings of the two most prominent early-twentieth-century obstetricians—J. Whitridge Williams, a nonoperator from Johns Hopkins University in Baltimore, and Joseph B. DeLee, an operator from Northwestern University in Chicago—exemplified the contrasting approaches.[51]

Williams argued that birth was a physiological process that required an attentive birth attendant able to offer consummate medical treatment in the unlikely event treatment was necessary. DeLee argued that birth was a potentially pathological process that required prophylactic medical intervention to avert the inevitable pathologies. His proposed interventions included injections of morphine and scopolamine (occasionally supplemented with chloral and sodium bromide by rectum) during first-stage labor, followed at the end of second-stage labor by ether, an episiotomy, removal of the infant via forceps, and manual removal of the placenta. DeLee famously recommended those measures in 1920, in an article, "The Prophylactic Forceps Operation," published in the inaugural issue of the *American Journal of Obstetrics and Gynecology*. In the article, he described childbirth as physically devastating to women. The passage from the article quoted (and condemned) most often by contemporary scholars reads, "So frequent are these bad effects that I often wonder whether nature did not deliberately intend women to be used up in the process of reproduction, in a manner analogous to that of salmon, which dies after spawning." DeLee also mentioned cesareans in the article to bolster his case for the trauma inherent in birth: "Women clamor for relief from the dangers and disabilities of childbirth and we have to afford them relief . . . they have backache, rectal and bladder trouble. . . . They even beg for Cesarean section to escape the dangers and pain of childbirth."[52]

Before publication of the article, DeLee read the paper aloud at a professional meeting. Williams, who was in the audience, rose to denounce the recommendations, chiding, "If his practice were to become general and widely adopted, women would be worse off eventually than had their labors been conducted by midwives." This was harsh indictment in an era when obstetricians rarely missed an opportunity to disparage midwives. DeLee had publicly characterized them as "a relic of barbarism." Without invoking his name, Williams continued to criticize DeLee in writing: "if a gifted obstetrical teacher inculcates his pupils with the idea that every labor is pathological he inevitably opens the door to every sort of abuse, for if students become convinced that labor is ordinarily not a physiological function, they will be tempted to relieve the pathologic process by every variety of interference."[53]

Despite their public enmity, the two men were friends, with more in common philosophically than their published words indicated. "Operators" and "nonoperators" shared the same goal—to prevent obstetric emergencies and the resulting damage to women. And DeLee, in fact, often practiced much like Williams. His home-birth dispensary in Chicago employed precisely the approach Williams promulgated: basic, aseptic, and nonintrusive care despite "adverse conditions with a group of patients physically below par." One observer enthusiastically described the bare-bones nature of the treatment provided by the Chicago Maternity Center (the moniker eventually bestowed on DeLee's dispensary, known informally as the CMC): "No instruments are used to bring a baby unless the life and health of mother and babe demand it. . . . The cleanliness organized in the dirtiest homes is before godliness." The enthusiastic admirer also commented on the rarity of cesarean sections performed by CMC obstetricians in the 1930s: "excepting in the most remote rural regions, it would be hard to find a smaller number of the so-often deadly Caesarean operations done than the Center does among its mothers."[54]

Doctors working for the CMC served Chicago for more than 80 years. They consciously sought to avoid the dangerous path of emergency cesareans—the mother, removed hastily from the home by ambulance, "brought under the knife, exhausted, often infected, and on the verge of dying." In one rare case in the 1930s, a CMC physician was summoned "sleepy-eyed" in the middle of the night to the home of a 40-year-old, first-time mother with a misshapen pelvis caused by rickets in childhood. Compounding the problem, the fetus presented as a footling breech. Making "a quick calculation," the doctor washed the baby's foot with an antiseptic, placed the foot back in the uterus, and administered general anesthesia "to soothe the mother's agony, but most of all to keep the baby from killing itself trying to be born again." The ambulance arrived. "With the siren . . . shrieking for a right-of-way," the doctor remained at the mother's side, "keeping her deep under the ether," during the "wild journey to the maternity hospital." At the hospital, waiting obstetricians performed a Porro cesarean because the baby's foot "having been in the outside world, infection of the mother's womb was certain." Both mother and baby survived the ordeal.[55]

DeLee was well aware that his home-birth dispensary, employing nonoperator techniques despite his published operator philosophy, saw spectacular results. While maternal mortality was 0.59 percent nationwide in the early twentieth century, the death rate at DeLee's home-birth Lying-In Dispensary charity was less than one-fourth that—0.14 percent. Even European physicians characterized DeLee's venture as the best of its kind in the world.[56]

Why DeLee's published writings contradict what archival records reveal of his actual practice is unclear. Pressure from paying patients seems to have been one factor. DeLee's concerted attempts to garner respect for his specialty seem to have been another. In fact, the two were often hard to distinguish. In 1922, the husband of one of DeLee's wealthy patients protested the $1,500 bill he had received for his wife's birth, which, indeed, was an outlandishly high charge for the era. Given an annual inflation rate of 2.81 percent, DeLee was demanding almost $21,000 (in 2017 dollars) from the new father. Yet DeLee declared the bill reasonable: "The labor began at three in the morning and I was in almost continuous attendance until noon. . . . The amount of mental and physical strain was many times that of an ordinary labor." He lectured the husband on the value of obstetricians: "The

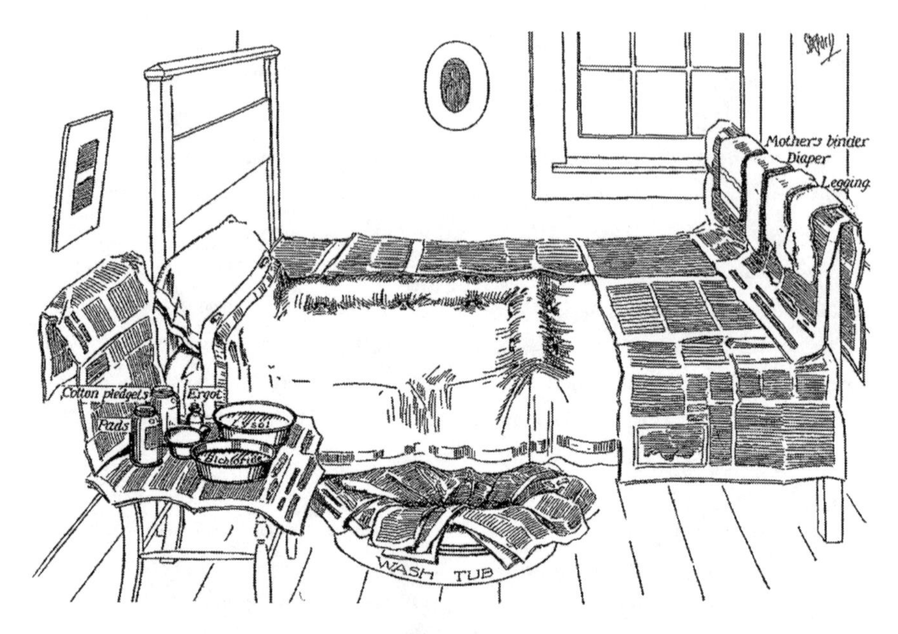

Illustration of a "bed prepared for [a home] delivery" according to the strict guidelines of the Chicago Maternity Center, the home birth dispensary that Joseph DeLee opened in 1895. An observer said of the CMC standards, "The cleanliness organized in the dirtiest homes is before godliness."

Source: *Technic of the Chicago Maternity Center Formerly the Chicago Lying-In Hospital Maxwell Street Dispensary* (Chicago Lying-In Hospital and Dispensary, 1921), 11. The *Technic* was the little red book carried by all dispensary physicians to home births.

work is hard and burdensome, it restricts one's liberty, robs one of rest at night, requires exceptional skill, and withal, it does not pay."[57]

DeLee was not alone in fielding this type of complaint. An assistant professor of obstetrics at the University of Minnesota attended the birth of a patient who similarly balked at paying her medical bill. He had done nothing, she protested, other than "stand around and let nature do the work!" The exasperated physician grumbled later to colleagues, "Her labor was long and tedious, and I spent hours encouraging her to bear with womanly fortitude a process that was essentially physiological. I admonished, I cheered, I held her hands, I did everything I could, except to put her to sleep and take the baby away." He noted that given this type of ingratitude, no one should be quick to condemn the obstetrician who decided to "do something" during labor to justify his bill.[58]

Precisely what an obstetrician did, however, seemed to depend on a woman's social and economic status. DeLee and Williams toiled in the unapologetically class-based, early-twentieth-century United States. While in the nineteenth century, poor women and women of color underwent the majority of cesarean births, DeLee seems to have bowed to very different class expectations and stereotypes in the twentieth century by practicing as a nonoperator among impoverished women and as an operator among women of means. As his profession's quintessential operator, he developed complex, prophylactic techniques to service the wealthy, even as he gained international renown for his successful, no-frills practices at his home-birth dispensary. His contrasting treatment of Alice Roosevelt Longworth, the oldest child of President Theodore Roosevelt, was indicative of his approach to well-to-do pregnant patients.[59]

In 1924, at the age of 40, Longworth became pregnant with her first child. As a resident of Washington, DC, she initially sought Williams's medical expertise in Baltimore. Eventually, she traveled to Chicago to consult with DeLee, apparently at Williams's behest. In a letter to Williams, DeLee complained, "while her pelvis is normal she insists upon a cesarean section." Although acquiescing to such a demand from a patient would have been virtually unprecedented at the time, DeLee told Williams, "In view of her aged primiparity and the necessity of preserving this very important baby I am inclined to grant her request." As one of the first American obstetricians to embrace the European method of cesarean incision, DeLee added, "I am also more favorable to this in view of the safety of the low or cervical cesarean." At some point, however, DeLee likely convinced Longworth that her demand was a foolhardy one; ultimately, her baby was born vaginally, although not without drama. DeLee noted, "the ether was taken badly, patient choked and turned blue etc., giving me much concern." He went on to perform an episiotomy, apply forceps, and manually remove the placenta—precisely as his 1920 article recommended. Then he packed her uterus to staunch an unexpected hemorrhage. DeLee characterized her postpartum condition as "very satisfactory, likewise that of the baby." Ultimately, Longworth recovered beautifully.[60]

DeLee's ability to embrace both the methods of the operator—for his wealthy, private patients—and the methods of the nonoperator—for the working-class women who frequented his home-birth dispensary—indicate that the two obstetric camps had more in common than their rancorous, published debates indicated. Garnering professional respect was a priority for both factions. Both denounced the poor outcomes of doctors who lacked sufficient training. Both called for a concerted effort to lower maternal mortality. In the early decades of the twentieth century, DeLee wrote often of his concern for the estimated 20,000 mothers who died annually in the United States during or shortly after childbirth, and the "hundreds of thousands" of women who "date lifelong invalidism from apparently normal confinement."

Williams, too, lamented the rise in the maternal death rate when every other cause of premature death was dropping. He dismissed the inherent dangers of childbirth as wildly exaggerated, however, and instead blamed high maternal mortality on the generalist physicians who practiced obstetrics as a mere sideline. "Doctors," he complained, "kill far more patients throughout the country by ill-judged operative procedures than do the midwives by puerperal infection." Both Williams and DeLee would have characterized their ostensibly opposing approaches in the same way—as measures intended to ensure healthy mothers and babies by the safest possible means. On occasion, they simply disagreed about the means.[61]

Operators and nonoperators agreed on another point; both condemned any inordinate use of cesarean section. DeLee avoided cesareans by implementing the series of procedures that he described in the inaugural issue of the *American Journal of Obstetrics and Gynecology*—the same procedures he employed during Longworth's birth. Williams sidestepped the surgery by letting "nature" take its course, unless a rare condition demanded his intervention. Planning ahead in order to avoid an emergency action was so important to both men, and their respective camps, that each considered an insignificant cesarean rate to be a hallmark of their professional success.

Avoiding cesareans was so important to these two leading American obstetricians of the first half of the twentieth century that, in what appeared to be an undeclared contest between the two, DeLee and Williams exchanged a series of letters in which each repeatedly claimed to have the lowest cesarean rate. Ultimately, Williams triumphed. At slightly less than 1 percent, his 213 cesareans in the 22,000 births he had attended or supervised represented about half the 1 in 50 births ending in a cesarean that DeLee saw in his combined lying-in hospital and home-birth service. DeLee prevailed in a far more significant way, however. His published protocol during labor eventually held sway. It is DeLee after all, not Williams, who is known today as "the father of modern obstetrics."[62]

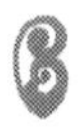

In 1922, J. Whitridge Williams criticized "certain tendencies" in modern American obstetrics that, he charged, led to "great abuse." While he did not want to be so conservative as to join the ranks of obstetricians who decades earlier had ignored warnings about the infectious nature of postpartum infection, neither did he want to succumb to the "furor operativus" that afflicted some of his colleagues. Williams lamented they were in danger of forgetting that the "great majority" of women were capable of spontaneous vaginal delivery. He was particularly critical of the prophylactic use of forceps and "the abuse of Cæsarean section." Edwin Cragin urged similar restraint. He asked colleagues, "Are we in our enthusiasm over radical obstetric surgery neglecting the fundamentals of obstetrics; the routine precautionary methods which may make the resort to radical obstetric surgery unnecessary?" Others agreed, warning that a cesarean section "*always carries with it a certain risk to the life of the patient*, even in the most competent hands and under the best conditions."[63]

The discussion indicated that physicians remained wary of cesarean surgery well into the twentieth century. When deaths after a cesarean rose from 11 percent of all maternal deaths in 1927 to 33 percent in 1934, a year when only 0.76 percent of births in the United States were by cesarean, obstetricians' ongoing caution seemed to be justified. Critics of increasing the number of cesarean sections could now argue with conviction that the indications for cesareans had, indeed, "dangerously" widened.[64]

Yet the debate, and the use of cesarean section, led to medical innovations as well—some, although not all, beneficial. Faith in the predictive value of pelvimetry, however useless that "science" would eventually prove to be, prompted doctors to appreciate the benefits of prenatal care. Pelvimetry demonstrated to obstetricians that when a mother did not consult any medical authority—midwife or doctor—until she was in labor, serious medical conditions might go undetected. With prenatal care, doctors could mitigate the conditions that might derail vaginal birth. Without prenatal care, birth could become a series of hastily planned, emergency actions likely to end badly—precisely what all obstetricians sought to avoid. By the 1920s, doctors tended to agree that prenatal "study and care" provided information that minimized the need for invasive examination and treatment during labor.[65]

While their devotion to pelvimetry persuaded doctors of the benefit of prenatal examinations, two federal programs helped to persuade mothers. The Sheppard-Towner Act, passed by the US Congress in late 1921, offered myriad benefits to pregnant women until its repeal in 1929. The federal dollars generated by the act (to be matched by participating states, and all but three accepted the money) were used to pay visiting nurses to dispense prenatal advice to women in their homes and produce and distribute informational pamphlets that primed women to seek regular prenatal care. If women had any lingering doubts about the efficacy of prenatal care after Sheppard-Towner, the Emergency Maternal and Infant Care Program (EMIC), funded by Congress from 1943 to 1949, erased the qualms. Through the Social Security Act, the EMIC paid all prenatal and maternity care expenses for the wives of servicemen in the military's four lowest pay grades, covering the medical expenses of more than 1.2 million women—one in every seven births in the United States during the years the EMIC was in effect. The EMIC also was instrumental in completing the move of the primary site of birth from home to hospital—92 percent of EMIC-funded births occurred in the hospital at a time when only 79 percent of births in the United States overall occurred there.[66]

Labor induction was a more ambiguous consequence of the early-twentieth-century cesarean controversy. If a mother had a major pelvic deformity, some physicians began to induce labor at 36 weeks, hoping that a smaller-than-normal baby would permit a vaginal birth. Thus cesareans, or more precisely the desire to avoid them, were an entrée to the chemical induction of labor that would become routine decades later. Of course, induction in the hopes of avoiding a cesarean then subjected the infant to the suffering and uncertain outcome inherent in premature birth. Yet that, too, led to innovation—techniques and technologies for the care of premature infants.[67]

Cesareans also helped physicians solve some longtime mysteries. Williams observed that "from the time of Hippocrates," doctors and scientists had theorized that the right ovary produced eggs that became boys, while eggs emanating from the left ovary produced girls. Cesarean surgery helped Williams and his team disprove the theory by allowing them to see which ovary contained the corpus luteum. Thus, cesarean sections, albeit indirectly, added to doctors' knowledge of human reproduction.[68]

At the time, though, few saw any connection between the contentious debate about cesareans and medical innovation. The discussion seemed esoteric, limited to a distinct few in the medical world. The mothers affected by the long-running polemics knew nothing of it. That was about to change, however. Beginning in the 1930s, and widely by the 1960s, cesareans would go public.

Chapter Three

Risk or Remedy?

1930s–1970

Even as obstetricians discussed the appropriate indications for a cesarean section, the operation remained so rare that the public was largely unaware that the surgery, let alone the contentious debate, existed. Only 2 to 2.5 percent of births overall ended in a cesarean in the 1930s, 1940s, and early 1950s, and that number did not reflect how few cesareans were performed at most hospitals. Ranging from less than 0.5 percent at many institutions to as much as 6 percent at a few large, urban hospitals, a birth by cesarean continued to be an extraordinary event in the professional life of physicians and the personal experience of mothers. Given the small numbers, the surgery was simply not on the public's radar.[1]

As late as the 1960s, physicians still belittled colleagues who performed cesareans with any regularity. J. P. Greenhill, the longtime editor of the *Yearbook of Obstetrics and Gynecology* and a protégé of both J. Whitridge Williams and Joseph B. DeLee, was typical. He intimated that only doctors who lacked sufficient training relied on cesareans: "In fact for many there is but one way out of a difficult obstetric situation, suprapubic [i.e., cesarean] delivery." In listing the "*legitimate indications*" for a cesarean, Greenhill used typographic emphasis to imply that, despite the surgery's growing safety, too many "illegitimate" surgeries were being performed. The ability of an obstetrician to execute a difficult delivery "from below"—obstetricians' chummy vernacular for vaginal birth—continued to be a source of professional pride.[2]

If the scorn of colleagues failed to persuade a doctor to change his habits, the recommendations of hospitals and professional organizations usually succeeded. In the 1950s, the Joint Commission on Accreditation of Hospitals advised in their "Standards for Hospital Accreditation" that obstetricians consult at least one colleague before performing a cesarean. Hospital administrators adhered to the suggestion so assiduously that when Francis Bayard Carter, the chair of the Obstetrics Department at Duke University Hospital, failed to ensure that all obstetricians under his supervision observed the recommendation, he received a stern letter from a hospital bureaucrat: "I noticed a total of 22 cesareans [for the year, out of about 1,500 births] but . . . there is a record of only 13 consultations." Lest Carter underestimate the seriousness of the oversight, the administrator quoted directly from hospital accreditation standards: "Except in emergency, consultation with a member of the Consulting or of the Active medical staff shall be required in all . . . cesarean sections . . . or other operations which may interrupt a known, suspected, or possible pregnancy." In this case, however, failure to document consultations rather than failure to conduct them was the likely error. Carter, who was fastidious about keeping the cesarean section rate low at Duke, regularly advised colleagues working outside his institution to consult not one but two colleagues before performing a cesarean. He also believed oral communication alone was insufficient: "it is always good to have written signed consultations for Cesareans, repeat Cesareans etc."[3]

It was in this atmosphere, with obstetricians still wary of cesareans, that the public caught its first glimpse of the surgery, courtesy of the American press, particularly women's magazines. American women's magazines were singularly influential immediately after World War II, helping to redefine and inform consumerism, family life, and health. Indeed, those publications helped link the three. While mothers had always been responsible for the health of their children, with the help of their favorite magazines in the 1950s they became educated consumers of medical services. Offering information about cesarean section was a small component of the educational effort. Thus, even as social and institutional pressures kept the rate low, the surgery was coming to public attention. As early as the 1930s, and in earnest by the 1960s, newspapers and magazines explained cesarean surgery, its causes, and its effects. These types of articles helped to establish a climate of heightened awareness and vigilance around childbirth—the stirrings of a zeitgeist that would eventually, in later decades, foster acceptance of a much higher cesarean rate.[4]

Newspapers and Magazines Depict a Rare Surgery

Given how rare the surgery was before World War II, women had few opportunities to familiarize themselves directly with cesarean sections, or even vicariously through friends and relatives. What little the public did know usually came from outlandish depictions in newspapers. Through the 1940s, when a newspaper did allude to the surgery, it was often in a sensationalist context—a freak incident rather than a carefully considered medical procedure.

Typically, a newspaper relayed the story of a young woman, eight or nine months pregnant, who died suddenly. Immediately after her death, an intrepid physician, in the unlikely event one happened to be nearby with access to anything akin to a scalpel, intervened to ensure that good came from the tragedy—the delivery of a healthy baby via an emergency cesarean section. In short, the popular press tended to depict the surgery as a combination of ghastly curiosity and the act of a superhero.

In a standard rendition, the *Los Angeles Times* ran a story in 1932 about a pregnant woman who died of a heart attack in her physician's office. Within seconds, colleagues rushed in from adjoining rooms to assist the woman's doctor. Unable to save the mother, the quickly assembled team succeeded in surgically removing a healthy baby girl from her deceased mother's body. In an even more macabre story reported almost 20 years later, an Alabama woman was eight months pregnant when her mother accidentally shot her in the eye with a newly purchased gun. The dying woman's husband sprinted to the nearby home of a former flight surgeon seeking help. Unable to save his pregnant neighbor, the valiant physician saved her son, using a pocketknife to perform a cesarean section.[5]

With public knowledge of the surgery largely limited to descriptions of freak incidents, whenever reporters did mention a cesarean section in an ordinary medical context, they assumed most readers would not know the meaning of the term. Thus, when *Time* magazine ran a photo essay in 1935 featuring a cesarean section performed in a bustling Houston hospital, a footnote appeared in the accompanying text defining the foreign-sounding phrase: "removal of a baby from the womb by means of abdominal incision when normal delivery is dangerous or impossible." Yet even this largely staid, educational article ultimately reverted to sensationalism. Appended to the sober definition was this commentary: "one of the most . . . spectacular of major operations."[6]

On the rare occasion that a woman's magazine in the 1940s discussed cesareans in an ordinary medical context, an article most often described a woman over the age of 35 who was pregnant for the first time. In 1941, *Good Housekeeping* told the story of "Sally Cummings," an apparent amalgamation of several "older," first-time pregnant mothers. In Sally's case, her doctor determined that her pelvis was too small to accommodate a full-term infant. He told her, "We'll have to take the baby by a Caesarean section." Several factors, in addition to Sally's pelvis, had contributed to his evaluation. Married for 10 years before conceiving, Sally was considerably older than the conventional primipara, and, equally importantly, she wanted the baby "badly." Thus, her doctor told her, a cesarean would be key to realizing her dream: "very little chance that the baby will die or be marred or in any way injured." His assurance implied that vaginal birth posed risks that cesarean section did not. Other magazine articles describing the benefits of cesarean birth for older, first-time mothers seemed to confirm that if the fictional Sally had been younger, married less than five years, and ambivalent or unhappy about her pregnancy, a trial of labor would have been appropriate, despite her problematic pelvis. As one physician noted, doctors only chose cesarean surgery "as the lesser of two evils," and the most common example of the greater evil was "a woman approaching the change of life with her first pregnancy and a pelvis of borderline size" attempting to give birth vaginally. Doctors calculated slim odds that these women would bear more than one child, and so the apparent benefit of the surgery—at least one living child—outweighed its risks. As two prominent obstetricians said of such a scenario, "an increased premium is placed on the infant while less attention is given to the maternal risk in subsequent pregnancies."[7]

The link between cesarean section and hope for an "elderly primigravida" was one of the first examples of a purely positive public portrayal of the surgery. The argument that cesarean section offered a first-time mother "in the later-than-average years" her sole opportunity to have a much-wanted infant had become so compelling by the 1950s that a first-time mother over the age of 35 was four times more likely to give birth by cesarean than a younger woman with identical anatomy or pathology.[8]

The articles portraying cesarean section as a rare but beneficial medical procedure were part of a new genre—informational pieces, aimed at the public, about the benefits of medical care during childbirth. The articles touted a new, "streamlined" way of birth that targeted "white-collar and professional groups, where at present the low birth rate is causing grave alarm," reflecting the ongoing racial and class prejudices supported by eugenic theory. The birth rate was low during the Great Depression, and anxiety about the "right" women bearing a sufficient number of children became a refrain of women's magazines. The class-based, racist messages were overt. "Race Suicide of the Intelligent" was the title of one *Ladies' Home Journal* article. The article's author scolded educated white women for "violating their own biological natures" rather than "leaven[ing] and lift[ing] the level of the masses, who never can lift themselves alone." An earlier *Journal* editorial admonished women, "potentially [the] mothers of children with greater native ability," who had, on average, only one child (as opposed to the mothers with only a fourth-grade education who had, on average, four children) for "squandering their genetic inheritance."[9]

The hope that easier births would increase the birth rate among culturally desirable women put medical interventions in a new light. Doctors started to recast the maligned "meddlesome midwifery" of the nineteenth century as a beneficial social measure. If only women understood how much easier childbirth had become—thanks to assorted analgesics and anesthetics and the ability to induce labor or speed up a spontaneous labor—perhaps the country's birth rate would increase. Descriptions of these modern births were thus deliberately tantalizing. The account of one woman's experience, appearing in *Reader's Digest* in 1938, included a description of an induced labor, accompanied by the wonders of Nembutal and scopolamine, and the benefits of unconsciousness. Eventually the new mother awoke to ask a nurse when she would have her baby. The nurse responded breezily, "You've had it, hours ago. It's a little girl."[10]

Not every physician approved of the interventions or the magazines describing them, however. One eminent obstetrician denounced mothers who "want quick, painless delivery—the present *Hurryitis Americanus* has affected them, and some of the doctors too." Others complained that the articles touting these measures encroached on their professional territory. An exasperated Kansas City obstetrician complained of being forced to cater to "American women in accordance with what they read in magazines." Another, equally annoyed doctor charged that the articles imparted a knowledge to women that was "little more valid than that of a chronic sufferer from toothache who would set up as authority on dentistry." The denunciations did not staunch the flow of information, however. Technological developments in obstetrics constantly provided hooks for women's magazines to hang stories on.[11]

Although doctors did not recognize it at the time, the articles ultimately benefited the medical community. By the 1930s, women were giving birth in hospitals with increasing frequency. The move from home to hospital would not have occurred as rapidly if pregnant women, and women hoping to become pregnant, had not learned from magazines and newspapers of the treatments available only in institutional settings. These treatments included labor induction, analgesics and anesthetics, and even the occasional cesarean surgery. In this sense, despite physicians' indignation, the lay press had been helpful to them. Hospital births were not an easy sell. Traditionally, only the most desperate and impoverished women gave birth there. Not until 1914, when women's magazines showcased the stories of a few wealthy Americans who traveled to Freiburg, Germany, to give birth painlessly in a hospital under the influence of "twilight sleep," did hospital birth begin to acquire a measure of cultural respectability. Although the popularity of twilight sleep proved fleeting, the nationwide coverage of the treatment portrayed hospital birth for the first time as an acceptable option for women of all classes.[12]

Even with news of painless birth, however, women did not flock immediately to hospitals in significant numbers. Not until 1936 did the *Ladies' Home Journal*, the most widely read women's magazine in the United States, attest directly to the benefits of hospital birth: "who denies the many lifesaving advantages of hospitals, with their expert nurses, their laboratories, their apparatus for transfusions, their operating rooms for emergencies?" By 1938, half of all births in the United States took place in hospitals.[13]

"Sit Tight and Be Conservative"

By 1950, the safety of both vaginal and cesarean birth had increased markedly. Maternal mortality had fallen steeply, from 70 deaths per 10,000 births in 1930 to 10 deaths per 10,000 births in 1950. The death rate after a cesarean had fallen even more dramatically, from 50 percent or more in the nineteenth century to less than 2 maternal deaths per 1,000 cesareans in the 1950s. The lowered death rates in both vaginal and cesarean births could not be attributed to any innovations specific to obstetrics, however. Rather, antibiotics and blood transfusions, made available to the public after World War II, deserved the credit. They quelled the two biggest killers of new mothers: postpartum infection and hemorrhage. Antibiotics and blood transfusions were so effective that, for the first time, they rendered the pathologies that a cesarean could alleviate—placental abruption, severe placenta previa, and eclampsia, for example—significantly more life-threatening than the surgery.[14]

Cesarean sections nevertheless remained rare; experienced obstetricians still considered the surgery to be more a risk than a remedy. They continued to use their skill to avoid the surgery; medical students thus had few opportunities even to observe the operation. When younger doctors did have a chance to perform the surgery, they reported the experience with palpable excitement. "The mother and baby are in good shape two days later," one obstetrician explained enthusiastically to the doctor who had been his mentor during his residency, while also admitting that his "*lack* of experience in going after babies from the abdominal route didn't help my extraction of the fetus!" He struggled so mightily to remove the fetus from the uterus that rather than the "pretty, smooth round head" cesarean babies were known for, this baby's head "had been moulded and actually had a caput!" His mentor responded by complimenting him on his approach ("you were right in rupturing membranes") but also by reminding him that forceps should always be the first option—"if you will practice . . . they will pull you out of many, many traps." As the seasoned physician's advice indicated, forceps remained the first recourse of the adept obstetrician despite the lowered cesarean death rate.[15]

A retired obstetrician, who completed his residency in 1969, described how determinedly he and his colleagues provided women with the opportunity to give birth vaginally. If a woman had placenta previa, for example, they constructed a "double set-up" in the delivery room—that is, they would prepare for anesthesia "and your nurses and all the instruments laid out for the cesarean and you also had a vaginal delivery table in the room." Another retired obstetrician described how thoroughly his superiors scrutinized any decision-making leading to a cesarean. "You had instruments where you could actually measure true pelvic measurements . . . and [if] the measurements turned out to be ok, you know you were looked down upon" if a cesarean had been performed. The minutest details of every primary cesarean, whether performed by a resident or a private physician, had to be presented to the hospital's entire obstetric department—"and the history, the labor management, the pelvic measurements" were all included in the presentation. "Cesareans were a super big deal."[16]

A physician in New York learned in the early 1950s just how big a deal they were. The American Board of Examiners rejected his application for certification in obstetrics and gynecology. During the oral portion of his examination he had provided an unsatisfactory explanation for his cesarean rate—deemed too high by examiners. Colleagues approved of the denial. One noted, "It has been very distressing to all of us at times to try to put into intelligent terms the indications for many of . . . [his] sections. They are often obscure and shrouded in mysticism." As their reaction attests, obstetricians were outraged far more often than they were comforted by cesareans in the 1950s. One California obstetrician described a woman who had delivered five children vaginally only to be told she must deliver her sixth child by cesarean due to a preoperative diagnosis of cephalopelvic disproportion. "I don't understand," he wrote to a colleague, "how in the hell she could deliver a 9+ lb baby previously & then have cephalopelvic disproportion . . . with this pregnancy."[17]

The ability to help a woman avoid a cesarean remained a genuine point of pride among physicians in the 1940s, '50s, and '60s. Even in the face of a well-accepted indication for the surgery, obstetricians leaned toward vaginal birth. A North Carolina doctor described two difficult births that ended vaginally in 1952, one with an abrupted placenta ("handled from below inspite [*sic*] of some elements desirous of section") and a mother with a "very small" pelvis ("again the pressure was quite high for section"). Another obstetrician practicing in Virginia in 1949 assured a colleague that during the 10 months he was in charge of the obstetrics section of an army hospital, only 1 of the 300 babies born there had been delivered by cesarean—"and that for proven cephalo-pelvic disproportion." Another doctor, angered in 1952 because his hospital had seen "well over" 50 cesareans in 1,700 births, bet a colleague five dollars that the hospital where he had done his residency had not seen more than five cesareans that year despite a similar number of births. He wrote to the chair of his former department only to learn that he was wrong. The hospital had seen not five, but "roughly . . . 12 or 13 Cesareans in 1534 deliveries or 1 in 118 patients." His former colleague apologized for the high number: "Sorry if you lose the bet but we still think too many Cesareans are done for no real indication."[18]

Just as doctors had recommended patience during labor in the nineteenth century, so, too, did their professional descendants in the mid-twentieth century. Even an unusually lengthy labor was no excuse for performing a cesarean. In 1951, one obstetrician described a 92-hour labor caused by "much inertia" of the uterus. Rather than consider a cesarean, he focused on the dilemma posed by the patient's "intolerance to pain." He knew anesthesia would slow labor even further, yet, without pain relief, the patient had become "quite obnoxious on the ward." He found the solution in neither a cesarean nor general anesthesia but in caudal analgesia: "With this she went ahead and delivered spontaneously."[19]

Francis Bayard Carter, chair of the Duke University Department of Obstetrics and Gynecology for more than 30 years beginning in 1931, was president at various times of the most prominent professional organizations in his field during his career—the American Academy of Obstetrics and Gynecology, the American Board of Obstetrics and Gynecology, the American College of Obstetricians and Gynecologists, and the American Association of Obstetricians and Gynecologists.

He was also typical of the older, experienced obstetricians who taught their students to avoid cesarean sections. When one of his former students, now a practicing obstetrician in Tennessee, wrote to remind Carter about a promised gift—a pair of Kielland forceps—the student also asked Carter for "a little inscription from you on them." Carter told his young colleague to order the forceps with the inscription, "Learn to wait, get good anesthetic and use them well," and to send him the bill. He similarly advised in subsequent correspondence, "Sit tight and be conservative."[20]

Yet, as some of these complaints attest, a few obstetricians were becoming quicker to perform cesareans. In the late 1950s, one physician applying for board certification satirized obstetric practice in a letter to the president of the American Board of Obstetrics and Gynecology. Under the heading, "A Candidate's Comments," the letter described a fictional birth: "Her cervix was RIPE, in fact it was rotten, and I was AT MY WIT'S END so I SADDLED HER [i.e., administered saddle block anesthesia] AND SECTIONED HER [i.e., performed a cesarean]. I guess I should have CLEANED HER OUT [likely a reference to performing a hysterectomy], because she WENT DOWN HILL." He added a terse sign-off—"Well THAT'S THAT . . . NO COMMENT."—and a phony signature—"Frankly, I. M. Wright"—an apparent backhanded reference to arrogant colleagues. His parody was an indication of the increasingly divergent approaches to birth among obstetricians.[21]

Pairing Obstetrics and Gynecology

Obstetricians had ample reason to be more quarrelsome than other specialists. Their fight for professional respect still had not been won. As late as the 1930s, obstetrics remained so undervalued that on the rare occasion a midwife did seek help from a physician during a home birth, virtually no one thought to summon an obstetrician. Aid usually came from a general practitioner, but midwives called upon whoever happened to be nearby—pediatrician, otolaryngologist, dermatologist, ophthalmologist, urologist, gastroenterologist, neurologist, gynecologist. The specialty was irrelevant—to the specialist as well as the midwife and laboring woman.[22]

While a gynecologist might seem to be the most logical choice on this list, in an era when obstetrics and gynecology were distinct fields, gynecologists were no more adept than otolaryngologists at delivering babies. One obstetrician recounted the story of an "eminent gynecologist" who performed a cesarean on "a multiparous woman who always had had easy labors," simply because her baby was in the breech position. Not knowing how to execute a successful delivery, the gynecologist surgically removed the full-term infant from its mother's womb.[23]

Rather than having significant knowledge of, or respect for, each other's fields, gynecologists tended to belittle the work of obstetricians, and vice versa. After a patient's husband complained about the bill for his wife's birth, Joseph DeLee berated the man: "I, myself, could make much more money, with infiinitely [*sic*] less trouble, doing simple gynecological operations, and the temptation to quit obstetrics is very strong."[24]

J. Whitridge Williams was atypical in this sense. Although his titles—professor of obstetrics and obstetrician-in-chief at Johns Hopkins University and Hospital—bore no mention of gynecology, he identified with both specialties and blamed the mutual animosity on obstetricians and gynecologists in equal measure. Long before there was any widespread discussion of conjoining the specialties, he told an audience of gynecologists in 1914 that he looked forward to the day when obstetrics and gynecology were unified into what he referred to as "a broader gynecology, instead of being divided as at present into knife-loving gynecologists and equally narrow-minded obstetricians, who are frequently little more than trained man midwives."[25]

As Williams intimated, the fundamental difference between obstetrics and gynecology was that gynecology was a surgical specialty and obstetrics was not. In the nineteenth century, American gynecology was borne of surgical experiments on distinct groups suffering from very different conditions—slaves and poor white immigrants suffering from vesico-vaginal fistulas, and wealthy, white, Protestant women exhibiting debilitating nervous symptoms. In the case of the latter, gynecologists often identified women's reproductive organs as the source of their mental illness, a finding that called for removal of the uterus or ovaries or both. The practice became so common that decades later, in 1915, one Chicago physician likened the current "furor operativus" (a reference to cesarean sections—a "makeshift for real obstetric practice") to gynecologists' earlier penchant for oophorectomies. In short, the work of obstetricians centered on nurturing a physiological process, as opposed to gynecologists, who often resorted to surgery when treating a pathological process.[26]

Surgery was so foreign to obstetricians that in the nineteenth and early twentieth centuries they customarily viewed cesarean birth as distinct from obstetrics. Max Sänger, the German physician who was the first to suture the uterus after performing a cesarean, illustrated the division between obstetrics and gynecology in an 1890 letter written in imperfect English to an American colleague: "My duty is now main gynecological, as I never had a peculiar obstetrical service, excepted the time of Assistantship and later as Operator on the Leipzig Maternity. I am on the point of building a new gynecological private clinic upon aseptic principles and I hope many American confrier will guest me to show it after the accomplishment." And in a letter the following year, Sänger seemed to suggest that cesarean surgery was more akin to gynecology than obstetrics: "Myself, I have no obstetric ward at all, nearly no obstetric practice. I get in my private clinic only cases urging Caesarean operation."[27]

Well into the twentieth century, obstetricians and gynecologists acknowledged the division between their specialties. In 1929, a New Orleans doctor reminded colleagues that obstetrics was "not an adjunct of general surgery" and that pregnant women and their children were "not safe in the hands of men who so regard it." His statement was both a swipe at gynecology and a denunciation of the obstetricians who advocated broadening the indications for cesarean sections. The only feature that obstetrics, the medical oversight of a physiological process, and gynecology, the surgical management of pathological processes, had in common was that both restricted treatment to women.[28]

Yet while conjoining the two specialties did not make medical sense, the coupling did make professional sense. Indeed, rendering the two specialties one became a cornerstone of obstetricians' effort to elevate the status of their field.[29] With poor obstetric training still a serious problem in medical schools, in 1921 the American Medical Association's (AMA) Council of Medical Education sought to remedy the deficiency by appointing J. Whitridge Williams to head the organization's new Committee on Graduate Training in Gynecology and Obstetrics. The committee ultimately made two recommendations: (1) merge the department of obstetrics and the department of gynecology at all teaching hospitals in the United States and (2) establish three-year, hospital-based residencies in the newly combined specialty. The resulting American Board of Obstetrics and Gynecology (ABOG), founded in 1930, became the third medical specialty examining board in the United States, after ophthalmology, in 1916, and otolaryngology, in 1924.[30]

For the obstetricians who had worked so long to little avail to portray their abilities as a necessity for all pregnant women, coupling their title with "gynecologist" became a selling point. With that addition to their professional identity, the medical and lay communities no longer perceived obstetricians as mere bedside-sitters and hand-holders. Now, they were also surgeons capable of treating an array of illnesses and conditions, from fistulas to cancers. Equally beneficial to the traditionally denigrated field of obstetrics, one of the first acts of the ABOG was to limit certification in the new specialty to physicians who restricted their practice to women. That move effectively barred general practitioners from the birthing business, although some generalists fought back. The battle waged in the 1940s by the Indiana Academy of General Practitioners against their exclusion from attending hospital births led to a new medical specialty in family practice. Board-certified family physicians became the only specialists, other than obstetrician/gynecologists, permitted to attend hospital births. Unlike obstetrician/gynecologists, however, they were not permitted to perform cesarean sections.[31]

Obstetrician/gynecologists also sought to exclude from the baby-delivery business the surgeons who occasionally performed cesareans. The move against surgeons began on the local level. When obstetricians at a Schenectady, New York, hospital mandated in 1941 that all cesareans had to be performed using the safer lower transverse cut, as opposed to the prone-to-rupture but easier-to-perform classic cut, they simultaneously ruled that surgeons at the hospital would no longer be permitted to perform cesareans. As one obstetrician explained at the time, "General surgeons do not like the low segment section." In a more sweeping defense of obstetricians' turf, an Arkansas obstetrician wrote to the president of the American Academy of Obstetrics and Gynecology in the 1950s to object to the fact that members of the American College of Surgeons were permitted to represent obstetricians on the AMA's newly established Resident Review Committee. He complained, "As a sop to the Academy, these representatives of the American College of Surgeons would also be members of the American Academy [of Obstetrics and Gynecology] but I should like to point out that they will be representing the American College of Surgeons, not vice versa." Thanks to this type of territorial vigilance, obstetrician/gynecologists eventually eliminated their competition. By the 1960s, they were the uncontested, and highly respected, experts on childbirth in the United States.[32]

In the aftermath of the ABOG's founding and the consolidation of the new specialty, the growth of residencies in obstetrics and gynecology was impressive—from 104 slots at 48 hospitals in 1935 to 773 positions in 255 hospitals in 1945. By 1954, 438 American hospitals housed residency training programs in the dual specialty. The melding of the specialties signified comprehensive expertise in women's health and medicine. As an officer of the American Board of Obstetrics and Gynecology explained to a colleague, "a man cannot be fully qualified to practice either branch, as he chooses, if he has not acquired at least a fundamental knowledge of the other in which he may be less interested."[33]

Training was rigorous. Duke University Hospital in Durham, North Carolina required would-be residents to serve one year as an intern at a teaching hospital before joining Duke as an intern in obstetrics and gynecology. Then, after a year at Duke, candidates allowed to continue in the program served as a junior assistant resident in obstetrics and gynecology for an additional year, followed by three years as a senior assistant resident. Only then, "if he [was chosen for further] . . . advancement," was the candidate allowed to finish the program by serving as a resident instructor for a year before seeking board certification. "In short," said the director of Duke's residency program in obstetrics and gynecology, "the training schedule is 6 years and the competition is keen."[34]

Perhaps most significantly for American birth practices, the merger of obstetrics and gynecology portended the triumph of the operator camp. The sensibility of the gynecologist, a specialist accustomed to surgically treating a host of gender-related pathologies, would eventually overpower the instincts of the physiologically oriented obstetrician. This was evident in a letter written by the chairman of the Department of Gynecology and Obstetrics at the University of Kansas Medical Center in 1970 in response to an inquiry about a residency position there. In his reply, he listed the daily classes offered to residents in obstetrics and gynecology: "Gynecology, Pathology, Case Conference, Tumor, Perinatal Problems, Dystocia, Journal Review, and Basic Science." While the basic science classes included placental physiology and physiology of reproduction, the bulk of classes leaned toward pathology, including further training in surgery, urology, and "special cancer work."[35]

The generation of obstetricians who engineered the melding of the two specialties ultimately recognized the loss for obstetricians. Even DeLee, the de facto leader of the operator camp who has long been excoriated by birth reformers and feminists for championing a host of routine medical interventions during labor and birth, came to regret the approach to childbirth that his recommendations fostered. Two years before his death in 1942, he told a lay audience that 95 percent of births required "only good obstetric treatment," which he defined precisely as his friend and professional nemesis J. Whitridge Williams always had: prenatal care, treatment of complications before they endangered mother or infant, aseptic practice, and the presence of a skilled physician who avoided attempts to "streamline" birth. DeLee, who has been credited with doing more than any other obstetrician in US history to foster streamlined birth, told his audience: "Mother nature's methods of bringing babies are still the best." The medical interventions DeLee was witnessing by the early 1940s seemed to have driven him squarely into the nonoperator camp, even as operators triumphed.[36]

Delivering the Baby Boomers

While neither the melding of obstetrics and gynecology nor the post–World War II ability to treat postpartum infection and hemorrhage immediately inspired obstetricians to view a cesarean as a ready solution to a problematic birth, the flood of births dubbed "the baby boom" pointed them in that direction. As veterans returned home after World War II, marrying young and having a large family came to be seen as primary components of postwar contentment. In this atmosphere, childlessness, or having only one child, was characterized as both personal tragedy and public treason. Large families were considered happy families, and happy families created productive, socially responsible citizens who would contribute to the nation's stability, growth, and ability to defend itself. While the Great Depression had seen an average 18.4 births annually per 1,000 women of childbearing age, by 1957 births had increased to an annual 25.3 per 1,000 women of childbearing age. In other words, between 1940 and 1960, when a record-breaking 59.4 million children were born in the United States, birth rates doubled for third children and tripled for fourth.[37]

This surge in births posed unique challenges—many physicians were still on active duty in the armed forces. Given the inadequate staffing, handling even a routine number of hospital births would have been daunting. The postwar increase was an entirely different challenge; the temporary hardship became an ongoing crisis. Compounding the problem, most births in the decade after the war were to first-time mothers, whose labors lasted longest and who, due to their inexperience, required the most attention. Medical intervention became a way to address the problem—a coping mechanism for overworked obstetricians as well as their patients.[38]

In lieu of an adequate number of staff members to comfort and encourage mothers, nurses and doctors used sedatives and painkillers. Obstetricians spoke frankly about this use of drugs, jocularly referring to the powerful narcotic Nisentil as "nice 'n' still." As one obstetrician noted approvingly: "A good labor floor has been a quiet labor floor." Gene Lawrence, who delivered babies in the Chicago area from 1946 to 1988, gave all his laboring patients an updated version of twilight sleep—scopolamine and Demerol. Not only did the drug combination diminish women's need for attention, Lawrence theorized that his treatment was a patriotic service. "I felt," he explained years later, "that the less the patient knew about their labor the more willing they would be to have more kids." He recalled proudly, "And that gave rise to the boomers really. Because I delivered the boomers."[39]

Given the pressures of the baby boom, coupled with the miracle of antibiotics and blood banking, the medical perception of cesarean section began to change. With some statisticians reporting an aggregate 1,000 cesareans without a single maternal death, one obstetrician explained to a women's magazine in 1960 that a vaginal birth demanding daunting maneuvers with forceps now presented a greater hazard than cesarean surgery. This type of claim not only primed reluctant obstetricians to think differently, it also educated the public about the benefits of the little-known surgery. The cesarean section rate rose accordingly—from about 2.5 to 4 percent of births in the decade and a half after World War II. Yet the numbers, just as they had during the first half of the twentieth century, varied widely from hospital to hospital. While some hospitals maintained traditionally low rates and others average rates, women's magazines reported that a few hospitals were seeing a remarkable one cesarean for every five births.[40]

A spokesperson for a prestigious New York City hospital with the city's highest cesarean rate explained the reasons for the institution's numbers. Local physicians steered their most difficult cases to the top-tier institution. Those referrals drove a 4.5 percent cesarean rate among "ward patients" and an almost 9 percent rate among private patients. His explanation was comforting. The obstetricians at hospitals with the highest rates were not practicing medicine haphazardly. They were simply the most adept at handling the toughest births.[41]

Celebrating Childbirth Technologies

Because birth and childrearing were at the center of so many women's lives during the baby boom, women's magazines showcased many more articles than they had in the past about medical advances in childbirth. Rather than the sporadic articles of the 1930s and 1940s, news about the medical treatment of childbirth became a staple in the 1950s. Some of those articles extolled the benefits of recently developed anesthetics. Mothers who had previously given birth under general anesthesia were reportedly enthusiastic about the new regionals, particularly caudals and saddle-blocks, "as were their families when the mothers returned to their rooms in a cheerful, wide-awake condition." Other articles celebrated the benefits of labor induction. As opposed to the uncertainties of spontaneous labor—no one knew precisely when it would begin or how long it would last—women learned that Pitocin rendered labor predictable. One doctor also explained in a *Better Homes and Gardens* article that induction served as a useful diagnostic for determining a woman's need for a cesarean section. "So dependable are these speed-up benefits, that if a woman fails to deliver in an hour, a serious impediment to normal birth is indicated." Rather than "subjecting mother and baby to [the] prolonged, injurious stresses of unproductive labor," a failed induction now served as a cue that a cesarean "or other emergency measures" might be needed. In addition to its alleged therapeutic and diagnostic benefits, doctors also claimed that Pitocin had palliative powers—it softened "the outlet . . . to permit easy passage" of the newborn. The black press customarily described the same innovations to its readers, including not only physician-approved caudal anesthesia but also consumer-advocated novelties such as hypnosis and natural childbirth.[42]

Collectively, these articles implied that mothers who wanted better pregnancies, births, and babies would embrace medical interventions. Labor was unpredictable by nature; medicine steadied the course. And both the mainstream and black presses delivered similar messages about medical intervention. A physician writing a lengthy story on childbirth for the *Chicago Defender*'s national edition wrote, "But how natural should birth be? This is the decision only an obstetrician can make, not an overeager patient and her friends. The criterion of good obstetrical care, in my opinion, is a live mother who is not damaged in any way that will require a future operation, or cause a chronic complaint." And there was no dearth of new postwar treatments to describe to mothers. Radioactive chromium-51 was described as "a safe, quick and accurate tracer for locating the site of the placenta" in the event of excessive bleeding late in pregnancy or during labor. In the early 1960s, the *Ladies' Home Journal* described "the birthsuit"—an "abdominal decompression chamber" designed to saturate the fetus with oxygen. The device consisted of a reclining chair inside an airtight suit that covered the body from neck to feet. Holes on either side freed a woman's arms, allowing her to eat or read during the 30 minutes of daily treatments that were recommended during the final months of pregnancy. Advocates for the birthsuit claimed it cut the duration of labor in half; vanquished labor pain; decreased the incidence of hemorrhage and perineal tears; eliminated stillbirths and fetal brain injuries, particularly cerebral palsy; and reduced fetal distress by 80 percent. The treatments also ensured that "highly gifted" parents would not run the risk of producing "mediocre" children. Readers of the *Ladies' Home Journal* learned that the "increasingly superior beings" ensured by prescribed use of the birthsuit heralded an "intelligence revolution" within a generation. Women

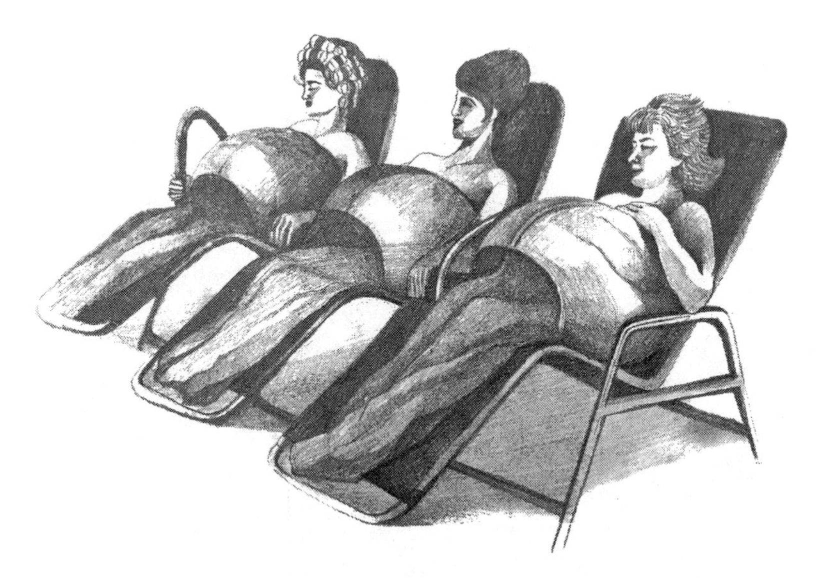

Three women undergoing a birthsuit treatment in the early 1960s. Proponents of the birthsuit, invented by South African obstetrician O. S. Heyns, claimed that 30-minute, daily treatments during the final months of pregnancy would prevent virtually every problem during labor plus boost children's intelligence. Heyns claimed that one typical woman who underwent treatments as directed bore an infant who amassed a 200-word vocabulary by 18 months of age.
Illustration by Maryam Khaleghi Yazdi, from a photograph in Heyns, *Abdominal Decompression*, 25.

praised the device. "It was bliss," said one second-time mother. "This time I really enjoyed [birth]."[43]

Magazines began to portray cesarean sections in the same laudatory light as other medical interventions. Cesarean birth was as "safe and uneventful as an appendectomy," according to one physician writing in *McCall's* in 1958. Another doctor assured mothers, "except for a simple vaginal birth," cesarean section had become the safest route into the world. And the surgery came with a bonus—it "unquestionably" produced the prettiest newborns. To forestall any frivolous demand for cesareans, the doctor making that observation was also quick to promise that "the pulchritude of the vaginally delivered infant catches up and all is equality." The black press likewise explained cesareans to their readers: "One woman may deliver a child normally through the birth canal. Another may require a Cesarean operation,—the opening of the abdomen and uterus to free the baby, because the bony structure of the normal birth canal will not permit passage of the child. Such individual problems must be left to the discretion of the doctor."

And, in an era when personal comportment was all important, mothers also learned about some of the fashion accoutrements demanded by cesarean delivery. "If a woman knows she will have a Caesarean section, she would be wise to get herself an extra supply of bed jackets."[44]

Articles promised women that a cesarean was neither to be feared nor avoided if a physician suggested that a mother have one. In 1960, a mother pregnant with her third child complained in a letter to a doctor's column in the *Ladies' Home Journal* that despite "two perfectly normal childbirths," her obstetrician inexplicably proposed delivering her third child by cesarean. "I can't understand it. I'm wondering if he is just one of those doctors who likes to cut!" The physician authoring the monthly column explained that times had changed. The "modern, low type of Caesarean" was akin to a vaginal delivery. "You might almost say that the uterus doesn't know the difference!" He reminded her of her duty to her child. "We doctors have learned more about conditions which might result in a baby who survives a hard delivery, but is brain-damaged, for instance." While doctors once avoided cesareans because they were likely to harm the mother, now mothers learned that cesareans protected their babies from harm, while any risks to themselves were inconsequential.[45]

The Kennedy Family and the Public Perception of Risk

With the birth of John F. Kennedy, Jr., in late 1960, followed by the birth of his brother Patrick in 1963, obstetricians' mid-twentieth-century penchant for medical intervention became headline news. Although the birth of a president's child would garner news coverage in any era, the attention paid by the press to obstetric innovations during the baby boom, coupled with the public's unrelenting interest in John and Jackie Kennedy, invited scrutiny of Jackie Kennedy's cesareans. John Jr.'s birth fostered a positive attitude toward the surgery. Three years later, the birth and death of his brother eroded that outlook. The contrasting births not only typified, but also seemed to justify, the contradictory messages that the lay press had relayed to the public for years—a cesarean was a heroic effort that preserved life and health; a cesarean was a macabre surgery associated more with death than life.[46]

What the public did not know before John Jr.'s birth was that Jackie Kennedy's reproductive history had been difficult from the start. Her first pregnancy in 1955 ended in a miscarriage; she gave birth by cesarean to a stillborn daughter, Arabella, in 1956; Caroline was born by cesarean in 1957. When Kennedy was pregnant again in 1960, her obstetrician, John Walsh, scheduled her third cesarean for mid-December. The operation occurred almost three weeks earlier, however—as an emergency, rather than as a long-planned surgery.[47]

When the country's newspapers announced John Jr.'s birth on November 25, however, reporters did not dwell on its emergency nature. Instead, they offered only a few procedural details in an upbeat tone. The baby's due date had been December 27; a cesarean was scheduled for December 12. Walsh explained why: "Two weeks early is a standard procedure" when planning a cesarean. Jackie Kennedy, however, either went into labor or began to bleed—newspapers were respectfully silent about the nature of the emergency—three weeks before the planned surgery, so Walsh ordered an ambulance to take her to a nearby hospital. Despite the unexpected turn of events, mother and baby were doing well according to published accounts. The *New York Times* reported that John Fitzgerald Kennedy, Jr., "basked" in his incubator. Walsh declared the birth complication-free "other than the fact that the baby arrived sooner than we expected." He was unprepared for the hoopla. When asked if the newborn resembled his father or mother, Walsh was dismissive: "Frankly, new babies look mostly like new babies." In contrast, Mrs. Kennedy's press secretary was prepared to gush. She described John Jr. as "healthy and beautiful, and just wonderful."[48]

The press and public were so ignorant of the risks for an infant born more than four weeks prematurely that news reports focused not on Mrs. Kennedy or her newborn son but on the drama of the president-elect, who was en route by air to Palm Beach when his wife was rushed unexpectedly to the hospital. Reports of the president-elect's experience were breathless: word of the imminent birth "was flashed by radio" midflight to Kennedy's "family-owned two-engined Convair." Immediately after landing, Kennedy "walk[ed] briskly" to an office inside the Palm Beach airport to speak on "an open line connected to the third-floor maternity ward" in Washington. After learning from a nurse that his wife was headed to surgery, he decided to return to Washington immediately, hoping to get there before the baby arrived. He abandoned the family-owned plane that had flown him to Palm Beach and essentially hijacked the "faster charter" American Airlines plane carrying the press corps. Kennedy boarded, looking "nervous and taut," learning en route by radio that the baby had been born. He now had a son. The news, announced on the plane's loudspeaker system, sparked "a burst of applause and cheers" among reporters. Kennedy appeared "coatless" at his compartment door to acknowledge the congratulations "with a wave and a broad smile."[49]

If most Americans remained largely ignorant of cesarean section despite the articles that had appeared in the lay press through the 1950s, after John Jr.'s birth no one could escape the torrent of information about the surgery. Within days, Americans knew what the phrase "cesarean section" meant and far more—why Jackie Kennedy had planned to have her baby by cesarean; what a "low cervical cesarean" was; when that form of the surgery had been invented, by whom, and why it had supplanted the "classic" cesarean. Articles provided step-by-step explanations of how doctors performed the operation and sutured the resulting wound. The public learned about the frequency of cesarean birth—2 to 6 percent of hospital births in the early 1960s—that one of every three cesareans was a repeat, and that many physicians recommended that a woman have a hysterectomy after three surgical births. Until the barrage of information, even women who had given birth by cesarean remained so ignorant of the consequences of that recommendation that one mother, a registered nurse no less, wrote to Francis Bayard Carter, the chair of the Duke University Department of Obstetrics, for help after giving birth three times by cesarean. As custom dictated, her doctor had advised, and she had consented to, a bilateral salpingectomy after her third birth to prevent further pregnancies. She wrote to Carter to ask, "Would it be possible for you to do a repair job, so I could become pregnant again? I am willing to take the chance, and would be happy with another baby. I am 35 years old and in excellent health, so the sooner the better." Carter responded tactfully, "Since you have had the fallopian tubes removed it is highly problematic that any plastic operation to restore your fertility could in anyway be guaranteed to be successful." He nevertheless suggested she see an obstetrician/gynecologist in New York, where she lived.[50]

Two years later Jackie Kennedy was pregnant again, and the press used the opportunity to demystify cesarean sections even further. Rather than the traditional limit of three cesareans per mother, now women learned they could safely have "eight (or even more)" babies by cesarean. Only obstetricians "still devoted to out-of-date ideas" rendered a woman infertile after three cesarean surgeries. The low transverse cut, "carrying far less risk of damage to the womb itself or to other organs" than the classic cut, allowed women to have as many children as they wished by cesarean. Indeed, mothers learned, low transverse cesarean surgery was so minor that it "leaves the woman free to wear a bikini afterward without embarrassment." The association between cesarean section and one of the most glamorous women in the world transformed the surgery's image. Virtually overnight, the rare, risky procedure that befell only the most unfortunate women became a straightforward, trouble-free, trifling process that all women were fortunate to have available to them if they needed it.[51]

The wholly positive image suffered a dramatic setback, however, after the birth of Patrick Bouvier Kennedy on August 7, 1963. Born via emergency cesarean nearly six weeks before his due date, weighing only 4 pounds 10½ ounces, and suffering from hyaline membrane disease, he lived less than two days. The press, likely emboldened by the intense interest in the Kennedys and the image of youth and attractiveness that the couple had carefully cultivated, provided more medical details with this birth than they had with John Jr.'s. At the time, physicians and scientists did not know the cause of hyaline membrane disease, and newspapers speculated ominously that the illness likely sprang "from factors that necessitate Caesarean section." Doctors theorized (wrongly) that a mother's hemorrhage, for example, which was exactly what had prompted Kennedy's latest emergency cesarean according to the now forthright news accounts, probably interfered with the circulation of oxygen to the placenta, impacting the neonate's ability to breathe.[52]

The news articles negated the positive publicity about cesareans that had accompanied the birth of Patrick's older brother. While baby John had "basked" in his incubator, Patrick "was trundled down in an incubator . . . and rushed to Boston by ambulance" from the Otis Air Force Base Hospital near Falmouth, Massachusetts, where he had been born. While the public had not been offered any descriptions of the risks faced by John Jr. after his premature birth by emergency cesarean, the description of Patrick's ordeal was grim. The baby was in a "submarine-like" high-pressure oxygen chamber. Two events suggested the baby had a poor prognosis: his move by air force ambulance to the Children's Hospital Medical Center in suburban Boston and the president's request that his son be baptized shortly after his birth. After her baby's death, Jackie Kennedy's obstetric history became public knowledge. For those who did not care to absorb every detail, the press summed it up—the first lady had endured a miscarriage followed by four cesarean births resulting in only two living children.[53]

The week after Patrick Kennedy's death, *Newsweek* published a two-page examination of what had gone wrong with his birth, noting that while the baby's death had been traumatic for the entire nation, it was potentially terrifying for many American women who might worry that they, too, would one day face a cesarean section. The magazine attempted to subdue those women's fears, explaining that the condition that necessitated Jackie Kennedy's most recent emergency cesarean was rare. Placental abruption had caused a profuse hemorrhage, sparking the crisis. For Kennedy, the condition seemed to be chronic. The placenta had also abrupted in two of her earlier pregnancies—her stillborn daughter's and

John's. The overriding message seemed to be that the condition was peculiar to a few unlucky women, and so the vast majority of women need not worry.[54]

In subsequent years, newspapers and magazines attempted to recoup the loss of faith in cesareans sparked by Patrick's death. *Time* magazine told the public that cesarean birth per se was not a threat. In planned cesareans, the mortality rate of babies was "almost the same as for natural deliveries." Only when the surgery was "an emergency measure," as it had been in Patrick Kennedy's case, was infant mortality 10 times higher than in vaginal deliveries. While the birth of Jackie Kennedy's first son effectively mainstreamed cesarean section, the birth and death of her second son became the prototypical example of the worst consequence of the surgery. In providing an example of the surgery's benefit and, soon after, a particularly vivid example of the surgery's risk, the two births created a fault line between the anxiety and loathing provoked by the surgery for much of its history and the normalization of the surgery that would come to predominate less than 20 years after Patrick's death.[55]

Cigarettes and Cesareans

The placental abruptions that caused bleeding in three of Jackie Kennedy's five pregnancies were likely caused by something other than terrible luck, however. Today, the medical community recognizes that an abrupted placenta can be one of many smoking-related complications of pregnancy. Although it is impossible to pinpoint the precise cause of Kennedy's difficult pregnancies, she was a chain smoker throughout her adult life, including during her five pregnancies. She first took up the habit at the elite prep school in Connecticut she attended as a teenager. By the time Patrick was born in 1963, when Kennedy was 32, she had smoked heavily for more than 15 years. She hid her habit well, directing aides to confiscate any photos taken of her with a cigarette in hand. After her husband's death, she instructed the Kennedy Presidential Library not to reproduce any photographs of her smoking.[56]

Although Kennedy was obviously embarrassed by her addiction, smoking was an acceptable activity for American women well before the 1960s. In 1944, a Gallup poll revealed that 48 percent of men and 36 percent of women smoked, with urban women far more likely to be smokers than women living in rural areas.[57] Among educated women, smoking rates were even higher; by the late 1930s, the majority of students at women's colleges were smokers.[58] The tobacco industry deliberately targeted women; ads for Chesterfield cigarettes regularly featured "Chesterfield's Girl of the Month."[59]

The widespread custom consequently became one of the many indirect contributors to the eventual normalization of cesareans. In causing many problem pregnancies, cigarette smoking helped to justify the penchant during the baby boom years for medical intervention during childbirth. And while the relationships between smoking and premature birth, smoking and fetal loss, and smoking and neonatal morbidity were unknown during those years, Jackie Kennedy's problematic pregnancies ensured that cesarean surgery was on the cultural radar.[60]

The few articles about pregnancy and smoking that appeared in obstetric journals before 1964 tended to be polemical and thus easily ignored. "It is my conviction that excessive cigaret [*sic*] smoking has a degenerating influence in many ways upon every woman and that is prejudicial to her highest efficiency as a sweetheart, a wife, or a mother," wrote one Michigan physician in a 1936 article on smoking and maternal health. Even the US surgeon general's report on the effects of smoking, issued the year after Patrick Kennedy's death, barely mentioned the effects of maternal smoking, stating only that the babies of smokers had lower birth weights than average. Given the paucity of information available to either the medical community or the public when Kennedy was pregnant, it is unlikely any physician told her, or even knew, that her addiction to nicotine might have triggered her pregnancy outcomes. Thus, Jackie Kennedy's secret smoking habit, rather than fostering awareness of the damage smoking could do to a fetus, instead advanced public knowledge of the need for birth by cesarean section.[61]

Not until 1979, when the US surgeon general issued "The Health Consequences of Smoking for Women," did the public learn the costs of smoking during pregnancy. The report explained that smoking "significantly affects" the fetus by depriving it of oxygen in two ways—via the carbon monoxide produced by cigarette consumption and by reduction of blood flow to the placenta. The decreased blood flow, in turn, caused miscarriage, placental abruption, and stillbirth. One or more of those conditions afflicted at least four of Jackie Kennedy's five pregnancies.[62]

Owing to the popularity of cigarettes, Jackie Kennedy was by no means the only woman in the public eye who smoked throughout her pregnancies. Marie Killilea, the author of two best-selling books about her family life, was another heavy smoker who, like Kennedy, had a series of problematic pregnancies. Killilea described the birth of her fourth living child—her only birth by cesarean section—in her second book published in 1963. The birth occurred in 1956, after Killilea had experienced 11 pregnancies resulting in only three living children. One of those children, a daughter, Karen, was born in 1941, almost three months prematurely, weighing less than 2 pounds. Eventually, doctors diagnosed Karen with cerebral palsy.[63]

Likely due to the combination of Killilea's many fetal losses and her age—she was 43 at the time of her last birth—when she became pregnant for the final time, her doctor decided well in advance of labor to deliver the baby by cesarean section. Killilea shared with her readers the appealing metaphor her physician used to describe his plan: "I shall pluck the baby like a rose." After the doctor "plucked" the newborn—and Killilea used the verb when she described the birth—she reported that her daughter, Kristin, was "healthy, howling and beautiful."[64]

Unlike Kennedy, however, Killilea made no effort to hide her cigarette smoking from the public. Quite the contrary: in her two best-selling books, cigarettes were omnipresent. As she lay in her hospital bed soon after Karen's birth, "Jimmy [her husband] lit a cigarette and put it between my lips." One doctor was "snuffing out his cigarette" as he told Marie and Jimmy that he was sure Karen's case was hopeless. During a visit with another physician, Jimmy lit one cigarette from another. In her second book, when her obstetrician imparted the good news that she was pregnant for the twelfth time at the age of 43, Killilea reported that, in celebratory spirit, "he offered me a cigarette and lit it up for me."[65]

When Killilea was pregnant with her last child, her obstetrician was so concerned about her having yet another miscarriage or stillbirth that he ordered her to remain in bed throughout the pregnancy. So strictly did she adhere to his orders that even casual visitors to her home knew to treat her "with inordinate solicitude." She wrote, "I had only to glance at a table to have one . . . leap to get cigarettes, matches, a newspaper." Although her baby was not due until May, she stayed in her upstairs bedroom through the winter, leaving only twice (with her doctor's permission), to join her family downstairs during Christmas. Someone carried her downstairs both times, and while downstairs she "stay[ed] put until I was carried back up to my room."[66]

Doctors commonly ordered women with Killilea's reproductive history to remain bedridden during pregnancy. Equally ordinary was not to issue any recommendation to quit smoking. Indeed, prevailing wisdom in the medical community often prompted the opposite recommendation. As one obstetrician noted in 1964, "To force a thoroughly addicted [pregnant] cigarette smoker to cease would, in the first place, probably not work, and, in the second place, might create, from the increased tension and eating problems, increased fetal hazards."[67]

In the late 1950s and early 1960s, when Jackie Kennedy was giving birth and Marie Killilea's books were national best sellers, the cesarean section rate rose from its longtime 2.5 percent average to about 4 percent of births. In addition to antibiotics and blood banking making cesarean birth safer, if the reproductive histories of Kennedy and Killilea are any indication, the increase in female smokers after World War II might also have contributed to that rise by increasing the number of problematic pregnancies leading to emergency cesareans. Indeed, given the widespread attention paid to Kennedy's births, and the likely role cigarettes played in their outcomes, normalizing smoking for women was probably yet another of the many factors leading to the rise in, and greater acceptance of, cesarean sections in the 1970s and 1980s.[68]

Questioning Childbirth Technologies

After the death of Patrick Kennedy, although magazines still employed soothing platitudes when discussing birth by cesarean ("Caesarean section today is one of the safest of major operations"; "think of the Caesarean section as one of the two major paths of delivery"), caveats once again outnumbered assurances. The public learned that although cesareans were considerably safer than they had been 30 years earlier, the maternal death rate was nevertheless five times higher after sectioned births than vaginal ones. Magazines advised mothers to get a second opinion before agreeing to a first cesarean. Doctors ceased claiming that babies born by cesarean fared better than babies born by a difficult vaginal delivery. Even given an indication that a woman's first cesarean might be necessary, many doctors reverted to the old custom of allowing a mother to experience at least four or five hours of "good labor" before making any definitive decision about how to proceed.[69]

After the Kennedy baby died, all obstetrical interventions—not just cesareans—came under scrutiny. Rather than the celebratory accounts of "streamlined" birth that had appeared a few years earlier, *Good Housekeeping* linked labor induction to rising infant mortality. "Even more shockingly," the magazine told readers, doctors suspected that inducing labor might be the cause of the "dramatically" increased rate of mental illness and "retardation" among American children. Periodicals began to tell tales of birth interventions gone awry. A Chicago woman, whose obstetrician had induced her labor to avoid missing a golf tournament, suffered a "tetanic contraction" caused by too much Pitocin. The contraction cut off oxygen to the woman's daughter, who was born in severe respiratory distress. As the child grew, she exhibited an array of behavioral problems—she did not get along with other children, and she was slow in school.[70]

Instead of induction bestowing benefits, women's magazines now portrayed the practice as "possible elective tragedy." A Harvard University obstetrician characterized induction as "difficult, dangerous and . . . foolish," a medical procedure that rendered the vicissitudes of labor and delivery riskier and more strenuous, not easier and safer, as previously claimed. Women learned that 0.6 percent of babies died after an induced labor—"a significant price to pay for convenience." In contrast to the largely laudatory stances taken by newspapers and magazines through the 1950s, after Patrick Kennedy's death the lay press was more willing to be critical of modern childbirth practices, even to the point of fearmongering. The fear would prompt a hunt for, and an embrace of, diagnostic tools designed to alleviate risk—tools that would lead to more cesarean sections.[71]

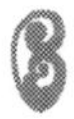

Between 1930 and 1965, newspapers and magazines offered many, often contradictory, perspectives on cesarean section. Cesareans were a deadly peril, a freak oddity, a safe albeit still rare option, a surgery bordering on the glamorous, a perfectly normal way to give birth, safer than vaginal birth, and then, once again, a risky business. During this 35-year period, however, cesareans remained infrequent enough that the transmutations did not have a particularly profound impact on public thinking. Cesareans were still outside the experience of the vast majority of women. The births of John and Patrick Kennedy brought the surgery into sharper public focus. Even then, though, the portrayals remained inconsistent.

Depictions of other birth interventions were similarly contradictory. Some magazines ran articles applauding the benefits for babies of labor induction. Other articles warned that induction threatened children's well-being. According to one magazine, medical technology promised miraculous outcomes. According to another, it was to be avoided if possible. While public health workers had instructed pregnant women since the 1920s to seek out prenatal care early and to follow their doctors' orders to the letter to ensure a healthy infant, in the 1960s and 1970s women learned that the medical technologies and treatments recommended by doctors—anesthetics, analgesics, some medications, and all x-rays—threatened the new lives their bodies were sustaining. At first glance the back-to-back sentiments—medical technologies benefit newborns, medical technologies harm newborns—seemed incongruous, but both stemmed from the desire to mitigate risk in the most emotional of medical arenas: childbirth.

A change in the medical view of labor was at the heart of these inconsistencies. As nineteenth-century medical records attest, nurses and doctors had long described labor in positive terms. Strong contractions signaled systematic, desirable progress. "Pains very good," "pains constant and good," "pains very good & effective," "pains strong & good," were phrases doctors peppered throughout nineteenth-century obstetric logs. Mothers often described their labors using equally positive terms: "easy," "easy and rapid," "not long or hard," "short and normal."[72]

By the last quarter of the twentieth century, medical assessment of labor was starkly different. Labor might be required to achieve most births, but labor was a necessary evil. Doctors practicing in the 1950s and 1960s customarily administered analgesics throughout first-stage labor to prevent their laboring patients from feeling much of anything. During second-stage labor, physicians administered general anesthesia to ensure that patients not only felt nothing but did nothing. Doctors removed their babies with forceps. As obstetrician Gene Lawrence explained years after retiring, "I didn't want my patients to push. I didn't want them to do anything. Because I think they ruin their pelvic floor, they loosen all of their musculature, their critical musculature. To bladder control, to fecal control . . . pushing was one of the no-nos as far as my practice was concerned." This change in thinking—that labor was potentially harmful, to women and children alike, rather than primarily beneficial—would have profound effects on public and medical attitudes toward childbirth and definitions of desirable and necessary treatments during childbirth.[73]

Diagnostic tools developed in the 1950s and 1960s seemed to confirm what DeLee had claimed in 1920: labor was a pathological process. The Apgar score, the Friedman curve, the Bishop score, ultrasound, and the electronic fetal monitor, described in the next two chapters, bolstered the culture of risk surrounding childbirth. And as these tools identified seemingly burgeoning risks, the number of cesarean sections skyrocketed.

Chapter Four

Assessing Risk

1950s–1970s

By the middle of the twentieth century, the long-running disagreements among obstetricians had ended in a victory for the operator camp. Just as Joseph DeLee had suggested in 1920, the physicians practicing in American hospitals were treating childbirth as "a decidedly pathological process." Every treatment DeLee had called for, and more, had become a component of maternity ward protocol. Obstetricians shaved pubic hair and administered an enema, a ritual known as "the prep"; they induced or augmented contractions by puncturing the amniotic sac and/or administering Pitocin subcutaneously or intravenously; they dispensed assorted analgesics throughout first-stage labor; they administered general, pudendal-block, or saddle-block anesthesia throughout second-stage labor; and they performed an episiotomy. By the 1950s, forceps had become mandatory in virtually every birth; mothers were too heavily drugged to push. In short, birth in US hospitals in the 1950s and '60s was a prescribed, industrialized process governed wholly by the physician.[1]

A new focus on the fetus helped drive the protocol. As one retired obstetrician said of the medical culture when he first trained, "we didn't really think a whole lot, when I was a resident, about the outcome for the baby. We were focused more on the mother because that was right at the end of the period where we were getting to where maternal mortality was way down." Only after the maternal death rate dropped "tremendously," he explained, did obstetricians "become more and more focused on protecting the baby and making sure he or she is safe and healthy."[2]

With the well-being of the fetus now on a par with concern for mothers, physicians developed diagnostic tools to help them detect and prevent trouble. Three of the tools, developed in the 1950s and '60s to identify and mitigate risk during childbirth—the Friedman curve, the Bishop score, and the Apgar score—heightened obstetricians' perception of the risks of childbirth. Other developments amplified the public's perception of risk—namely, the horrifying birth defects that resulted from the use of thalidomide by pregnant women during their first trimester followed quickly by a German measles epidemic, both against the backdrop of a March of Dimes campaign against birth defects. The medical and lay views of risk shaped by these events would eventually help stoke the unprecedented increase in the cesarean rate that began in the early 1970s.

Laboring on the Friedman Curve

As hospital-based residencies in obstetrics and gynecology became the primary training ground for obstetricians, sitting by women's bedsides throughout labor became a significant component of residents' training. Both laboring women and obstetric residents benefited from the practice. Women enjoyed constant companionship in an era when their husbands and friends were barred from labor and delivery, while obstetricians-in-training were afforded many opportunities to witness the rhythms of labor. As one observer said approvingly in the 1930s: "They watch every mother from beginning to end of her ordeal . . . no matter how long or seemingly uneventful the travail. . . . So our young medicos and nurses have an unparalleled chance to learn the natural history of childbirth." An obstetrician trained in the 1950s recalled how his constant presence also helped ease mothers' fear and pain as they labored. "The doctor in the room," he quickly learned, "[was] worth 100 milligrams of Demerol."[3]

Emanuel Friedman was an obstetric resident in the 1950s, when this practice was in its heyday. He based his eponymous curve, a depiction of the average length of first-time labors in the form of a sigmoid curve, on 100 births, data he probably collected as he labor-sat. Quickly and widely adopted, the Friedman curve prompted the notion that if a first-time mother labored longer than the curve indicated was within the range of "normal," she and her baby were at heightened risk. The more a labor veered from the curve, the greater the risk.[4]

The longest portion of the curve represented the average number of hours spent by women in the first stage of labor, that is, from their initial contractions to full cervical dilation. Friedman then subdivided the first stage into four phases. He found that phase one, the "latent period," before appreciable cervical dilation

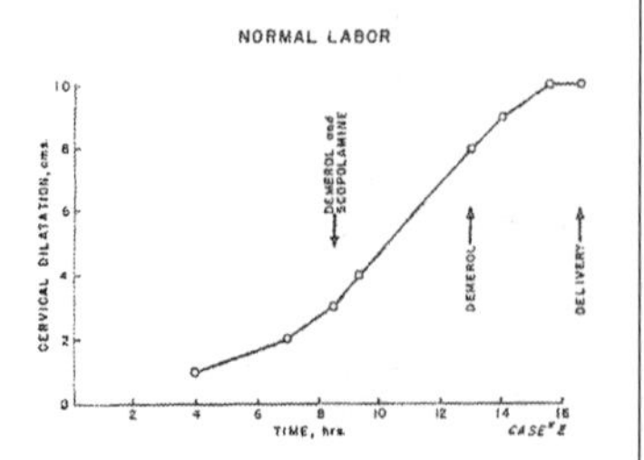

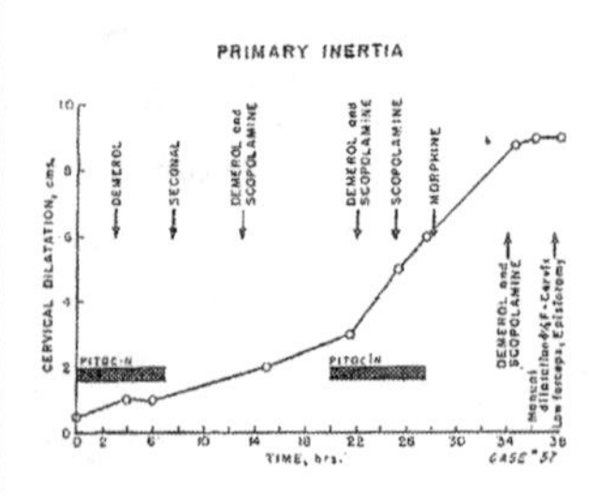

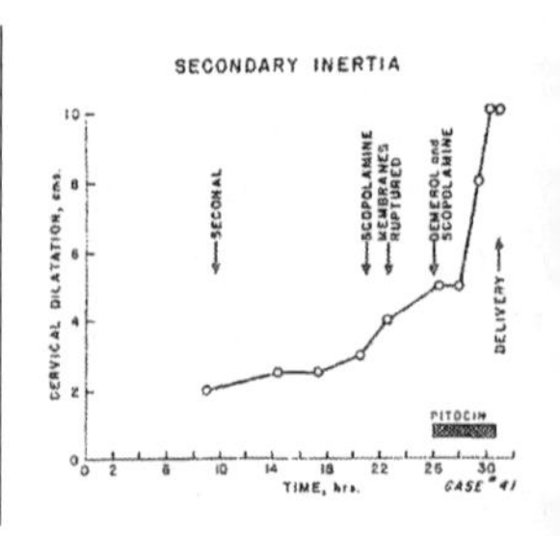

Examples of Emanuel Friedman's early "graphic analysis" of normal and abnormal primiparous labors. Note the use of drugs in all labors being charted. Soon, the sigmoid curve representing "normal" labor would become known as the Friedman curve. *Left*: A curve representing normal labor. *Center*: A curve indicating primary inertia—ineffective uterine contractions due to a mechanical, genetic, or hormonal defect. *Right*: A curve indicating secondary inertia—a slowdown in labor often caused by exhaustion, medical interference, and/or the parturient's anxiety and fear.
Source: Friedman, "The Graphic Analysis of Labor," 1572, 1573.

occurred, lasted from 1.7 to 15 hours—a mean 7.3 hours. During the latent phase, the cervix softened, effaced, and dilated about 2 centimeters. During phase two, the "acceleration period," the cervix dilated, usually relatively rapidly, from 2 to 4 centimeters. If the acceleration phase was appreciably slower than average, he found that a long labor was likely. During the third phase, the "steady period," the cervix continued to open—from 4 to 8.5 or 9 centimeters. Then, as the first stage of labor ended, it entered the "deceleration period," dilating a full 10 centimeters.[5]

Friedman formally introduced his curve in a 1954 article published by the *American Journal of Obstetrics and Gynecology*. He did not characterize his findings as sacrosanct. Rather, Friedman readily acknowledged the capriciousness of labor, noting that "the causes for the extreme variations in the lengths of labor so commonly encountered" had long interested doctors. He also recognized that the numerous medical interventions that had become common in American maternity wards since the end of World War II either extended the "normal" length of labor or truncated it, depending on the intervention. This observation was important because the majority of labors graphed by Friedman were not what a subsequent generation of mothers and physicians would have termed "natural." Rather, the labors that he observed and meticulously recorded were subject to what he characterized as "routine labor care"—enema, amniotomy, Pitocin infusion, sedation, and regional or general anesthesia. He noted that the latent period was especially "sensitive to this type of interference, prolonged with heavy sedation, and shortened with stimulation." He did not explain the potentially contradictory effects of the use of both stimulation (stripping the membranes and/or using Pitocin) and sedation (the continual use of analgesics) on the length of labors. Not until half a century later did studies show that first-time mothers undergoing spontaneous, unmedicated labors have slower cervical dilation rates than the Friedman curve indicates. As one obstetrician, who completed her residency in 2003, observed, "It's like looking at growth charts for babies and using the ones the formula companies come up with when breastfed babies don't grow that way." Yet for decades, obstetricians based their medical decision-making, including whether a cesarean was necessary, on the Friedman curve.[6]

Despite Friedman's recognition that variation in the length of labor was normal and that medical treatment often caused unusually long labors (and uncommonly short ones for that matter), by the early 1960s American physicians had adopted the Friedman curve for use at every birth. As time passed, Friedman, too, seemed to take his "graphicostatistical evaluations" more seriously, announcing in 1961 that the data he had accumulated represented a reliable definition of "the limits of normal progress in labor." Most notably, he stated that cervical dilation slower than 1.2 centimeters an hour represented a "critical limit." As alarming as the descriptor "critical" sounded, Friedman did not suggest that failure to achieve the "limit" called for extreme medical action. He proposed benign remedies for hastening labor instead, like those used by nineteenth-century obstetricians who rallied flagging "uterine energies" by providing mothers with a warm drink or urging them to change position. Friedman called for similarly supportive care (provision of "nutrition, fluids, electrolytes, rest, antibiotics, and encouragement to the patient") during the "long harassing hours" of labor. He assured his colleagues that "primary dysfunctional labor per se," now defined as a labor falling off his curve, posed no real risks to either mother or baby.[7]

That the labors of first-time mothers were considerably longer than the labors of women who had previously given birth was so well accepted that Friedman soon developed two curves—the one for primiparas he introduced in 1954, and another for multiparas the following year. In the explanatory text accompanying his second curve, Friedman still exhibited flexibility. Although doctors had long defined the average duration of labor as 24 hours for the first-time mother and 18 for the multipara, he explained that even a multiparous labor lasting 24 hours was "not an abnormality."[8]

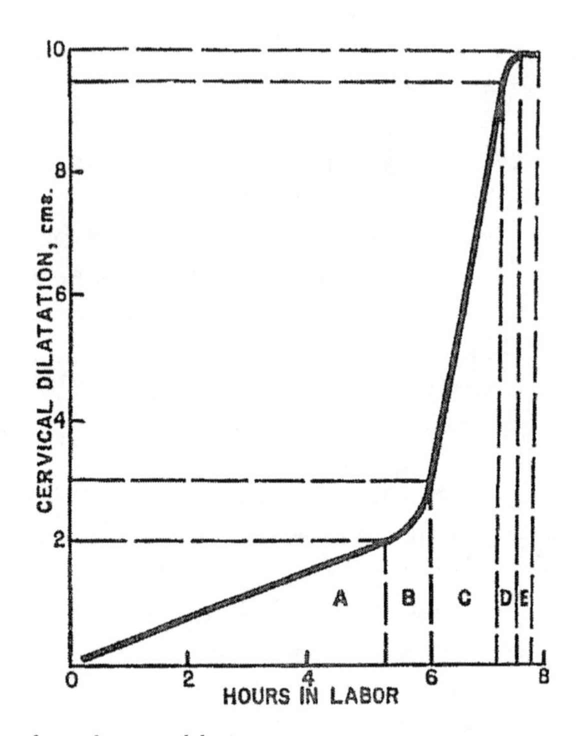

Friedman curve for multiparous labors.
Source: Friedman, "Labor in Multiparas," 692.

For years after he introduced the two curves, Friedman continued to refine both based on additional data. One of his residents, who began his residency in 1966, explained that immediately after every birth "we submitted a punch card form to his office" containing the details of that particular birth. In addition to updating his curve according to the ongoing accumulation of statistics, his former resident recalled that Friedman developed unique protocols based on assorted scenarios: "whether it was a prolonged latent phase, or a primary dysfunction, or an activated phase arrest . . . we would act . . . according to his suggestions."[9]

Despite Friedman readily admitting to the limitations of his curve, the curve became inviolable. Generations of medical school professors used the Friedman curve to teach their students about the "normal" and "abnormal" temporal parameters of labor. In 1960, J. P. Greenhill, the obstetrician who updated Joseph DeLee's textbook after DeLee's death, described the sense of security the curve provided physicians, allowing them "to simplify and to view objectively the complex dynamic changes of the progress of labor, previously loosely defined." Obstetricians now had a metric that rendered the most vexing aspect of labor—its length—seemingly more certain. At least doctors knew how long it *should* take, if not how long it *would* take.[10]

Before the Friedman curve, physicians did not use time as a yardstick to determine the quality of a labor, nor did physicians necessarily measure the length of a labor in hours. "Desultory" contractions might appropriately continue for days. Their counterpart—regular, strong contractions—usually indicated labor was progressing nicely, however long it might last. Before Friedman, lengthy labors were little cause for alarm, especially for first-time mothers. As one Kansas City physician wrote in 1941, other than the temporary exhaustion experienced by both doctor and patient, and the anxiety experienced by waiting family members, long labors rarely harmed anyone.[11]

Nor was a lengthy labor alone cause for significant medical intervention. After embrace of the Friedman curve, however, the labors that physicians would have shrugged off previously as exemplifying the inherent unpredictability of childbirth earned a pathological label. One obstetrician, trained in the 1980s, explained that during her "fairly typical" training as a resident she learned that birth must be "accomplished within a reasonable time frame." She recalled, "When I went to do my high-risk rotations they actually had a transparency with the Friedman curve that they would put over the top of the patient's labor chart and if they were falling off the curve . . . you would start Pitocin."[12]

Not until long after epidural anesthesia came into widespread use did obstetricians and anesthesiologists recognize that it too, like the analgesics before it, prolonged the active phase of labor by an average of one hour when measured against the Friedman curve. Yet, epidural or no, residents learned that "falling off the curve" demanded medical intervention. And, by the 1980s, intervention often meant not just Pitocin but a cesarean section.

Labor Dystocia per the Curve

To the consternation of obstetricians trained in an earlier era, the use of cesarean surgery to "cure" a long labor was increasing. One older physician described a typical scene in the 1980s: "Some patients have been 4 centimeters for a couple of hours and the residents say, 'We're done, let's do a c-section.' " Whenever she overheard that sort of pronouncement, she intervened. "Hey," she would tell the residents, "give her a chance, the baby's fine." She treated those episodes as teachable moments. After the patient delivered vaginally, she reminded residents " 'Hey, what was the rush a few hours ago?' And they [would] say, 'Well, by the book, [the patient had the] same [cervical] exam [result] for this many hours.'" An obstetrician who completed his residency in 1969 remembered the identical phenomenon. He and his cohorts would chart a patient's progress at two-hour intervals, "and then actually map on the Friedman grid her progress in labor." If a mother was not progressing appropriately, that is, "by the book" according to the dictates of the Friedman curve, they treated her with oxytocin. After that, if she still "didn't make any progress over two hours . . . we would then deliver by cesarean section."[13]

Although dystocia—traditionally defined as blocked labor caused by a rare physical anomaly—had always been considered a serious, even life-threatening, condition, only rarely had a long labor been diagnosed as dystocia. Traditionally, dystocia was an extremely long labor plus something else—an anatomical abnormality so severe that it prevented a woman from giving birth vaginally. The first published account of a cesarean section in the United States, described in the first chapter of this book, is an example of a nineteenth-century dystocia—the labor had gone on for days because the mother had no discernable cervical opening.[14]

That remarkable condition typified the unusual physical irregularity that prompted a diagnosis of labor dystocia through the first decades of the twentieth century. Other causes of dystocia included cervical stenosis, often triggered by either syphilis or a self-induced abortion using a corrosive substance that scarred the vagina and cervix; vaginal atresia; and an extremely large uterine, cervical, bladder, or vaginal tumor. Dystocias were so rare that obstetric texts assured physicians that even the birth of a "double monster" (an early-twentieth-century term for conjoined twins) could be "readily accomplished" vaginally. J. Whitridge Williams said of a merely long labor—uterine inertia in early-twentieth-century parlance—if "the patient is in good condition, the delay may be regarded with equanimity." He even assured colleagues that virtually any "obstruction is gradually overcome by the pressure exerted by the presenting part," the "presenting part" being the baby. After introduction of the Friedman curve, however, the medical view changed. A long labor was "sluggish, indolent, and inherently powerless," a problem in need of a medical remedy.[15]

As these adjectives attest, with adoption of the curve, the definition of dystocia changed markedly, becoming any labor falling outside the parameters of the curve. The American College of Obstetricians and Gynecologists (ACOG) coined several vague descriptors for the new dystocia: "failure to progress in labor," "difficult labor or childbirth," and "the slow, abnormal progression of labor." Under the new meanings, dystocia, a previously rare diagnosis, became commonplace. By the 1970s, Friedman himself had compiled 65 terms used by physicians to describe pathologic "labor variants," all falling under the dystocia rubric, including arrested labor, desultory labor, disordered labor, difficult labor, dysfunctional inertia, functional inertia, protracted labor, uterine asynchrony, uterine exhaustion, uterine inertia, and, the most commonly used descriptor, failure to progress.[16]

Although the new dystocia had little in common with the old, both shared a crucial characteristic: The diagnosis called for drastic medical intervention. One obstetrician recalled that when she began her residency in 1991, she learned to define a "prolonged labor" as "two hours with no change in the [dilation of the] cervix" during the active phase of labor. The cure was cesarean section. A Chicago-area obstetrician who started her residency in 1997 likewise remembered learning that a common indication for cesarean section was "arrest of labor," defined as "failure to dilate [any further] over a period of time . . . a couple of hours." Her original supervisors insisted that laboring women must "stick to a pre-defined curve and if they fall off the curve you're very quick to call c-sections." Critics of the practice, who were usually older obstetricians, characterized the new definition of dystocia as meaningless. They described "failure to progress" as an observation, not a medical condition needing a remedy. Yet the diagnosis remained common. An obstetrician who delivered his last baby in the mid-1980s said of his much younger counterparts in the late 1990s, "They do sections, sections, sections on the slightest provocation. If a mother is stuck at 4 centimeters dilation for 3 hours they go ahead and do a cesarean section. If they were to stop and realize what it takes for a cesarean section to occur—loss of blood, the inhalation anesthesia, the anesthetic risk, the operative risk. It's appalling. It's appalling to me anyway."[17]

Eventually recognizing that the burgeoning number of dystocia diagnoses had played a role in tripling the cesarean rate between 1972 and 1982—from 5.5 to 16.5 percent—ACOG officials urged their members to reassess their management of dystocia, suggesting they focus on identifying and correcting abnormal contraction patterns, fetal malposition, and inadequate pushing, rather than turning to cesarean delivery as the solution. The directive might have come too late, however. As one obstetrician observed prophetically in 1955, he and his colleagues increasingly faced "condemnations" for "intelligent restraint," while intervention earned them accolades. That atmosphere, far more pronounced 30 years later, likely made it easy to ignore the advice from their professional organization.[18]

Popularizing Induction with the Bishop Score

With the Friedman curve identifying so many cases of dystocia and most physicians still wary of cesarean section, doctors needed a nonsurgical treatment for the condition. As if in response, in 1955 magazines heralded "the recent mastering" of oxytocin, the hormone that stimulates labor. Mothers vouched for the advantages of chemically induced labor: "I was rested, ready for labor both physically and mentally, had arrangements made for the family at home, and we had an unhurried and pleasant daylight trip to the hospital."[19]

Women learned that synthetic oxytocin, developed and marketed under the trade name Pitocin, had other benefits as well. If a pregnant woman was carrying a large baby, rather than plan for cesarean surgery, "a few minute drops" of "purified, standardized" oxytocin could be counted on to instigate an early labor, and ensure a pre-term baby weighing several pounds less than it would have at full term, in order to guarantee a vaginal birth. Physicians did not necessarily need a medical reason to administer oxytocin, however. *Newsweek*, in recommending induction purely for convenience, likened an intravenous Pitocin drip to a spa treatment—"almost as easily arranged as a visit to the hairdresser." Women's magazines assured mothers that not only was induction safer than ever, thanks to Pitocin, it was "at times sounder and more conservative than allowing the patient to be caught up by ill-timed labor which may be more hazardous to the baby and may have to end in a Caesarean operation."[20]

Yet the belief that Pitocin promised fewer cesareans was illusory. Doctors soon found that chemically induced labors increased, rather than decreased, the likelihood of cesarean birth. That a poorly timed induction might end in a cesarean section had become so well known by the early twenty-first century that one seasoned obstetrician instructed her residents to avoid inducing first-time mothers. "If you want to keep your c-section rate low," she advised them, "you don't induce a primip unless you have an indication." That sort of advice had little effect, however. As another obstetrician said of the chemical induction of labor, "People want it. People like to plan."[21]

Failed inductions ending in cesareans was the problem that Edward Bishop, an obstetrician at Pennsylvania Hospital in Philadelphia, designed his score to solve. He unveiled it in 1964. The Bishop score, based on data from 1,000 Pitocin-induced births, helped physicians judge when a mother was ready to go into labor, that is, when Pitocin was most likely to work. The score allotted zero to three points to

Determining the Bishop score

Cervix	Score			
	0	1	2	3
Dilatation	Closed	1-2 cm	3-4 cm	>5 cm
Effacement	0–30%	30–50%	60–70%	>80%
Station	−3	−2	−1	+1, +2
Consistency	Firm	Medium	Soft	
Position	Posterior	Midposition	Anterior	

The Bishop score allots 0 to 3 points to each of five cervical and pelvic characteristics—dilatation, effacement, station, consistency, and position—in order to assess a woman's readiness for labor. A score of 9 or above, provided the pregnancy was at least 36 weeks along and was not the woman's first, indicated that induction was likely to be effective and that the infant would not be dangerously premature.
Illustration adapted from Bishop, "Pelvic Scoring for Elective Induction."

each of five cervical and pelvic characteristics: dilatation, effacement, station, consistency, and position. A score of nine or above, provided the pregnancy was at least 36 weeks along and not the woman's first, indicated that induction was likely to be effective. The score became so integral to obstetric safety that 40 years after its introduction, obstetricians still pointed to it as a landmark achievement.[22]

In the wake of the Bishop score, labor induction became more common while spontaneous labor became correspondingly less common, contributing to the growing unease with spontaneous vaginal birth and the relative comfort with methodical cesarean surgery. In 2012, looking back on her career, an obstetrician who graduated from medical school in 1973 blamed the growing incidence of induction, now encouraged by the existence of the Bishop score and the assurance it seemed to provide, for distorting the medical and lay view of labor. Only spontaneous labor, she contended, was normal labor. And why, she asked, "would you want anything on your side other than normal labor? Normal labor is the best thing to have on your side if you're trying to have a normal birth." Yet with the increasing number of induced labors, cesarean surgery not only became more likely, it became more acceptable.[23]

Focusing on the Neonate with the Apgar Score

While a clear line can be drawn from the work of Friedman and Bishop to more cesarean surgeries, the high-profile work of Virginia Apgar had a less direct, but equally profound, effect on the increase. As an anesthesiologist who often worked in labor and delivery during the 1940s and '50s, Apgar developed a method to assess the health status of an infant immediately after birth. Quickly dubbed the Apgar score, her diagnostic tool was soon adopted worldwide, becoming as well known to parents as to physicians. Less than a decade later, Apgar embarked on another career, spearheading a nationwide campaign to prevent birth defects under the auspices of the March of Dimes. Her work in anesthesiology and public health became so widely recognized for its contribution to pediatrics that many in the medical community credited her with initiating the pediatric subspecialty of neonatology. Yet the profound effect of her work on obstetric practice has been largely ignored.[24]

Because the Apgar score forced obstetricians to focus immediate attention on the neonate, they began to connect their own worth as physicians to individual and aggregate scores. Apgar's later work in public health prompted mothers and fathers to similarly fixate on the notion of the perfect newborn. Obstetricians' and parents' focus on perfection, in turn, contributed to medical and public complacency toward the burgeoning cesarean rate; increasingly, cesareans were deemed an avenue to perfection.

Yet Apgar developed her score out of medical necessity. As an anesthesiologist during the post–World War II baby boom, she observed daily the consequences for newborns of the analgesics and anesthetics given to their mothers during labor. By the time she invented her score in the early 1950s, the list of drugs used in assorted combinations to control labor pain was long. Morphine, Demerol, Seconal, Nisentil, and Thorazine represented only a partial inventory of the smorgasbord of medications used in assorted combinations to control labor pain. The practice of administering varied drugs throughout first-stage labor, followed by general anesthesia in the delivery room, was so commonplace by the 1930s that one obstetrician complained in 1937 that obstetric practice had largely become "treatment of drug confusion." One typical mid-twentieth-century mother, who gave birth to four children over 14 years, in 1951, 1953, 1957, and 1965, received a steady dose of unspecified analgesics in the labor room during her last three births and general anesthesia in the delivery room for all four births. She explained, "I didn't really experience the delivery itself" for any of her children.

Indeed, each successive birth, she recalled, was more heavily drugged than the previous one. And her fourth labor was also induced.[25]

Apgar witnessed these developments firsthand. After mothers entered the second stage of labor, she was often called to the delivery room to administer general anesthesia to the women who had already spent many hours under the influence of a mix of narcotic, barbiturate, opioid, and/or antipsychotic medications. She was especially troubled by the breathing difficulties of their newborns. Although most in the medical community denied that the respiratory distress seen in neonates was iatrogenic, Apgar suspected that the analgesics and anesthetics given to mothers during labor were triggering their newborns' struggle to breathe. She became the first physician to prove that the drugs given to mothers did indeed enter the umbilical vein within two minutes.[26]

Apgar's discovery did not alter established obstetric protocol, however; the drug regimens remained in place. Perhaps the boundaries set long ago by medical specialists to protect their turf were so powerful that an anesthesiologist's discovery could not inform the practice of obstetricians. In any event, unable to convince obstetricians to give fewer and less powerful drugs to laboring mothers, Apgar developed a workaround—an objective, rapid means of assessing the condition of newborns to determine their need for resuscitation in the delivery room.[27]

Ingenious in its simplicity, the Apgar score represented a neonate's health status as a numerical appraisal of the five signs monitored by anesthesiologists throughout surgery to evaluate a patient's well-being: heart rate, respiration effort, muscle tone, reflex irritability, and skin color. To compose the score, a nurse or doctor in the delivery room examined every infant one minute after birth and assigned a 0, 1, or 2 to each of the five signs. A doctor or nurse then added the five figures together. Initially, Apgar deemed babies with a total score of 0 to 2 in dire trouble and in need of immediate resuscitation, 3 to 7 in need of medical surveillance until they were out of the woods, and 8 to 10 unambiguously healthy and vigorous. A few years later, after studying biochemical analyses of many infants, she shifted the demarcations somewhat: babies who received one-minute scores of 0 to 3 were seriously depressed and in need of immediate medical attention, 4 to 6 moderately depressed and in need of monitoring, and 7 to 10 healthy and vigorous.[28]

After Apgar described her method in a medical journal in 1953, physicians worldwide recognized its utility. Formulating an Apgar score became standard procedure at births, a ritual that continues to this day. Eventually, Apgar advised that the score be calculated twice—not only one minute but also five minutes

Determining the Apgar score

Sign	0	1	2
Heart rate	Absent	<100 / minute	>100 / minute
Respiration effort	Absent	Weak cry	Good cry
Muscle tone	Limp	Some flexion	Active motion
Reflex irribility	No response	Grimace	Cry or cough
Color	Blue or pale	Blue extremities	Completely pink

Virginia Apgar's score signifies the health status of a newborn in the form of a numerical appraisal of the five signs monitored by anesthesiologists during surgery to evaluate a patient's well-being: heart rate, respiration effort, muscle tone, reflex irritability, and skin color. Alarmed by the narcotized neonates who were affected by the drugs given to their mothers during labor, Apgar devised the score to alert medical personnel to an infant's need for resuscitation immediately after birth.
Illustration adapted from ACOG Committee Opinion, "The Apgar Score."

after birth. The first number became the "one-minute Apgar," the second the "five-minute Apgar"; collectively, the two scores became known as an infant's "Apgars."[29]

Apgars soon became not just an indicator of the immediate medical needs of the newborn but also a predictor of neonatal outcome. Regardless of birth weight, physicians observed a two- to threefold increase in neurological abnormalities in children with a five-minute Apgar in the 0–3 range. In the mid-1960s, a study of 17,000 scores collected at 13 major medical centers found that an infant with a five-minute Apgar of 0 to 1 had only a 50 percent chance of surviving the first 28 days of life; a baby with a five-minute Apgar of 9 to 10 had a 99.5 percent chance. For a time, the one-minute score came to be associated with how much medical attention a newborn needed immediately after birth and the five-minute score with the odds faced by an infant for significant morbidity and death. Only decades later, after some grammar schools requested a child's Apgar scores upon entry, did the ACOG issue a series of committee "statements" and "opinions" declaring that Apgar scores did not reflect long-term outcomes nor constitute evidence of permanent neurological damage but rather were simply a convenient shorthand for a newborn's status and the effectiveness of resuscitation efforts immediately after birth.[30]

Apgar touted her tool as serving two purposes. Before the score, not until a pediatrician performed a systematic examination of the infant in the hospital nursery, usually 48 hours after birth, did any member of the medical team do much more than confirm that a newborn breathed, cried, and displayed all the anticipated, visible body parts. In requiring a member of the delivery room team to methodically examine and assess every infant immediately after birth, Apgar scores focused immediate attention on the neonate. Virginia Apgar also heralded her score's ability to enhance communication among the anesthesiologist, obstetrician, delivery room nurse, and pediatrician. As one member of the medical team handed off a baby to another, the score served as a cryptic, mutually understood language that provided each medical caretaker in turn a means of sharing the identical evaluation of the newborn's status.[31]

An indication of the score's influence was its inclusion in 1961 in the twenty-fourth edition of *Dorland's Illustrated Medical Dictionary.* Apgar wrote to the dictionary's editor, thanking her for the honor, one she had expected only posthumously, if ever. *Dorland's* editor responded that the entry was not intended as a tribute: "We are only recording history which has already been made."[32]

By the early 1970s, the score had become as familiar to the public as to the medical community. In a note to her former Lamaze instructor, one mother celebrated her son's recent birth by invoking the magic number. "He was . . . very bright eyed and alert and registered 9 out of 10." The proud mother felt no need to explain 9 out of 10 *what.* Less than two decades after Virginia Apgar introduced her score, not only physicians but also parents knew exactly what the numbers meant. This recognition of the meaning of Apgars, and parents' occasional delight in a score, was further evidence of medical attention switching from mother to baby. While medical intervention during birth had always been about recognizing and alleviating risk, and effecting rescue, efforts had focused almost exclusively on maternal risk and rescue. The Apgar score helped to transfer the primary focus from maternal to neonatal outcomes.[33]

Evaluating Performance, Not Babies

Initially, obstetricians' quick adoption of her score gratified Apgar. In the article introducing her innovation to a wide medical audience, she expressed appreciation for "the enthusiastic interest and competitive spirit displayed by the obstetric house staff who took great pride in a baby with a high score." She interpreted their keen interest as a sign of the score's ability to aid newborns. She issued her thanks during the score's early days, when she advised that anyone present in the delivery room—the obstetrician, anesthesiologist, nurse, or occasional pediatrician—was qualified to issue the score. It did not matter who formulated it, as long as the assessment necessitated by the score had spurred someone to examine the baby promptly.[34]

She eventually realized, however, that obstetricians perceived the score's meaning differently than other delivery room personnel. As L. Stanley James, one of Apgar's closest associates, observed, obstetricians viewed the score not just as a means of assessing the neonate but also as an appraisal of their own skills—the higher the score, the better the obstetrician. The conflict of interest inherent in such a view manifested almost immediately. Given the opportunity to issue what they thought of as an evaluation of their own work, obstetricians handed themselves the highest possible grade. The "competitive spirit" Apgar originally relished ensured inaccurate scores.[35]

Apgar discovered the problem after many hospitals reported a plethora of perfect scores, which should have been rare. In the original article describing her technique, Apgar explained that babies almost never receive a perfect ten at one minute because the score's fifth sign, color, rarely earned the maximum two points. Due to their high capacity for carrying oxygen and their low oxygen saturation level at birth after enduring the long, slow squeeze through the birth canal, infants are born only infrequently with fully oxygenated skin color. In other words, newborns are typically cyanotic at birth.[36]

Yet hospitals were reporting a sizeable number of perfect scores. At Sloane Hospital in New York City, for example, 13 percent of infants were receiving one-minute scores of 10. Apgar wanted to know why. On a hunch, she forbade obstetricians at Sloane to evaluate newborns and assigned that task instead to other delivery room personnel. Perfect one-minute scores tumbled 70 percent—to 3.9 percent. Later, Apgar was "appalled" to learn that the number of perfect 10s at some other institutions was far higher than at Sloane. At one hospital, where only obstetricians (or midwives, if they had delivered the baby) issued the scores, an extraordinary 83.9 percent of newborns received a perfect one-minute Apgar. Disheartened, Apgar considered advocating for elimination of the score. If professional egos overstated the score, it was of little use.[37]

Her colleagues rallied, however, insisting the score had value despite what could be characterized as grade inflation. Apgar switched gears and called for a broad change in protocol, as she had at Sloane, advising that no one responsible for delivering the baby be permitted to assign the score. Hospitals soon adopted the recommendation that only "trained impartial observers" issue scores. Now the duty fell either to the anesthesiologist, the pediatrician (generally unrealistic because, Apgar noted, he is "hardly ever present for the actual delivery"), or the circulating nurse ("these nurses are *excellent*, with much experience and no personal involvement with that particular baby").[38]

Apgar had solved the problem, although she might have misjudged obstetricians' motivation for inflating scores—hubris was not necessarily their primary incentive. Many doctors were actually justified in thinking the score represented an evaluation of their work. During internal hospital audits, hospital administrators had begun to use average, aggregate Apgar scores as one way of appraising the quality of their hospitals' services. Wanting to look their best before parents and peers, obstetricians gave themselves, and indirectly their hospitals, undeservedly high marks.[39]

Apgar scores came to have a similar meaning for parents, too. Mothers equated a perfect Apgar with a flawless baby, and so maternal pride probably magnified obstetricians' sense of what was at stake when formulating an Apgar. One woman reported enthusiastically in 1973, "Our wonderful little son cried before being completely out, and had a perfect 10 Apgar rating!" Another mother used the score in two ways—to boast about her daughter's perfection and to spotlight her own heroic conduct during the birth. "You can imagine my pride," she wrote, "at being told she had an Apgar rating of ten—the highest possible and most probably due, they all said, to the fact I was given no medications through labor." Fathers likewise used their children's scores to showcase their pride. One new dad reported, "The baby's Apgar checked out among the highest of all deliveries in the hospital."[40]

Inflating scores also provided obstetricians with a means of tempering an uncomfortable reality. Although infant mortality had steadily declined in the United States since the last quarter of the nineteenth century, the perinatal subset of that mortality—the number of infants who died in the first two weeks of life—had shown far less improvement. In corresponding with a colleague, one physician lamented the country's "perinatal wastage," terming it "the darkest frontier of medicine." Thus, low Apgar scores were also a reminder of a medical and public health failure. The striving for perfection that manifested as too many perfect Apgar scores would, within two decades, appear in a different form—a steeply higher cesarean section rate as cesareans came to be seen as less risky than many vaginal births.[41]

A Mother's Duty to Avoid Risks

Following the success of her neonatal scoring system, Virginia Apgar embarked on a second career. In 1959, she left her longtime jobs as professor of anesthesiology at Columbia University and director of the Columbia-Presbyterian Medical Center Division of Anesthesiology to accept a position with the March of Dimes—a public health foundation entering its third decade. Originally established as the National Foundation for Infantile Paralysis in 1938 to find a cure for polio, the organization was renamed the March of Dimes in response to a clever fundraising effort. In the 1950s, after successful testing of the polio vaccine, the March of Dimes shifted its focus to the prevention of birth defects. As the organization's senior vice president for medical affairs and director of the Division of Congenital Malformations Research, Apgar, by then a household name, proved to be an unparalleled spokesperson. Advice on how to prevent birth defects was soon ubiquitous—as influential as later public health efforts to lower smoking and drunk driving rates.[42]

Only recently had scientists begun to characterize birth defects as preventable, mainly by pinpointing rubella—a virus popularly known as German measles—as one cause. In the 1940s, the public learned that rubella contracted during the first trimester of pregnancy put the developing fetus at significant risk for blindness, deafness, microcephaly, and other disabling conditions. That discovery prompted a hunt for other causes of congenital abnormalities, paving the way for Apgar's second career. Researchers soon learned that Rh-factor incompatibility, maternal diets deficient in protein, and some drugs and all x-rays taken during pregnancy could have consequences for a fetus at least as serious as rubella. Those discoveries prompted the March of Dimes' second crusade.[43]

Apgar's job was to convince the public that prevention was key to diminishing birth defects. As the indefatigable face of the campaign, she toiled doggedly to transform women's behavior during pregnancy. In an era when airline travel was far less common than today, she logged 100,000 miles annually. Just as the term "Apgar score" became popular vernacular in the 1950s, Virginia Apgar's work for the March of Dimes a decade later was similarly recognized beyond the insular world of medicine. As a colleague observed in a tribute to Apgar after her death in 1974, "she lifted birth defects from a secret closet and put them firmly on the map."[44]

Newspapers, magazines, radio, and television all provided Apgar with a forum for her message. She told the *New York Times Magazine* that 250,000 American babies—7 percent of the infants born annually—were "born damaged." No family was immune. She took special care to explain that a child's birth defect should never become any parent's secret shame. In one of the hundreds of letters she wrote in response to queries from distraught mothers, Apgar told a heartsick woman whose son had spina bifida, "After being in this field for ten years, I am astonished that young couples take for granted that each baby will be normal. . . . You were unfortunate in being the one couple in 16 to have a less than perfect baby. Please do not harbor any feelings of guilt." Education, prevention, and reassurance were Apgar's watchwords.[45]

Articles promulgating her messages bore the promising titles, "How to Have a Perfect Baby," "New Ways to Save Your Unborn Child," and "They're Solving the Mysteries of Birth Defects." The last article described "simple, common-sense precautions" that pregnant women could take to increase their chances of a good outcome—seeking prenatal care; eating a balanced diet; knowing their own and their husband's blood type to prevent the effects of Rh-factor incompatibility; and avoiding drugs, x-rays, and exposure to infectious diseases, especially German measles. Additional "Rules for Childbearing," published by *Woman's Day*, included become pregnant only between the ages of 18 and 40; follow doctors' instructions during pregnancy; familiarize yourself with your own and your husband's medical history; consider adoption in light of a family history of birth defects; avoid "heavy" smoking; and keep pain medications to a minimum during labor.[46]

Other magazines and newspapers delved into an array of additional topics related to the March of Dimes' crusade: inherited diseases and conditions; "mongoloid idiocy"; and the "science of fetology," a new discipline established to "end the personal heartache and social tragedy of birth defects." Most articles mentioned, and many highlighted, Virginia Apgar. *Woman's Day* dubbed her "guardian of the newborn" and described her in superhuman terms—as "larger than life," a "fireball" who "does not walk: she gallops." Apgar, "an international synonym for the care of the newly born baby," had become a crusader for preventive obstetrics. In 1973, even the era's premiere television talk show, *Donahue*, hosted Apgar and relayed her messages.[47]

Because the campaign to prevent birth defects focused on threats to the developing fetus and how to mitigate them, the March of Dimes aimed its messages at women. Women learned to actively avoid a number of "culprits" during pregnancy to ensure development of a healthy fetus. High on the list were viral and bacterial infections (such as rubella and syphilis), medical treatments (such as x-rays and certain drugs), and an array of behaviors (such as succumbing to emotional distress and eating poorly). While doctors might prevent mishaps during the birth process, over the nine months of a pregnancy a mother's responsibility to prevent problems was far greater than a doctor's. The overriding message of the campaign was that maternal vigilance was the cornerstone of prevention.[48]

Apgar instructed married women of childbearing age to always behave as if they were pregnant during the second half of their menstrual cycles because "if that baby really *is*, he is in the most crucial weeks of his life." Women's magazines echoed Apgar, telling readers that not only pregnant women but women with even the remotest potential to become pregnant should be on constant guard. The ubiquitous admonitions, rather than empower mothers and alleviate their guilt, as intended, presented them instead with an all-consuming task that was nearly impossible to fulfill, especially in the 1950s and '60s when women only rarely learned in a timely fashion that they were pregnant.[49]

When the March of Dimes hired Apgar, home pregnancy tests were almost two decades away from store shelves—women's magazines did not advertise the first home test kits until 1978. Until then, only a visit to the doctor could confirm a suspected pregnancy. Yet during the 1950s, 1960s, and much of the 1970s, women frequently postponed their first prenatal visit because health insurance seldom covered prenatal care—the US Congress did not pass the Pregnancy Discrimination Act until 1978. This act required employers in all states to cover maternity care as they would any other medical condition if they offered health insurance to employees. Before the law's passage, to avoid unnecessary out-of-pocket expenses, women ordinarily waited until they had missed at least two periods before consulting a physician. Apgar chided women about the dangers inherent in that practice. By the end of the first trimester of pregnancy, she warned, "The baby is completely formed. He has a brain, a heart that beats. He is either off to a good start—or he isn't." Early awareness of pregnancy, she implied, encouraged beneficial, and quashed harmful, health behaviors.[50]

While Apgar cast birth defects as a public health crisis to be remedied by societal and political initiatives, rather than a tragedy to be borne in isolation by individual women and their families, she simultaneously intimated that pregnant, and potentially pregnant, women nevertheless bore a disproportionate share of the burden of prevention. Mothers were thus the recipients of conflicting messages: birth defects were neither their fault nor their individual responsibility to thwart. Nevertheless, mothers bore the primary responsibility to prevent birth defects.

Along with the medications, viruses, and x-rays to be avoided; the blood types to be checked; the stormy emotions to be subdued; and the prenatal diets to be adhered to, the birth process was to be approached with special trepidation. Even Apgar, despite her encouraging messages of prevention, referred to birth as "the most risky time" of a person's life. A 1967 *New York Times* article describing "the world of the unborn" offered a harrowing description of birth from the perspective of the tiny, defenseless, beleaguered fetus forced to "endure the 50-pound pressures of labor."[51]

Birth was cast as a menace to the very fetus that a mother had been vigilantly protecting from defects for nine months. The "watchful waiting" during labor advocated long ago by nonoperators now appeared to be quaint at best, irresponsible at worst. By the early 1970s, Apgar, who had become one of the most well-recognized and revered physician figures in the country, said publicly what obstetricians were telling patients privately—that certain diagnostics and treatments must be employed during childbirth, for the sake of the fetus. In addition to all the personal measures women should take daily before and during pregnancy, Apgar specifically advised that planned cesareans and the recently developed electronic fetal monitor promised to aid in decreasing the incidence and severity of several types of birth defects.[52]

At the height of her messaging, two public health crises—one on the international, the other on the national, stage—aided Apgar's efforts in a particularly graphic and compelling way. First came news in 1962 of the effects of thalidomide on the developing fetus, a story emanating largely from Europe. Then, from 1963 to 1965, the United States saw a German measles epidemic. Both the drug and the disease injured tens of thousands of infants. If Americans had not yet recognized the threat of birth defects and the importance of preventing them, the horrifying nature of the injuries inflicted by thalidomide and German measles made a convincing case for prevention. The death of Patrick Kennedy in 1963 added to the mix.

The twin public health catastrophes reinforced Apgar's contradictory messages. While thalidomide and German measles were compelling proof of her claim that birth defects are often both arbitrary and preventable, the horrifying effects of the drug and the disease also seemed to render more imperative than ever a mother's obligation to protect her developing fetus from risk. Thus, even as Apgar reassured women that birth defects were avoidable, thalidomide and German measles signaled not only that pregnancy was more dangerous than ever but that mothers' responsibility to thwart danger was more imperative than ever.

Thalidomide in particular magnified mothers' sense of both powerlessness and grave responsibility because originally women had been assured the drug was harmless. Chemie Grünenthal, the German pharmaceutical company and developer of thalidomide, marketed the drug in the 1950s as a safe sedative, so safe that in Germany it was sold over the counter. Distributed around the world under assorted trade names (Contergan, Softenon, and Distaval, to name a few), thalidomide was soon given to newly pregnant women, a group doctors thought to be uniquely in need of sedation. In some countries, including the United States, "anxiety of pregnancy" was a common postwar diagnosis, and pharmaceutical companies often ran advertisements for tranquilizers in obstetric journals.[53]

Yet what Chemie Grünenthal had claimed was a sedative so harmless that scientists could not find any dose large enough to cause side effects in rats became an international public health nightmare. Only much later did scientists learn that rats do not metabolize the drug. In humans, if ingested during the first trimester of pregnancy—precisely the crucial time Apgar was warning American mothers about—just one dose of thalidomide caused any one of a wide variety of fetal deformities. Which defect depended on which day during fetal development a mother ingested the drug; defects included malformation of the anus, genitals, ears, eyes, and internal organs—especially the intestines, kidney, and heart. The drug became best known, however, for one visible defect, an epidemic of phocomelia among infants. A condition known in lay terms as "seal limbs"—hands growing directly from shoulders and feet from hips—phocomelia was the most tangible, and horrifying, symbol of the risks facing a developing fetus. Thalidomide thus became the prototypical example of the consequence of ignoring Apgar's weightiest admonition: sexually active women of childbearing age should always assume pregnancy during the second half of their menstrual cycle in order to proactively protect a developing fetus, even a theoretical one, from harm.[54]

Fortunately, Frances Kelsey, a pharmacologist at the US Food and Drug Administration (FDA), largely spared American babies the effects of thalidomide. She resisted enormous pressure from Richardson Merrell, the pharmaceutical company seeking to market thalidomide in the United States. Alarmed by reports of nerve damage in adults who had taken the drug, Kelsey demanded that Richardson Merrell provide the FDA with proof that the drug would not even more readily damage a fetus. Yet despite few American infants being directly affected by the calamity, thanks to Kelsey's obstinance, Americans nevertheless experienced the crisis alongside the citizens of affected countries—via the American newspapers and magazines that carried unsparing photographs of damaged infants.[55]

A German measles epidemic following on the heels of the thalidomide disaster ensured that Apgar's message of maternal responsibility for prevention would become gospel. Doctors had known for more than 20 years that the childhood illness that was so mild it did not even warrant a doctor's visit was nevertheless the cause of a host of congenital defects if contracted during the first trimester of pregnancy, the crucial time Apgar continually warned about. With that discovery, a diagnosis of German measles during pregnancy became so dire that, long before the US Supreme Court handed down the *Roe v. Wade* decision ensuring abortion would be a legally available medical procedure, doctors routinely offered an abortion to any pregnant woman who contracted the disease during the first three months of pregnancy. Indeed, the laws permitting "therapeutic abortions," available in every state if the pregnancy threatened the life or health (including the mental health) of the mother, were also known informally as "German measles laws."[56]

News about thalidomide, followed almost immediately by the rubella epidemic, sparked new rounds of media focus on Apgar and the March of Dimes campaign. The similarities of the two crises were not lost on the magazines and newspapers that likened the outbreak of German measles to the earlier thalidomide disaster. "Rubella virus is as deadly as thalidomide for the unborn" was one media refrain.[57]

The Nation Responds to Anxieties about Birth Defects

Governmental reactions to the threats to fetal development were swift and comprehensive. In 1962, the Kennedy administration established an Institute of Child Health and Human Development to be housed in the National Institutes of Health. The Johnson administration followed a few years later with a "Bill of Rights for Children" that listed as one of its foci protection of fetal development. That bill of rights reiterated the weighty message conveyed by Apgar, reading in part, "Despite the highly controlled nature of the intra-uterine environments of mammalian embryos, the belief that they are completely uninfluenced by the condition of the maternal host is no longer tenable."[58]

In the private sphere, mothers' heightened sense of responsibility for neonatal outcome was evident in the many letters they wrote to Apgar. Mothers asked how to prevent miscarriage. They wondered if the newly invented birth control pill would harm a future baby. One mother worried that spacing her children too far apart might increase a younger child's chances for defects. Another woman feared that her use of a microwave oven during pregnancy had caused the "emotional disturbance" and inability to concentrate in school suffered by her 9-year-old son.[59]

Apgar had expected women to be comforted by the knowledge that they could prevent birth defects. Instead, the traditional worry of mothers, and women hoping to become mothers, that every undesirable physical and behavioral trait their child might eventually exhibit was in their power to thwart, loomed even larger. One woman, terrified of childbirth, wrote to Apgar to inquire, "Will my fear ingure [*sic*] or hurt the baby in any way when I do have one?" She also fretted that her future children might inherit her poor eyesight and turned-in feet. She implored Apgar, "Would you kindly answer my questions and help me to understand I have no reason to be afraid?" Apgar assured the distraught woman that her worries would not harm her baby "at all," although it was impossible to predict if her eye and foot troubles would be inherited by her offspring. "But," Apgar reminded her, "as you note, you overcame both these difficulties. None of us is perfect." Another mother, whose doctor had x-rayed her numerous times during her pregnancy because he mistakenly suspected she was carrying twins, worried that her now 19-month-old baby would soon have cancer. She wrote, "These thoughts are disturbing me to such a degree that I find I cannot function normally." Apgar instructed her to "relax," and urged, "Please start functioning 'supernormally' to make up for lost time!" Even what might have been a trivial concern in an earlier era was now momentous. One woman wrote to ask Apgar, "if two people with allergies to pollen, certain foods, dust and molds etc. marry, is it advisable for them to have children?" Apgar answered every query with her trademark reassurance, telling the woman concerned about inherited allergies, "There are so many allergies in this world that if only non-allergic people married, there would be very few families!" Apgar's attempts at light-hearted comfort were only marginally successful. Concerns now overwhelmed mothers.[60]

In 1964, *Harper's* magazine ran an article encapsulating the national anxieties about the perils of pregnancy and childbirth. The article warned, "A soldier in wartime has a better chance for survival than a baby during birth." The author of the article, the "gynecologist-obstetrician-in-chief" at Johns Hopkins Hospital (he was also the editor of the *American Journal of Obstetrics and Gynecology*), offered statistics rivaling Apgar's: "dead, damaged, and defective" babies numbered 300,000 each year in the United States. For every 1,000 babies born, 35 died shortly after birth, 35 had damaged brains, and 35 had a "hereditary defect."[61]

Antithetical to Apgar's original intentions, by the mid-1960s hospitals in both the western and eastern United States began issuing the urgent call, "Paging

Dr. Apgar!" over hospital loudspeaker systems to signify an obstetric emergency and the need for immediate assistance in the delivery room. Virginia Apgar, whose name should have been synonymous with childbirth safety due to her universally accepted neonatal assessment score and her untiring crusade to prevent birth defects, was now irrevocably linked to childbirth disasters. It was a sign of the times. Birth as a process necessitating medical intervention from beginning to end was about to come to full fruition.[62]

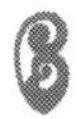

As the first physician to connect neonatal respiratory depression with the drugs administered to laboring mothers, Virginia Apgar developed her eponymous score. Then, as the face of a nationwide campaign to prevent birth defects, she conveyed messages of prevention to American mothers, warning them away from certain medications, treatments, and behaviors during pregnancy. Yet in alerting medical personnel in the delivery room to the neonates who required prompt medical attention, the Apgar score paradoxically permitted obstetricians to perpetuate, even enhance with impunity, the elaborate drug regimens that prompted the need for the score in the first place. A decade later, Apgar's nationwide campaign to prevent birth defects prompted women to view the risks of pregnancy and birth in new and magnified ways. Ultimately, women found comfort in more medical treatments during childbirth rather than fewer.

Friedman's work triggered similar ironies. Although he developed the Friedman curve while practicing the traditional, hands-off method of care favored by nineteenth-century obstetricians—sitting by laboring women's bedsides, comforting them, and cheering them on—mid-twentieth-century obstetricians eventually used the curve to justify the intensive, hands-on treatment that came to characterize childbirth in the 1950s and 1960s. By inadvertently broadening the definition of labor dystocia to include any perceived slowdown in labor, the Friedman curve transformed what had been an exceedingly rare, serious condition that occasionally required surgical intervention into a commonplace, serious condition that always demanded chemical intervention and, increasingly, surgical intervention. By the 1980s, "failure to progress," as assessed by the Friedman curve, was the number-one reason for performing a primary cesarean section.[63]

The Bishop score, prompted in part by the need to hasten labors due to the epidemic of dystocia diagnoses created by obstetricians' adherence to the Friedman curve, similarly helped to ensure that the chemical induction of labor would become commonplace. Bishop designed his score to help obstetricians judge when induction was likely to be successful. Yet with labor induction normalized, the Bishop score became less important. "That's one thing that's really changed over the 40 years that I've been in the field," said an obstetrician trained in the early 1970s. "We did inductions of labor back then [but] we did it when a nullip was completely effaced and 4 centimeters dilated." Since then, the obstetrician noted, the practice had changed. "They are doing them now with a long, closed cervix," precisely the type of intervention that Bishop formulated his score to eliminate. "It's insane! . . . The fact that obstetricians are so willing to bend to that trend. It's almost like boutique medicine."[64]

Collectively, the Friedman curve, the Bishop score, and the Apgar score allowed doctors to measure every labor and neonate against a series of ideals. Given that ability, physicians became more willing to actively encourage medical intervention to increase the likelihood of good outcomes, as defined by the authoritative messages provided by curves and scores.

In the decades that followed, an inflated perception of risk, bolstered especially by Friedman's and Apgar's work, led the medical community and the public to embrace two new medical technologies: ultrasound to periodically track fetal development and electronic fetal monitoring to observe a fetus's response to labor. By the early 1970s, fetal monitors were so well accepted that the machine would wholly replace the labor-sitting that had been part of obstetric residents' traditional training. Some older obstetricians, knowing the value of the now discarded practice of sitting by women's bedsides throughout entire labors, responded with alarm. In his ACOG presidential address in 1981, J. Robert Willson worried that obstetric residents were "learning to rely more and more on fetal monitors as they learn less and less about labor." His observation proved to be prescient. The link between use of the fetal monitor, changes in the way residents were trained, the deskilling of obstetricians, and a soaring cesarean section rate would soon be manifest.[65]

Chapter Five

Inflating Risk

1960s–1980s

News stories in the 1960s related to pregnancy and childbirth—including stories about thalidomide and the March of Dimes campaign—alarmed the public. Although childbirth was measurably safer than it had ever been in the United States (maternal mortality had plummeted from a high of 670 deaths per 100,000 live births in the 1930s to 10 deaths per 100,000 live births by the 1970s), anxieties surrounding childbirth were as powerful as ever—a byproduct of both a better-informed populace and the high hopes for medical treatment that came with the antibiotic age. Expectant parents had come to believe that medicine offered guarantees; one effect of their faith was the acceptance of diagnostic tools that seemed to mitigate the perceived risks of childbirth.[1]

The obstetricians' diagnostic arsenal, which included the Friedman curve and Apgar score by the early 1950s, and the Bishop score by the early 1960s, was soon augmented by machines. Ultrasound equipment changed the experience of pregnancy; obstetricians and parents could now view the previously invisible fetus. And just as sonography changed the experience of pregnancy, the electronic fetal monitor changed the experience of labor. Obstetricians and mothers had been primed to accept the monitor by the ongoing news about threats to the fetus, including a 1967 article in *Newsweek* describing labor as "the most perilous hours in an infant's life." A year later, the fetal monitor appeared to keep constant watch over the beleaguered fetus as a mother labored. Hospitals quickly adopted the device.[2]

While ultrasound equipment and fetal monitors alleviated medical and lay anxiety by ostensibly placing childbirth under medical control in previously unimagined ways, the machines also had their downsides. Ultrasound weakened obstetricians' hands-on skills. After describing the once-essential art of externally palpating a pregnant woman's belly to gather vital information, an obstetrician trained in the early 1970s lamented, "Oh, that art is gone . . . in labor and delivery now routinely, on every patient who comes into labor, residents do an ultrasound to make sure the baby is headfirst." Another obstetrician, trained in the early 1990s, marveled that the obstetrician who mentored her during her residency "could tell twins' positions just by hands on. And it was a very impressive thing to watch his clinical skills." She, on the other hand, is typical of more recently trained obstetricians—"reluctant to rely on my hands-on if the ultrasound is right there and I can know for sure. Because I wouldn't want to put this patient at risk."[3]

The electronic fetal monitor likewise came with unanticipated downsides, most notably an increase in the cesarean rate. The immobility imposed by the monitor made labors longer, leading to more diagnoses of dystocia to be remedied by cesarean surgery. And in a particularly frustrating development, the machine's messages were so difficult to interpret that false positives for fetal hypoxia became epidemic nationwide, prompting the largest spike in c-sections yet.

As obstetric residents shifted their attention from mother to machine, the monitor substituted for frequent physician-patient contact and greatly diminished the amount of time residents spent with laboring women. Spurred by the women's rights movement, a vocal group of mothers, including many who proved adept at garnering the attention of mass media, began to object to what they viewed as an inhumane, mechanical, isolating approach to birth. Once again, childbirth was in the news. This time, however, rather than celebrate the latest medical innovations, newspapers and magazines offered a view on American birth practices through the eyes of angry mothers. The great irony of the nationwide crusade for a more humane, "natural" approach to birth, however, was that just as feminist activists were seeing the most positive, concrete responses to their demands for birth reform, the cesarean section rate was seeing its most precipitous rise.

Ultrasound Makes an Appearance

In the 1970s, as the nascent birth reform movement came to public attention, ultrasound equipment was making its first appearance in the United States. Developed in Glasgow beginning in 1956, the machine was in use throughout the British hospital system by the mid-1970s, almost a decade before its firm establish-

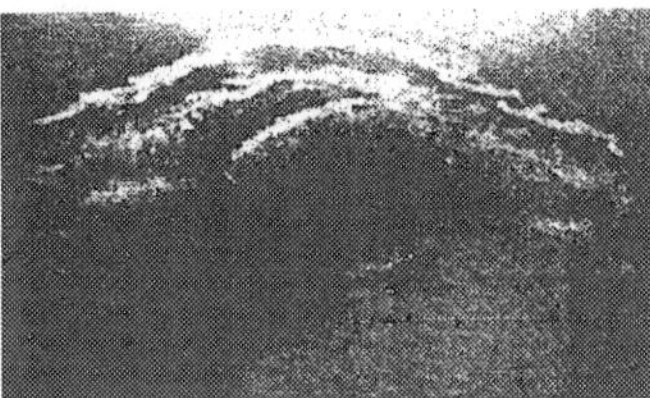
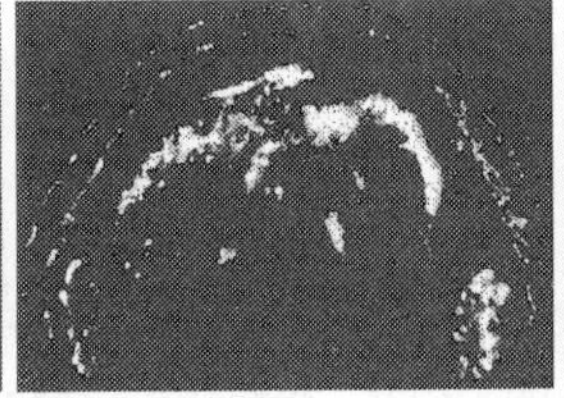
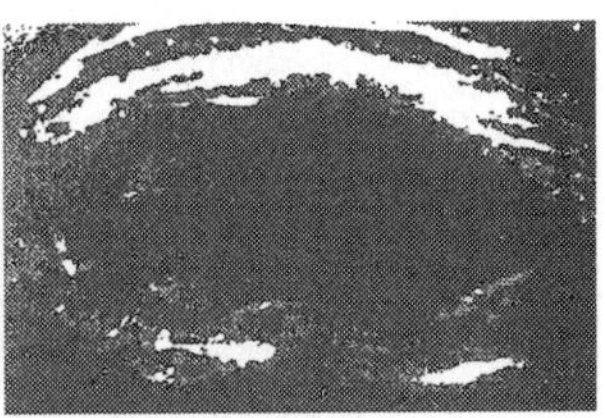

The earliest ultrasound images published in a medical journal. One unimpressed obstetrician described them as looking like "a cloud cover over Florida on the weather map." *Left*: Outline of a fetal skull in utero at 34 weeks' gestation. *Center*: Image of twins. *Right*: Uterus at 14 weeks' gestation.
Source: Donald, MacVicar, and Brown, "Investigation of Abdominal Masses by Pulsed Ultrasound," 1192, 1193. Quote from interview of Dr. Charles Hammond by Jessica Roseberry, June 2, 2004, Duke University Medical Center Archives, Durham, NC.

ment in the United States. To gain a foothold in the lucrative American market, one ultrasound manufacturer, Advanced Diagnostic Research Corporation (ADR), pitched the equipment directly to obstetricians, to virtually no avail. American doctors saw little use for the machine. Not until ADR developed a different ploy—pitching the machine directly to the pregnant women sitting in obstetricians' waiting rooms—did they make significant sales. Pregnant women's delight at seeing their developing fetus essentially sold the equipment for ADR. It did not seem to matter that early ultrasound images were essentially indecipherable—one obstetrician described them as looking like "a cloud cover over Florida on the weather map."[4]

The medical world first learned of ultrasound technology in an article written by its developer, Ian Donald, and published in the *Lancet* in 1958. Donald's stance against abortion inspired his invention. Although he supported therapeutic abortions and criticized the Catholic Church for its inflexible condemnation of all abortions, he initially envisioned ultrasound as a tool to persuade unhappily pregnant women to continue their pregnancies. Later, as the technology improved, the development of high-resolution 2D, and then 3D, images prompted the claim that ultrasound improved maternal-fetal bonding for all women, not just the unhappily pregnant. Eventually, the equipment became so sophisticated that one obstetrician described sonographic imagery as "just absolutely magnificent . . . like a photograph."[5]

Ultrasound exams became the highlight of prenatal care. As one typical woman marveled, "They did an ultrasound. You could see the little guy!" Fathers were equally entranced. A woman said of her husband's reaction to an amniocentesis,

"It was especially exciting for him to see the baby on the ultrasound and helped him feel closer to the baby." Another mother similarly focused on the sonogram during her amniocentesis: "The best part about the test . . . was actually seeing the baby on the ultrasound, watching it move." Ultrasound images became family keepsakes, appearing on refrigerator doors and in wallets alongside other family photos. Long before a woman could feel fetal movement, her fetus became a social being.[6]

By the early 1990s, 70 percent of pregnancies in the United States were undergoing ultrasound evaluation, even though the American College of Obstetricians and Gynecologists (ACOG) warned its members that benefits of the technology had not been established. Even in 2009, when virtually every pregnant woman in the United States had at least one ultrasound exam, an ACOG *Bulletin* listed only four, circumscribed benefits of the machine: the device could determine gestational age, number of fetuses, viability of the fetus, and location of the placenta. By then, however, the social value of ultrasound far outweighed its limited diagnostic value.[7]

In yet another example of shifting focus from mother to fetus, the now-visible fetus became a patient in its own right. While birth, or perhaps the first fetal movement that mothers are able to sense midway through a pregnancy, had once signaled the beginning of parents' relationship with their child, now the first sonogram served that purpose. An obstetrician trained in the early 1970s, who described herself as "probably the last maternal-fetal medicine expert in the country who did not routinely do ultrasounds in pregnancy," tried for a time to explain to her patients "that routine ultrasounds . . . do not change the outcome of pregnancy." She quickly discovered, however, that attempting to dissuade mothers from an unnecessary ultrasound was futile—"like fighting City Hall." She lamented, "to say they can't have their ultrasound . . . you can't go there."[8]

While most parents cherished their ultrasound experience and the permanent images it produced, a few did worry about its safety. Others questioned its accuracy. One woman (her first birth had been by cesarean) learned of the device during her second pregnancy when her doctor told her about the "wonderful new machine they just installed in the hospital . . . accurate within seven days of telling your due date." Pinpointing the due date was essential in her case because her doctor wanted to perform her second cesarean at precisely 38 weeks and feared a premature delivery. But three months after the ultrasound, her physician told her she needed an amniocentesis because he was skeptical that the due date determined by the machine was correct. "Great new ultrasound!" she groused.[9]

Despite the delight expressed by most parents, the technology also had a disquieting effect. The now visible but still unreachable infant rendered the potential dangers of pregnancy even more pressing. In 1991, Volvo, a car manufacturer with one of the best reputations for safety in the industry, exploited what had become the well-recognized association between ultrasound imagery and ubiquitous risk. An ad in *Harper's* magazine, showcasing an ultrasound image of a near-term fetus, posed the query: "Is something inside telling you to buy a Volvo?" No further explanation of the stark image was necessary; by the early 1990s, everyone recognized, and could appreciate the meaning of, a sonogram. The at-risk fetus, soon to be an at-risk babe-in-arms, urgently needed protection. And parents could rest easier—despite the heightened risks their children now faced—that there were machines to help protect them, whether those machines were safe automobiles or ultrasound devices.[10]

Monitoring the Fetal Heart Rate

Just as monitoring pregnancy in some fashion had always been important (ultrasound was only the most recent surveillance method), monitoring labor was equally crucial. By the mid-nineteenth century, physicians were using a stethoscope to listen intermittently to the fetal heart rate (FHR) during labor, theorizing that changes in the FHR indicated distress and that, depending on the continuity and severity of any change, a quick delivery via forceps might be necessary. Use of the stethoscope became so integral to care during labor that, in the early twentieth century, obstetricians created the fetal stethoscope, or "fetoscope." By the 1950s, however, obstetricians had lost faith in their ability to accurately count the fetal heartbeat; the normal FHR, at times, can be twice that of an adult.[11]

To replace human fallibility with a machine's precision, Edward Hon, a Yale University obstetrician, began work in the late 1950s on electronic techniques to evaluate and record the FHR throughout labor. He unveiled his invention a decade later. The ability of the electronic fetal monitor to continually record every nuance of the fetal heartbeat seemed so demonstrably superior to intermittent use of the fetoscope that the fetal stethoscope disappeared from maternity wards. "Yeah," noted one obstetrician who began her residency in 1991, "nobody does that anymore. Zero. I have seen one in Africa."[12]

The theory behind Hon's device was convincing. If obstetricians continually monitored the fetal heartbeat, they would learn instantly of fetal distress and thereby spare a child, through a timely cesarean, the lifelong neurological consequences of asphyxia. So certain were some leading obstetricians of the inherent value of the monitor that, before conducting any study of the machine's efficacy, they confidently predicted its universal use would reduce by half intrapartum deaths, "mental retardation," and cerebral palsy.[13]

Hon also hoped that the objective data provided by the electronic monitor would lower what was then a 4.5 percent cesarean section rate. He theorized that an obstetrician would no longer have to make an educated guess about the need for an emergency cesarean—with the monitor he would know for sure. *Life* magazine presented Hon's hope as fact, telling readers that a group of 400 mothers who had volunteered to test the monitor saw a 75 percent decrease in cesareans. A community hospital in Baltimore similarly reported, "There is no better way to prevent too hasty interference than to depend on the monitor record." That the only test of the fetal monitor had been performed by three physicians on the board of directors of the company then marketing the device, and that researchers had never compared the machine's efficacy with the fetal stethoscope's, was not mentioned. On its face, comparing the fetoscope to the monitor seemed unnecessary anyway. Logic dictated that the electronic monitor was the superior tool.[14]

Physicians assumed the intermittent use of a fetal stethoscope during labor provided incomplete information. That belief had been bolstered over the years by stories of a fetoscope that disclosed an ominous FHR, followed by an emergency cesarean that turned out to be unnecessary—the infant exhibited no sign of distress at birth. One mother described just such an experience. Theresa, 20 years old when she gave birth to her first child in 1971, was one of 10 children. After going into spontaneous labor, she checked into the hospital at 2 a.m. She was not afraid—eight of her siblings, including full-term triplets, had been born vaginally. Only her youngest sibling had been born by cesarean section, after her mother suffered a placental abruption likely caused by her grandmultiparity. Given her mother's experience, Theresa assumed her own first birth would be "a pretty natural thing. . . . I wasn't anticipating problems. I just assumed that bodies would do what they do."[15]

Fetal monitors had not been introduced at that particular hospital yet; nurses periodically checked her baby's heartbeat with a fetal stethoscope. When Theresa was two centimeters dilated, one of the nurses could not find a heartbeat. She called in a colleague, who could not find the heartbeat either. At 10 a.m., doctors decided to perform a c-section. They did not disclose their plan to Theresa, however. Instead, they told her husband, who was sitting in the maternity ward waiting room. Someone asked Theresa to sign some papers, probably a consent form, without offering an explanation, and she did not ask for one. She was in labor; nothing going on around her, or being done to her, was ordinary. Someone asked her to sign something, so she did. When an orderly wheeled her into the operating room, she was baffled: "I'm going, like, 'What's happening?'" A doctor told her, "We're going to operate." She was flabbergasted. "Why?" Even then, no one described the plan. "They just ignored me." She assumed that either her baby had died or that she was dying. No one attempted to reassure her. "It was like I was a non-entity."[16]

Not until after the birth did Theresa learn that doctors had performed the cesarean because of the "fetal distress" indicated by the fetoscope. Learning of the diagnosis after the birth only added to her bewilderment. "He was big and he was healthy. . . . I didn't see any problem. So, I don't know why they thought he was in distress." Memories of her son's birth still evoked her ire as she told the story 42 years later. "My body was hijacked. I just felt like . . . I got into some system that had nothing to do with me."[17]

Doctors also made the opposite mistake when using a fetoscope—delivering a stillborn fetus despite a normal heart rate throughout labor. Clearly, they concluded, the information provided by the fetal stethoscope was insufficient. The tireless monitor, on the other hand, would miss nothing. Physicians so trusted the new equipment that it became their focal point during labor—"their eyes glued to the graph that showed every tiny variation in the beat of [the] child's heart." As one doctor explained, "When you look at anything that has lights and a digital readout and a paper drum turning and an instanteous [*sic*] fetal heart rate recording . . . it makes you feel like you're getting a lot of information."[18]

An article in *Life* magazine helped the public view the monitor in the same way. The 1969 article, one of the earliest to describe fetal monitoring in the lay press, appeared under the headline, "'Watching' the Unborn inside the Womb," and explained why it was vital to do just that. During labor, the fetus "struggle[d] to survive the strains and pressures being put upon it." The electronic monitor now guarded the fetus during this monumental struggle. A large photograph on the article's first page showcased a monitor in the foreground, a physician bent at the waist, staring at the screen. In the background, a mother lay on a bed, covered with a sheet. Another physician stood beside her. That doctor is ignoring her, however. His eyes are riveted on his colleague across the room—the doctor whose gaze is affixed to the monitor. The men's behavior illustrates the newfound centrality of the monitor to childbirth—any information the laboring mother might provide was insignificant compared to the information imparted by the machine.[19]

Despite obstetricians' confidence in the utility of the monitor, Hon did not recommend it be employed universally, at least not at first. Rather, he characterized

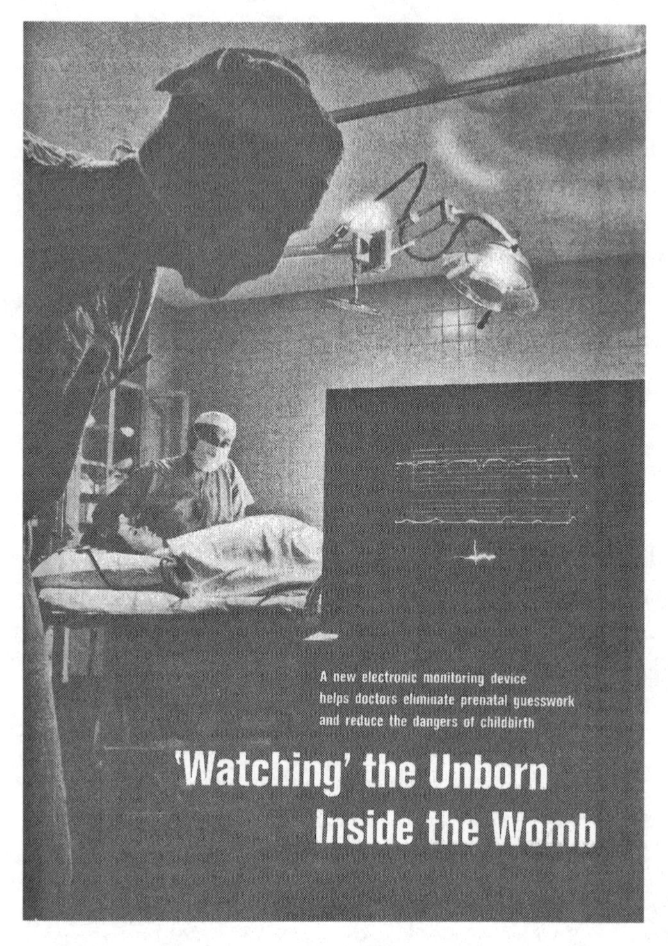

Life magazine helped to introduce the electronic fetal monitor to the public. Notice the centrality of the monitor to the birth. Even the physician standing beside the laboring woman has his eyes affixed on his colleague across the room, whose eyes are affixed to the monitor.

Source: "'Watching' the Unborn Inside the Womb."

his monitor as "fetal intensive care," implying it should be used only in situations identified as potentially dire. Hon's early articles listed the conditions that warranted continual monitoring. They included amnionitis, Rh sensitization, placental abruption, prolapsed cord, postmaturity, toxemia, and meconium staining. Many physicians immediately decided, however, that universal monitoring would ensure good outcomes for all fetuses, not just those facing tangible threats.[20]

Initially, the decision to adopt the monitor seemed brilliant. As monitor use increased nationwide through the 1970s, perinatal mortality decreased by more than half; individual institutions saw even greater declines. Many credited the monitor for the public health triumph. The medical community soon declared electronic fetal monitoring (EFM) an unparalleled success. The benefits of its ubiquitous employment appeared to be manifest, the harms nil.[21]

(Mis)Interpreting Monitor Patterns

There were skeptics, though. Unconvinced that EFM deserved credit for the lowered perinatal death rate, public health officials pointed out that hospitals not employing monitors were seeing identical decreases in infant death. These cynics attributed the universal declines to the revolution in pediatric care that coincided with the growth of monitoring. The pediatric subspecialties of neonatology and perinatology had recently made an appearance, prompting improvements in prenatal care, maternal nutrition, and neonatal care. Some hospitals opened neonatal intensive care units to accommodate their neonatal specialists. States were making their own unique efforts to transform infant healthcare. Illinois, for example, set up a statewide system of regional perinatal care centers. Nevertheless, most obstetricians believed that the monitor deserved at least as much credit for the improved statistics as the recent innovations in newborn care.[22]

The information conveyed by EFM appeared to be indisputably life-saving. The monitor indicated when there was a rapid fall in the FHR, as well as the FHR's "beat-to-beat variability"—changes in response to the normal stress of labor. Rapid decelerations could be a sign of fetal distress, while "short-term variability" evidenced a healthy fetal heart rate. The monitor's patterns did not necessarily lend themselves to reliable interpretation, however. While lack of short-term variability might indicate fetal hypoxia, it could also be a sign of normal activity, such as sleep. A few obstetricians did recognize the inherent difficulties in interpretation. One recalled that she "was quite vocal nationally" within a decade of the monitor's introduction, condemning use of the term "fetal distress" to describe the significance of deceleration patterns. She explained, "fetal distress describes the fetus" while the more appropriate term, "non-reassuring fetal status . . . describes your interpretation of what's going on. . . . Because the vast majority of babies with so-called 'fetal distress,' have perfectly normal gases and Apgars." Nevertheless, physicians began to err on the side of caution, intervening in the form of cesarean section after viewing an equivocal FHR pattern.[23]

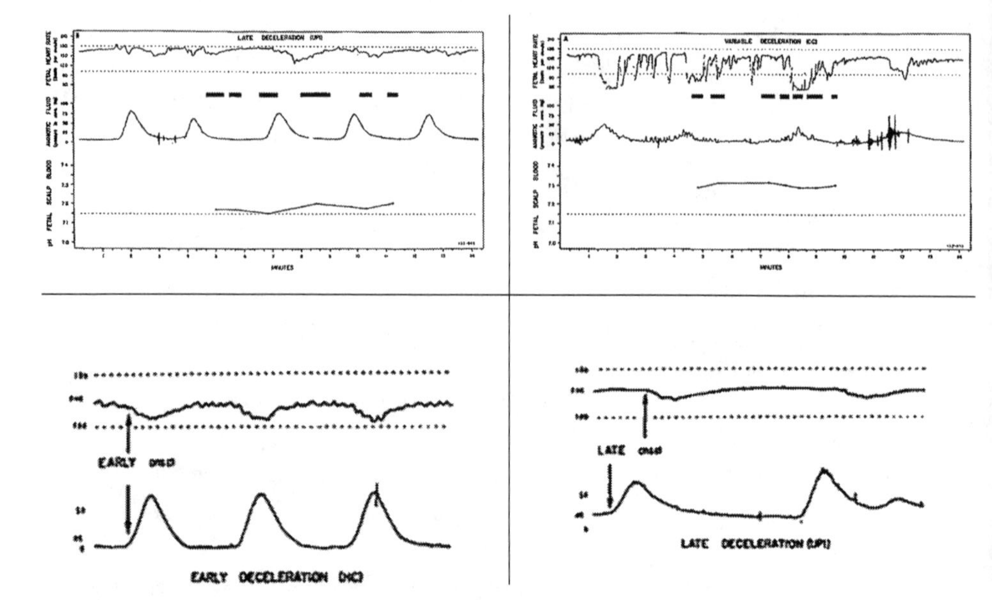

Edward Hon's early articles on his electronic fetal monitor contained numerous illustrations of fetal monitor strips and their meaning. The explanations of their meaning forewarned the difficulties for obstetricians of accurate diagnosis. *Upper left*: Hon explained, "Clinically, this FHR deceleration pattern would be considered normal. However, this degree of late deceleration probably indicates low margin of fetal reserve." *Upper right*: Hon explained, "Clinically, this degree of FHR irregularity and slowing would be considered diagnostic of fetal distress. However, since it is thought to be largely reflex in origin, variable deceleration of this degree appears to be innocuous." *Lower left*: FHR pattern associated with fetal head compression. *Lower right*: FHR pattern indicating uteroplacental insufficiency.
Source: Hon and Quilligan, "Electronic Evaluation of Fetal Heart Rate," 150, 160, 161.

That the meaning of a monitor strip was difficult to deduce should not have come as a surprise. Peppering Hon's first articles were dozens of FHR patterns, each accompanied by lengthy interpretations. "Naiveté and wishful thinking inspired our hope for a simple rule-of-thumb estimate of fetal distress," one group of early users admitted. "Obviously, the problem is much too complex for such an easy appraisal."[24]

Misinterpretations were numerous and widespread; some hospitals saw false positive rates for fetal hypoxia of 40 percent. To ensure greater accuracy, almost a decade before fax machines became workplace fixtures, some hospitals began to send monitor tracings by phone via a Xerox 400 Telecopier to experts standing at the ready to confirm a diagnosis. The endeavor failed to solve the problem, however. Even experts saw different meanings in identical patterns—these specialists were able to agree on the implication of a pattern only 68 percent of the time.[25]

One Chicago obstetrician who received her medical degree during the monitor's early days has witnessed more than four decades of attempts to make the device more reliable. "Please," she said in 2012, "there's no way! . . . It's like standing in front of a piece of modern art. Everyone interprets it differently. It's just crazy." Another obstetrician described the experience that confirmed for her the capriciousness of fetal monitor printout interpretation. She saw a fetus die "right under my surveillance. . . . I can't tell you how many other fetal heart tracings looked just like that one and the babies were just fine." Her experience was similar to obstetricians' earlier encounters with the fetal stethoscope. The misinterpretations also dashed Hon's hope that his device would lower the cesarean rate. Rather than avoiding unnecessary cesareans, Hon's colleagues were, in his words, "dropping the knife with each drop in the fetal heart rate."[26]

The rush to perform a cesarean based on doctors' interpretation of monitor strips profoundly altered the birth experience. Women giving birth in the 1970s, who were largely unacculturated to either EFM or a significant cesarean rate, were particularly distressed. Women's magazines had recently begun to carry positive descriptions of "natural" childbirth. These women were thus wholly unprepared for the machine's effects.[27]

Carol, 20 years old at her first birth in 1976, entered the hospital in spontaneous labor, feeling fine. A doctor ruptured her amniotic sac. "I went," she said, "from feeling nothing to being totally in excruciating pain." Medical personnel attached her to a fetal monitor, reviewed the monitor strip, and delivered frightening news. "They said I had to make a decision because they said either that I would die, or my baby would die, or both of us would die, if I didn't have a cesarean. . . . They said her heart was in distress." Carol was stunned. Her pregnancy had been trouble-free. "I walked. I exercised. I really felt good. And it just seemed like this diagnosis came out of nowhere." She tried to stay calm, "but I think I just felt disoriented to what was going on and I was feeling stress with the fetal monitor and the conversations." Some obstetricians were becoming well aware of this sort of monitor-induced anxiety. "We allow her to see the EM's chattering stylus and its winks," complained one doctor. The resulting "monitor-associated dystocia" then prompted "abnormal contractions and these in turn cause arrest of labor and sometimes diminished uteroplacental blood flow. . . . And we then apply the modern-day obstetric panacea—cesarean section."[28]

After Carol learned her baby would die if she did not agree to a cesarean, she signed the consent form, just as mothers almost always did in such a situation. "That's something I guess I'll never forget," she said years later, "that the baby would die, or I could die, or both of us . . . what they were saying, it just didn't seem right." The edict issued by doctors in 1976 seemed even less right to Carol when she described the birth 28 years later. "Since then, of course, I've read these books that said that half of [physicians] . . . don't know how to read" the monitors.[29]

Initially, obstetricians were not alarmed by the increase in cesareans. As one West Coast doctor told colleagues in the mid-1970s, "As an article of faith, I have adopted the policy that no intrapartum fetus is ever harmed by abdominal delivery." Rather than a procedure to avoid at almost all costs, as it had been during the first half of the twentieth century, a cesarean had become a remedy for the unpredictable risks of vaginal birth, risks identified increasingly often by the fetal monitor. Obstetricians' complacency was a sign of the times; when Hon introduced his device in 1968, medical technology in any form represented unalloyed progress.[30]

Consequently, the unexpected findings of the first randomized, controlled trial of EFM, released in 1976, did not diminish most obstetricians' faith in the monitor. The study, published in the *American Journal of Obstetrics and Gynecology*, compared an electronically monitored group of high-risk, laboring mothers with a similar group screened intermittently with a fetal stethoscope. Researchers found only one difference in outcome between the groups. The electronically monitored group had a cesarean section rate of 16.5 percent; the fetoscope group had a rate of 6.8 percent. Everything else about the two groups—Apgar scores; rates of neurological disability; admissions to the NICU, and numbers of stillbirths, neonatal, and perinatal deaths—were indistinguishable.[31]

Of the eight prospective, randomized trials conducted from 1976 through 1987—one involving almost 35,000 women—only one found any advantage to EFM over periodically listening to the fetal heart with a fetoscope. That study found neonatal seizures were twice as likely to occur in the fetoscope group. The significance of the finding became unclear, however, in a follow-up one year later. Of the babies who survived neonatal seizures, both groups had an identical number of abnormal infants. And all eight studies confirmed the findings of the original study: continual monitoring resulted in significantly higher cesarean rates than periodic use of a fetal stethoscope. Under the perpetual gaze of the monitor, fetal distress, once an infrequent diagnosis, had become commonplace, resulting in a precipitous increase in cesarean sections.[32]

Although a few obstetricians were beginning to disparage fetal monitors ("we call them feeble monitors," one said), most doctors had become uneasy attending a birth without the information the device provided. The monitor had served as obstetricians' eyes and ears for eight years before publication of the first study of the machine's efficacy, and most preferred to stick with their perception of the machine rather than adopt an objective evaluation of the machine. One obstetrician trained in the 1990s explained, "In medicine there's always what they call evidence-based practice and I think there's also practice-based evidence." And as early as the 1970s, the monitor had become an important component of the accrued experience of American obstetricians. Despite the initial research findings, one obstetrician insisted in 1979, "the benefits of monitoring have already been so great that it is unlikely that a truly objective double-blind study in either high- or low-risk patients will—or should—ever be completed."[33]

As the cesarean section rate rose throughout the 1970s and 1980s, rather than seriously consider abandoning, or decreasing their reliance on, EFM, obstetricians attempted to better train residents in reading monitor strips. In a typical effort, senior obstetricians at a large Chicago hospital ordered residents to measure umbilical cord blood gases after every delivery. Then obstetricians compared the results with residents' interpretation of monitor strips. An obstetrician described the process. "We got the pH, and the oxygen on the baby, and the carbon dioxide in the baby's blood . . . [then] we would compile [monitor] tracings and . . . force residents to analyze the tracings and try to predict the pH. And then we would pull out the pH and say whether or not they were right." Often, they were not. Senior obstetricians would then tell residents: "You didn't take in the whole picture. You did an emergency cesarean and the pH of the baby was perfectly normal. And it had Apgars of 9 and 9! So, the next time you see that pattern—think!" While the exercise did lower the cesarean section rate temporarily at that hospital, senior obstetricians eventually wearied of the exercise, and residents "got a little sloppier."[34]

When the cesarean rate at that hospital hit 20 percent, one senior obstetrician tried a different tactic. He began to post each physician's cesarean rate. "And the rate plummeted," remembered one of his colleagues. "There's nothing like peer pressure because back then the attitude was . . . 'oh my God, we've got to get our cesarean delivery rate down.' So, he published everyone's cesarean delivery rate. And those that were 30 percent plummeted over the next year."[35]

Another Chicago hospital decreased its cesarean rate from 17.5 percent in 1985 to 11 percent in 1987 by developing objective criteria for the four most common reasons for performing a cesarean. The hospital also required each obstetrician to obtain a second opinion before operating. Inspired by that hospital's success, the New York State Health Department established two rules of its own: (1) that all hospitals in the state maintain a record of the underlying cause of every cesarean birth, and (2) that the state's physicians document discussions with women about the consequences of repeat cesareans, in the hope of encouraging more vaginal births after a previous cesarean birth. The New York Health Department also established an independent committee of physicians to study any hospital that veered dramatically from the state's average cesarean rate. Yet even those measures failed to exert lasting effect. By 2010, despite New York's earlier three-pronged effort to lower their rate, the state's 34.7 percent c-section rate exceeded the nationwide average.[36]

Just as some obstetricians after World War II stuck to their original ethos and continued to avoid cesarean sections despite the availability of antibiotics and blood transfusions, more recently trained obstetricians had experienced residencies focusing in no small part on learning how to read fetal monitor strips. By 1976, when the first study of EFM appeared, half of all hospital births in the United States were electronically monitored. Even more significantly, all but one of the hospital-based obstetric residency programs in the country employed the technology. The newest generation of board-certified obstetricians was loath to abandon a tool that they had been taught was essential to their patients' wellbeing and their own success as physicians.[37]

The financial health of hospitals likewise ensured the technology's entrenchment. Childbirth is the most common reason for hospitalization in the United States, making maternity care vital to most hospitals' bottom line. And in the United States, where every component of medical care is customarily billed separately under the country's fee-for-service billing system, EFM became a singularly lucrative element of maternity care. Within a decade of its introduction in the late 1960s, payments received for EFM had become a mainstay of hospital budgets. The first 60 to 100 laboring women to use a machine paid its purchase cost. Afterward, the machine subsidized many other services—the perinatology staff, nurse specialists, research, and repair and maintenance workers. EFM also cut down on the need for costly personnel; as one Chicago obstetrician observed, the fetal stethoscope had required one-on-one patient care. "It is easier," he explained, "to buy 10 machines than pay 10 nurses." An obstetrician who completed her residency in 1977 added, "Institutions invested so much in the hardware that no matter what randomized trial came out showing the lack of benefit—and virtually all of them did . . . it was so engrained that we couldn't get rid of it." She characterized EFM as "a special type of tyranny. . . . You think it works, so you don't look for what will."[38]

Hospitals poured money into not only the machines but also infrastructure to accommodate the machines. Entire maternity wings were reconfigured so residents could observe many fetal heartbeats simultaneously. The resulting central monitoring stations, while convenient, altered residents' basic training. After her hospital consolidated its fetal monitor screens at the maternity floor nurses' station, one midwife complained: "They [obstetric residents] sit outside at the desk and watch the monitors. How do they ever learn about normal labor? . . . That's why I hate those monitors out at the desk, I just hate them." A resident at a large urban hospital in another state similarly described the "big conference room" where she and her cohorts gathered daily to watch "a bunch of computers and three big screens on the walls that can show you all the data for our patients, about 40 patients usually there at once." She explained that residents preferred those screens to the smaller ones at each patient's bedside because "it would be a little difficult to kind of see all the detail." But the resident also recognized the pitfall in the setup—"in a computerized age, we really feel like we don't spend enough time with the patient." But most felt helpless to do anything about it. "We just sort of throw up our hands," said another obstetrician.[39]

Over three decades, ACOG tried to address the changes in obstetric practice wrought by EFM. Initially, the organization's guidelines appeared to endorse the technology; subsequent guidelines were more cautionary. In an early advisory in 1975, ACOG recommended that internal placement of the monitor's measuring device "provides more precise data with less distortion than the external." In 1977, one year after the first randomized, controlled trial appeared in a medical journal, ACOG issued another bulletin advising, just as Hon originally recommended, that "at risk" patients be considered for monitoring, implying that monitoring not be universal. The advisory also described, for the first time, some deleterious side effects of internal monitoring—"fetal scalp infection at point of electrode entry," amnionitis, and uterine and/or placental perforation. In 1979, an *ACOG Committee Statement* described EFM as a "controversy" and warned that although it appeared to be useful in high-risk pregnancies, benefits had not been proven for low-risk patients. Indeed, in low-risk births, the organization advised, intermittent auscultation with a fetal stethoscope would suffice.[40]

Five years later, in a terse *Committee Statement* that seemed to signify ACOG's most profound doubt about the technology yet, the organization declared,

"Electronic fetal monitoring is highly sensitive but has low specificity." That is, the monitor strip was adept at indicating when a fetus was tolerating labor well (demonstrating high sensitivity) but did not do a good job of indicating when a fetus was compromised (exhibiting low specificity). The International Federation of Gynecologists and Obstetricians (FIGO) concurred, warning in 1987, "it cannot be emphasized enough that understanding and interpretation of a FHR record is not an easy matter." In 1989, another ACOG bulletin noted for the first time that a "significant increase" in the rate of abdominal deliveries had been reported in women electronically monitored on a randomized basis. Six years later, ACOG called the increase in cesareans the "primary risk" of EFM. The organization reiterated the problem in 2004: "increasing reliance on continuous electronic monitoring of fetal heart rate and uterine contraction patterns [has] led to an increase in the number of cesarean deliveries performed for *presumed* fetal compromise and dystocia, respectively [emphasis mine]," adding "with few exceptions, major improvement in newborn outcomes as a result of the increased cesarean delivery rate are yet to be proved." Nevertheless, in 2009, a record 85 percent of births in the United States were electronically monitored.[41]

In a bulletin released in 2010 and reaffirmed in 2015, ACOG's central message regarding EFM remained guarded. The organization (re)stated that the predictive value of an abnormal fetal heart tracing was poor and that the optimal time to effect delivery after such a tracing had never been established. "Honestly," said the obstetrician who supervised formulation of ACOG's 2010 EFM guidelines, "the technology rolled out [in the late 1960s] before we knew if it worked or not. Continuous monitoring became a standard obstetrical procedure before studies could show if the benefits outweighed the risks, and without clear-cut guidelines on how doctors should interpret findings."[42]

ACOG's reluctance to more directly and publicly confront the non-evidence-based use of the fetal monitor is perplexing. Perhaps ACOG officials, whose headquarters in Washington, DC, have round-the-clock guards with entrances locked to all except employees and invited guests, know better than anyone in the United States that changes in the policies and procedures affecting women's health and medicine generate firestorms. Abortion has created the most notable disputes, but lawsuits generated by passage of the Affordable Care Act demonstrated that even contraception remains fraught territory. ACOG officials are also likely aware of the negative public reaction to the attempt of the National Health Service in the United Kingdom to limit cesarean sections to medically necessary ones. Changing, or formulating, any policy affecting women's health and medicine requires the type of methodical, persistent public education that the ACOG might view as beyond its mission. Even changing their own members' use and perception of EFM would be a monumental task at this point. In looking back over his 40 years of practice, an obstetrician trained in the early 1970s could not think of any medical device that initiated a more drastic, and ultimately ingrained, transformation in the behavior and thinking of obstetricians than the fetal monitor. "It just changed the face of how we run labor and delivery units and how we practice obstetrics."[43]

The Toll of Technology on Laboring Mothers—and on Physicians

For women, electronic fetal monitoring exacerbated the physical travails of labor. Nurses placed the portion of the device attached to each patient either externally or internally. External monitoring required a pair of belts wrapped around the abdomen—one to measure uterine contractions, the other to measure the FHR. The belts not only confined women to bed throughout labor but also made a simple act, such as changing position, difficult. Internal monitoring, the method recommended by ACOG in its initial 1975 guidelines for EFM, was even more uncomfortable, necessitating rupture of the amniotic sac to place a pressure catheter in the uterus to measure contractions plus an electrode on the fetal scalp to measure the FHR. And during the first years of EFM use, another, even more uncomfortable procedure accompanied both the external and internal methods—doctors took blood samples from the fetal scalp to verify the meaning of monitor strips. One obstetrician described the process: "There was this cardboard cone . . . wider at the outlet and then narrower at the inlet, and you would put it into the woman's vagina . . . right up against the baby's skull and . . . make a little prick and then with the capillary action [blood] would come into this tube . . . then we would send that to respiratory and they would give us the baby's pH." Depending on the laboratory assessment, the obstetrician then either allowed labor to proceed or performed a cesarean.

Mothers who complained about EFM tended to focus their objections on immobility. "I had a belt around my abdomen to monitor my contractions and a monitor inserted into my vagina attached to my baby's head to monitor her heartbeat," protested one mother in the mid-1970s. "The belt kept slipping off and felt very uncomfortable. I felt like I couldn't move and was annoyed by that restriction." Another mother objected even more vociferously about her 1979 birth: "I was nearing the end of my rope. I couldn't get comfortable. I was in bed, strapped to that damn monitor, and lying almost completely flat on my back." Her

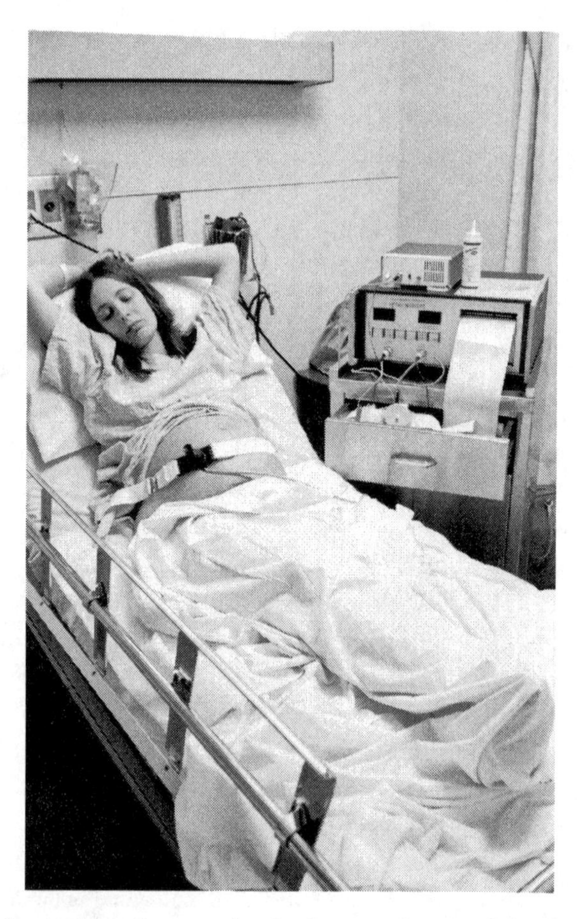

A woman in labor in the early 1970s, shortly after introduction of the electronic fetal monitor, attached externally to the monitor.
Photo courtesy of Sam Sweezy; © Sam Sweezy.

problems with the monitor increased as her labor progressed. "Every time I put the bed up someone would come in to check the monitor and crank it down again. I was becoming very vocal about my discomfort and I was told to 'shut up' quite a few times." Other mothers found the monitor reassuring, however. One woman who had been given epidural anesthesia explained, "It was nice to be able to know that everything was proceeding normally, since I couldn't feel what was happening." In a typical cascade effect, one medical technology had made a mother especially comfortable with, and grateful for, another.[44]

While a patient's right to refuse treatment is generally respected in American medicine, mothers' experiences with EFM demonstrated that laboring women fell into a unique category. One mother, who gave birth in Boston in 1979, attempted to decline fetal monitoring, "but the staff insisted I have this before I could use the birthing room." Because giving birth in the birthing room was of paramount importance to her, nurses' insistence that she consent to EFM as a condition for using the birthing room was tantamount to coercion. Compounding the unpleasantness, rather than the positive experience she had envisioned, the birthing room proved to be just as uncomfortable as the conventional labor room. She was still forced to labor on her back due to her attachment to the monitor. And her doctor performed an episiotomy, "even though I begged and pleaded not to have one." As another mother said of her hospital birth: "nobody even implied that I had a right to question or refuse these procedures."[45]

Electronically monitored mothers also received considerably less attention. An Indianapolis doctor observed: "we watch the monitor and not her. She dare not interrupt our silent vigil." One obstetrician contrasted that scenario with his residency in the late 1960s, before EFM. "I remember many a night I sat between two beds, with one hand on the right side and the other on the left side, on the bellies of two pregnant ladies, feeling for contractions and timing them." With the advent of EFM, however, that sort of hands-on doctoring became passé. "The fetal monitor . . . measure[d] contractions much better than you could by feel." Yet in acknowledging that gain, he also recognized the loss. "The patients feel something by you touching." Another obstetrician offered a similar observation: "The present day obstetrical resident is an electronic wizard. You go into a conference with them and nobody knows if the patient drinks or smokes or fights with her husband. But they know all about her A Scan and her B Scan. You get the feeling you're in a NASA conference."[46]

As EFM exacerbated many mothers' stress, the device placed physicians under considerable pressure as well. Reminiscing about the early days of the monitor, an obstetrician who started medical school in 1947 described how he first learned to monitor labor using a fetal stethoscope. "I would listen to the heart tones after contractions. And I may have done one, two that I can remember, cesarean sections because the heart tones went bad while I was listening." With the advent of EFM, however, he learned to respond quickly to the machine's ruling. "You see the abnormalities and you jump at it." Another obstetrician likewise recalled that the monitor "definitely" heightened his anxiety. "It made you realize that there were these wide variations that you did not expect to see, these decreases in heart rate that you don't pick up with a stethoscope. . . . As we started seeing these dips and things all over . . . it helped increase the section rate a lot."[47]

These sorts of reactions were soon apparent nationwide. "Every drop in the [fetal] heart rate precipitated a rush to the back to do a cesarean," one obstetrician remembered. "The rest is history." Obstetricians' interpretation of EFM messages—that far more fetuses than previously believed suffered hypoxia during labor—modulated physicians' previously negative attitudes toward cesareans.[48]

EFM, with its tangible fetal heart tracings as a byproduct, strengthened the understandable tendency of physicians to dwell on the infrequent bad outcome as opposed to the manifold good outcomes. One obstetrician explained, "I could have 10 deliveries which all have the same sort of fetal heart tracing in the last few minutes but one of them comes out with poor Apgars and goes to the NICU. That's going to be the one that I remember . . . not the other nine that did fine." And even if the baby in the NICU eventually did well, that would not matter either. "As the obstetrician, I'm seeing that baby be resuscitated in the delivery room, and I see that Mom be so scared. So that's what really emotionally sticks with you, and those are also the stories that you hear your colleagues getting sued for."[49]

Assembly Line Births during the Baby Boom

Physicians' embrace of, and reliance on, EFM beginning in the late 1960s was probably foreseeable. The regimented approach to birth that became popular after World War II helped pave the way for monitoring. Originally, obstetricians developed their rigid postwar protocols out of necessity, as a response to the baby boom, when women married younger and tended to give birth to several babies in quick succession. The pressure on obstetricians in the 1950s and 1960s, who almost always practiced without partners to share the workload, was, according to obstetrician Gene Lawrence, "terrible." Prescribed routine helped ease their arduous schedules.[50]

Lawrence, who practiced by himself for more than 40 years beginning in 1947, delivered an average of 40 babies a month through the 1960s. He explained that "to live some kind of life" he had to reliably "get rid of at least five or six pregnancies a week." He learned how that could be done during his residency at Chicago's behemoth Cook County Hospital where he "cleared out a labor line"—20 women, 10 on each side of a large room—"by just going along and giving each one a little stab [of Pitocin] . . . right under the skin, usually in any part—their hands, their butts, their thighs. . . . I would induce all these women into full labor and call a whole corps of interns down to deliver these kids. All of a sudden, seven births would take place at one time."[51]

After going into private practice—and as the father of two young children—Lawrence was even more pressed for time. To ensure both reliable office hours and family time on Sundays, he earmarked Wednesdays and Saturdays as his "delivery days." Although a patient occasionally defied the predetermined schedule by going into labor early, "basically you could get the bulk [of births] out of the way and not have to worry about never being home" or having to cancel other patients' prenatal and gynecologic appointments. This sort of regimentation was becoming common nationwide; in 1957, *McCall's* magazine denounced the "Tuesday-Thursday-and-Saturday obstetricians" who mostly attended planned births. Like those physicians, Lawrence's routine rarely varied. On delivery days, he performed gynecological surgeries in the early morning while nurses "prepped" his obstetric patients. "Then I would come from the operating room and would start them off with Pitocin. All of them." After administering "the pit," he "twilighted" mothers with "heavy doses of sedation," injections of scopolamine and Demerol throughout first-stage labor. As the first stage of labor ended, he gave the patient a dose of nalorphine to mitigate the inevitable respiratory distress about to be suffered by her newborn. "Because it was the scope," he explained, using the medical slang for scopolamine, "that really smothered the baby down." Afterward, in the delivery room, he administered either general or saddle-block anesthesia, greased the pelvic canal with an antiseptic, performed an episiotomy, and delivered the infant with forceps.[52]

Other long-retired obstetricians remembered a similar protocol: "when she was completely dilated and the head was well into the pelvis—engaged—then she would be put to sleep and prepped and draped and we used forceps and episiotomies were done." Later, when saddle-block anesthesia became more common than general anesthesia, the routine was the same: "when they got completely dilated, and the head was on the perineum, we would give them a saddle block, then deliver by forceps with an episiotomy."[53]

One woman was so traumatized by the rigid, invasive medical procedures common to births in the late 1950s that she postponed having a second baby for 15 years. Pregnant again at 39 in 1973, she wrote an angry letter posing assorted questions to a physician. Are women still subjected to "the degrading, humiliating pubic shaving ritual?" Does "every stranger, student, aide, nurse, or whoever is in sight exercise his ungodly right of finger exploration and other hand play?" Is "Demerol or Twilight Sleep" still in use, cutting off "all communication between patient and doctor" and ensuring "fears and hallucinations?" Were women still subjected to the "emotional torment of fighting to sit up while being told to lie flat but 'push down?'" Did doctors still enforce "the cruel strapping down and blackout at the moment of expectation for the questionable surgical procedure, episiotomy?" She did not mention the fetal monitor in her litany of complaints because it had not existed when she gave birth to her first child.[54]

Many women voiced similar unhappiness with postwar medical protocol. At the behest of the editors of the *Ladies' Home Journal* in 1958, women sent letters to the magazine describing their recent births. The result was an article published under the dramatic headline, "*Journal* Mothers Report on Cruelty in Maternity Wards." No respondent cast her experience in a favorable light. One woman described hospital birth as "a hell on earth." Another complained of "not [being] treated as . . . a human being." Still another characterized obstetric care as a series of "assembly line techniques." A mother from Georgia complained, "I was helpless and at their mercy." A Detroit mother, whose husband was a veterinarian, told *Journal* readers that her husband accorded animals greater respect during labor than obstetricians accorded their human patients.[55]

Increase in Cesareans Parallels Popularity of Birth Reform

In response to the mechanized approach to childbirth developed in the 1940s and '50s, a largely white, college-educated audience of pregnant or aspiring-to-be-pregnant women began purchasing books in the 1970s titled *Spiritual Midwifery* and *Immaculate Deception: A New Look at Women and Childbirth in America*. They attended childbirth education classes recommended by health reform activists. The classes, activists advised, would enable women "to resist the hospital routine of medication and interventions." Crusaders for reform characterized childbirth as a physiological event to be approached "matter-of-factly, instinctively, and without fear," "part of the natural order of things." Birth reform organizations burgeoned: Birth Day in Cambridge, Massachusetts, the International Childbirth Education Association headquartered in Seattle, the Midwives Alliance of North America, and the National Association of Parents & Professionals for Safe Alternatives in Childbirth were only a few.[56]

Inspired by second-wave feminism, this movement decrying the medical control of childbirth ironically coincided with the increase in cesarean sections. Indeed, the most precipitous increase in the surgery, between 1970 and 1985, paralleled a portion of the peak militancy, and greatest successes, of birth reformers. During this time, hospitals responded to women's complaints by offering homey "birthing rooms." After particularly bitter battles around the country, fathers, other family members, and friends were permitted to keep women company throughout labor and birth. Yet the c-section rate, unaffected by the militancy, kept rising—largely because the rapid increase was not initially on women's list of complaints. Even the 1976 second edition of the best-selling feminist health manifesto, *Our Bodies, Ourselves,* described the surgery as only "occasionally" performed "in the case of a very long, hard labor that seems to be accomplishing little." Although the cesarean rate had more than doubled (from 4.5 percent in 1965 to 11 percent in 1975) in the decade before release of the second edition of *Our Bodies, Ourselves,* the otherwise defiant Boston Women's Health Book Collective, the book's named author, commanded its readers, "If the doctor recommends a cesarean section, you must trust that judgment." Thus, even as birth reformers sought fewer medical interventions, and succeeded for a time to some degree, the rising cesarean rate prompted few objections.[57]

Only one grassroots organization focused on the burgeoning number of cesareans early on—Cesareans/Support, Education, and Concern (C/SEC) appeared in 1973. Other groups emerged only after the influence of birth reform organizations had begun to wane. The Cesarean Prevention Movement (later renamed the International Cesarean Awareness Network, or ICAN) appeared in 1982. Beginning in 2008, TheUnnecesarean.com provided a web forum for an unlimited number of mothers to voice their frustration over their unwanted surgeries. The website described itself as "pulling back the curtain on the unnecessary cesarean epidemic." Later, *The Unnecesarean* continued its educational activities on Facebook. In 2012, its founder, Jill Arnold, launched CesareanRates.com to educate the public about the wide variation in cesarean section rates among hospitals and to demonstrate how poor the obstetric data collecting and reporting was at the time. The organization's statistics have proven to be so unflinchingly helpful and accurate that in 2013 *Consumer Reports* licensed the data and in 2014 added a new criteria—cesarean section rates—to their ratings of hospitals.[58]

Arnold launched the original *Unnecesarean* site in reaction to her first pregnancy. When she was almost 38 weeks pregnant in 2005, her midwife suspected fetal macrosomia and advised that she give birth by c-section. Knowing that all the babies in her family had been born vaginally, despite their large size, but not wanting to put her baby at risk, Arnold began to "frantically" search the Internet for information to help her make a sound decision. Ultimately, she refused the planned cesarean. After going into labor spontaneously and arriving at the hospital, she

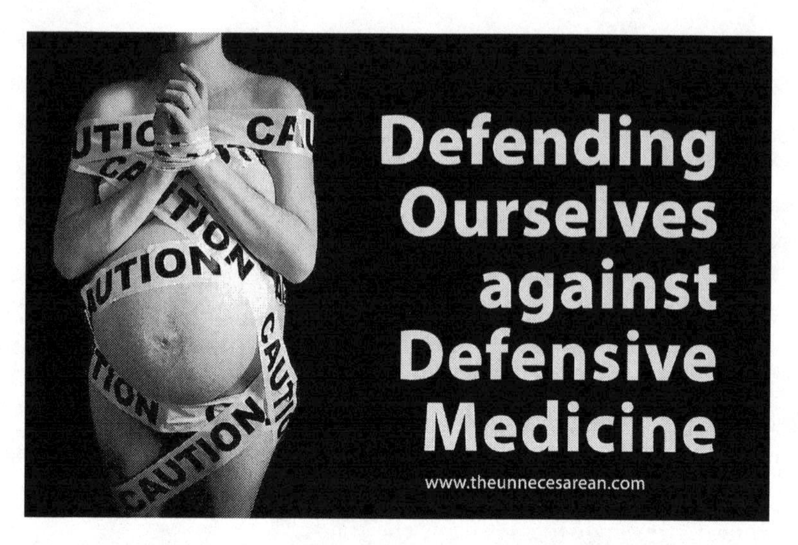

The Unnecesarean began as an online "maternity care digest" in 2008. The woman who posed for this photograph described in an e-mail exchange with the author the events that inspired the photograph: "I was pregnant very quickly after an incredibly traumatic, forced cesarean and the subsequent death of my child and felt that I had nowhere to go for support. Every care provider saw me as a walking bomb, and I felt I had no options but to either submit to a repeat cesarean I would not need, or give birth alone. The photo was part of a personal project I did to express that. . . . Both that pregnancy and the one after were successful VBACs." She offered the photo to *The Unnecesarean;* the website used it for a number of years as part of its crusade against defensive medicine.
Photo courtesy of Heather Armstrong, Amber Smith, and *The Unnecesarean* Maternity Care Digest, © Heather Armstrong and Amber Smith.

again refused the offer of a cesarean, ultimately giving birth vaginally to a healthy baby weighing 10 pounds. In 2007, she gave birth vaginally to her 11-pound second baby at a free-standing birth center.[59]

C/SEC, ICAN, and the assorted incarnations of *The Unnecesarean* provided information to women who hoped to avoid cesareans, proved cathartic for the women who were unable to escape the surgery, and offered a soapbox to mothers wanting to share their stories, many of whom condemned their surgeries as medically unnecessary. The foreword to the 1984 third edition of C/SEC's *Frankly Speaking: A Book for Cesarean Couples* was reminiscent of 1970s pro-birth-reform militancy: "C/SEC . . . believes that the increase in the number of cesareans being performed is nothing less than shocking and should be carefully studied to determine whether these burgeoning statistics represent a great leap ahead for medical science or a prime example of medical interference."[60]

Anti-cesarean activists even took to the airwaves. On January 20, 1988, the TV talk show *Geraldo* hosted members of the National Women's Health Network discussing cesarean prevention. After the show, pregnant women wrote to the organization requesting more information. "I am very concerned about how I will have my baby," wrote one mother. "I do not want Caesarian or Epidural, I want to have my baby normal without medication, if possible. I want to know how to prevent myself having a Caesarian Birth." A Michigan mother wrote, "If you have information on C-section & Natural Childbirth, please send both. I had one unnecessary C-section and hope to have my 2nd child natural." An Ohio woman was especially miffed after being told she might have to have a cesarean, "Please forward me the booklet shown on Geraldo's show . . . . I'm 8 months pregnant on second baby. They are now telling me that I might have to have a C-section. After delivering a 10 lbs 7½ baby vaginally the last time. Starving for more info, Thank you." Unfortunately, by the 1980s, when most of the anti-cesarean organizations appeared in response to the burgeoning cesarean rate, birth reformers were not getting the focused publicity they once had enjoyed. With fathers a routine presence in delivery rooms and "birth centers" appearing in urban areas, birth reform organizations seemed to have won the battle and any ongoing demands became less newsworthy. Despite some bursts of publicity, afforded by events like the *Geraldo* show, anti-cesarean voices went largely unheard in this environment.[61]

Yet the activists who did focus on lowering the cesarean rate connected the increase in cesareans with the rigid protocols, many still ongoing, that the original birth reform activists had objected to. One woman who opted for a vaginal birth at home after a previous cesarean wrote of her second birth, "There were no strangers, no IV's, no drugs, no monitors, no uncomfortable surroundings, no fear, no threats, no lies. Just a peaceful, caring atmosphere and a baby being born as nature intended." These mothers condemned both of the procedures that required cutting into women's flesh—cesarean section and episiotomy. A Michigan midwife, well known on the national birth reform scene, charged in 1984 that fewer than 8 percent of women giving birth in the United States managed to "avoid being cut in some way." She employed a male obstetrician's own words to condemn what feminists charged was the wanton mutilation of women. The physician had tried to justify the increasing number of cesareans, and the near-universal use of episiotomy, by explaining, "The vagina is not made for having babies anymore than the penis is." Anti-cesarean activists brandished the doctor's statement without editorializing.[62]

Ultimately, the changes wrought by the birth reform movement proved to be more cosmetic than systemic. Some nomenclature changed. Maternity "wards" became maternity "floors" or "wings," as part of the attempt to alter (cynics said "mask") the impersonal, routinized nature of maternity care. Women were permitted the company of their choice throughout labor, even in surgical suites during cesarean sections. Homey labor/delivery/recovery rooms hid medical equipment from view and ensured that women would no longer be trundled from a labor room to a brightly lit delivery room as they entered the second stage of labor. Nevertheless, without the counterweight of a vigorous, organized, nationwide birth reform movement, a movement that had largely disappeared by the mid-1980s, the cesarean section rate continued to rise largely unchecked.

In their quest for safer births, with better outcomes for women and children, both concerned mothers and their obstetricians sought to control birth—but in oppositional forms. Many women in the 1970s and 1980s, believing that medical interventions during birth were often unnecessary and dangerous, wanted fewer interventions and the right, which all other American patients customarily enjoyed, to refuse treatments and diagnostic tools as they saw fit. In contrast, most physicians believed medical treatments and diagnostics were means to safer births. Thus, while women were seeking control through "natural" births, obstetricians sought control in the form of more treatments and technologies, particularly use of the electronic fetal monitor, leading to more cesarean sections. The assertions of control by women and the assertions of control by doctors were at cross purposes. That is how and why, during the birth reform movement's peak of influence, the country was also seeing its steepest rise in the cesarean rate and the introduction and widespread acceptance of the fetal monitor. Hospitals were physicians' purview, not patients'.

Obstetricians Divided

Obstetricians did not hold a monolithic opinion during the era of birth reform any more than women did, however. Like the operator-nonoperator split half a century earlier, physicians' stances and their affinity for postwar birth protocols varied. A minority was sympathetic to the work of birth reformers. In Chicago, one obstetrician even filed a lawsuit on behalf of his patients who wanted fathers in delivery rooms, to the consternation of his colleagues. "I was totally opposed to the doctors that started it [the lawsuit]," recalled another Chicago physician. "And I knew them very well. I thought they were nuts!" And although most obstetricians vigorously opposed home birth, by the 1960s a few defended it. One even attempted to provide a balanced view: "I came up with a book of horrendioma on home birth . . . but if I'd been assigned the other side, I could have called hospitals and come up with horrendioma that would make us look sick."[63]

The cesarean section rate was another source of disagreement among obstetricians. Like many of his colleagues, Mortimer Rosen, director of obstetrics and gynecology at Columbia-Presbyterian Medical Center in New York City, deemed the rise in cesareans beneficial at first. A higher percentage of healthier babies was being born each year, and he assumed that the increase in cesarean births was one reason. By the late 1970s, however, as the cesarean section rate continued to soar, and infant morbidity and mortality leveled off, Rosen became one of the most vocal critics of the increase, arguing publicly that the cesarean section rate, then 16 percent, could not be justified medically. That a cesarean guaranteed a good outcome, he wrote in 1989, "was—is—nonsense." Roberto Caldeyro-Barcia, president-elect of the International Federation of Gynecologists and Obstetricians, agreed. *Good Housekeeping* magazine quoted him as saying, "many artificial practices have been introduced which have changed labor from a physiological event to a very complicated medical procedure in which unnecessary drugs and maneuvers are used, many of which are potentially damaging for the baby and for the mother."[64]

Yet despite their leadership positions, Rosen and Caldeyro-Barcia did not represent most obstetricians, who were affronted by birth reformers. Unaccustomed to being challenged, one obstetrician said of those days: "I would listen to them [women inspired by birth reform] but the 'birth plan' [presented by many pregnant patients seeking natural childbirth] would drive me crazy. And it was always third person singular. 'Dr. [X] is going to do this, Helen Jones is going to do this, John Jones is going to do this.' Not, 'I'm going to do this.'" On occasion, he would become annoyed enough to interrupt them. "I would take the fetoscope . . . put it on their abdomen and I said, 'You know I can hear your baby! Your baby is telling me don't listen to my mother! She doesn't know anything!'" Another obstetrician similarly recalled, "I would say most doctors were opposed to it [birth reformers' demands for fewer medical interventions], including me. I be the doctor. You be the patient. . . . We discouraged natural child birth." The chief of obstetrics at New York Hospital–Cornell Medical Center similarly decried any move away from medical intervention. "Babies die from natural childbirth," he warned.[65]

During his presidential address in 1979, the newly elected president of ACOG decried the "pressure cooker environment" he and his colleagues toiled in—"under siege from consumerists, environmentalists, women's liberationists, civil rightists and other special interest activists yet to be organized." By way of a satiric list, he singled out the desires of birth reform activists for special ridicule: "childbirth without fear, rooming in, husband in labor and delivery rooms, menu selection, free television, showers and bathtubs, improved admission procedures, no anesthesia or drugs, ad lib visiting hours, and ample parking." He urged his colleagues to "take the offensive against the faddists who would supplant proven excellence within the medical profession with popular mediocrity." He characterized "the trip through the birth canal" as "the most dangerous trip we ever take with the greatest chance of our dying of any one day in our lives." In a presidential address in 1983, another ACOG president charged that natural births harmed women: "Some of us are old enough to remember countless hours in the gynecologic operating rooms performing reconstructive vaginoplasties for these young women's grandmothers, who had pushed out their own babies naturally and laboriously many years before."[66]

An exchange sparked in the late 1980s by retired obstetrician/gynecologist Clayton T. Beecham typified the occasionally bitter disagreements among obstetricians about birth reform. In a commentary written for the journal *The Female Patient*, Beecham characterized natural childbirth as "a step backward," labeled feminists' calls for a less technocratic approach to birth "a short-sighted exploitation of nature," and associated birth reform with "maternal death, infant death, and maternal tissue destruction." He lauded cesarean sections, describing the surgery as "the ultimate in pelvic and birth-canal protection." A female physician countered: "Only a man who will never experience childbirth or a cesarean delivery could advocate major surgery to prevent the 'loss of vaginal sensation.' Perhaps he should experience 'a deep episiotomy' before he extolls its merits." Other obstetricians defended Beecham in equally forceful terms, expressing gratitude to the "quality leaders" in obstetrics, like Beecham, "who have their heads on right and have risen above the bilge and backwash going on in obstetrics today." These physicians offered what seemed to them to be the tangible benefits of EFM as de facto proof of the folly of birth reform.[67]

Given the widespread support for EFM in the medical community, obstetricians easily convinced most patients to use the electronic fetal monitor. While birth reformers persuaded many women in the 1970s to reject analgesics, anesthetics, and episiotomy as dangerous and unnecessary treatments, EFM seemed to be different. An article in *Newsweek* lauded the ability of the fetal monitor to "catch the first signs of any troubles."[68]

Doctors pointed to EFM as having revealed labor's manifold risks to the fetus and as proof that birth reformers' demands were irresponsible. "It is now widely accepted," wrote two obstetricians in 1975, just as the birth reform movement was reaching influential heights, "that uterine contractions are repetitive stresses to the fetus . . . labor and delivery are a hazardous time associated with a high degree of fetal risk." Faith in EFM was running so high in the medical community that few physicians had any patience for the women who objected to the physical discomforts of the machinery. One obstetrician suggested, "Our task is to help these patients recognize that they are introducing their own hedonism into a 12-hour event that may affect the 70–80 years of life of the infants they bear."[69]

Because of what ubiquitous monitoring implied—that labor posed omnipresent risk to fetuses—the device proved to be one of the most effective bulwarks against birth reform. In becoming the norm, electronic monitoring thwarted one of the main demands of reformers—intervention-free birth as the default. Instead, the monitor became a constant presence that often led to cesarean section.[70]

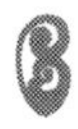

The electronic fetal monitor inadvertently served as an effective counterforce to birth reform. While the white, college-educated women who drove the narrative of birth reform had called for mothers to be given the option of remaining mobile during labor, monitors ensured that women would be relegated to their hospital beds. Even as activists called for less reliance on technology and more faith in women's bodies, EFM intimated that a mother's body threatened the fetus she carried. Although reformers called for a more humane approach to birth, the monitor became the focus of attention during labor rather than the laboring woman. The time obstetric residents once spent sitting by women's bedsides to comfort them, observe them, and learn from them was now spent watching machines housed far from patients' rooms. EFM created, in the words of one obstetrician, "more anxiety about bad things that could happen," intensifying the mechanical approach to labor "across the board." The appearance of the electronic fetal monitor, despite the visible birth reform movement, provided "a default invasiveness," ensuring that the average American birth experience would be more akin to an intensive care unit, rather than the homelike, supportive atmosphere that so many women in the 1970s said they wanted. The widespread acceptance of EFM ensured that obstetrics would remain mired in the very culture birth reformers wished to eradicate.[71] Consequently, wholesale public backlash against the normalization of cesarean section never materialized. The diagnostic tools and technologies introduced in obstetrics throughout the second half of the twentieth century—the Apgar score, the Friedman curve, the Bishop score, ultrasound, and finally the electronic fetal monitor—alongside some frightening news about pregnancy and childbirth, shaped public attitudes, creating the conditions for the normalization of surgical birth. Soon, malpractice costs and threats, the complexities of medical financing in the United States, further changes in the training of obstetric residents, and the growing number of female obstetricians would conspire alongside EFM to create an impenetrable wall around the culture of risk that obstetricians found themselves working in.

Chapter Six

Operating in a Culture of Risk

A Fraught Environment for Obstetricians

Twenty years after the introduction of the electronic fetal monitor, the influence of the birth reform movement had waned. Fallout from the movement nonetheless persisted; well into the 1980s, obstetricians complained of working in a fraught environment. Expected to accede to the contradictory demands of individual patients, consumer groups, insurance companies, the legal system, federal agencies, and their own professional organizations, they also were forced to contend with the risk culture created, in part, by the electronic fetal monitor.[1]

Thomas Sartwelle, an American trial lawyer specializing in birth injury, blames the monitor for what he terms a "phenomenon previously unseen in medicine's long history . . . defensive medicine." He contends that the seemingly irrefutable record of fetal distress provided by monitor strips was responsible for the excessive damage awards issued by juries beginning in the mid-1980s. The judgments, he writes, "not only substantially altered medical practice but medical ethics as well. Physicians' response to the rising claims was abandonment of the venerable 'first do no harm' principle, replacing it with the expedient self-serving ethics of 'do whatever is necessary to keep trial lawyers at bay.' "[2]

Although Sartwelle defines the rising number of cesareans as "harm," most physicians have not. An array of forces had converged by the mid-1980s to create a medical culture focused on the alleviation of risk during birth, however slight that risk might be. The forces included reluctance to sanction vaginal births after a previous cesarean (VBACs), a series of medical malpractice crisis points, the weaknesses of American healthcare financing, changes in the training of obstetric residents, and the counterintuitive effect of the dramatic increase in female obstetricians. In the cloistered world of obstetrics, these influences transformed doctors' perception of, and behaviors surrounding, cesarean section and vaginal birth. As a result, a medical procedure that was once dreaded and rare would become, by the early twenty-first century, the most frequently performed surgery in the United States.[3]

The Federal Government Weighs In

Initially, the public health community expressed the gravest discomfort with the spike in cesareans. The National Institutes of Health (NIH) called the rising rate "a matter of concern," while the Department of Health, Education, and Welfare (HEW) called for "controlled clinical trials" to assess the efficacy and safety of cesarean versus vaginal birth. The concern was significant enough that both federal agencies, the HEW in 1979 and the NIH in 1981, issued reports examining the causes of the increase in cesareans and providing suggestions to alleviate the rise.[4]

Between 1968, when the National Center for Health Statistics first began gathering data on cesareans, and 1977, the nation's cesarean rate rose 156 percent, even as the birth rate declined 12 percent. The HEW report noted that the increase did not appear to benefit either individuals or the healthcare system—cesarean sections saw a complication rate of at least 33 percent and a financial cost three times that of vaginal birth. As part of her data-gathering, Helen Marieskind, author of the HEW study, interviewed 100 obstetricians, granting interviews only to physicians willing to provide comprehensive data about their practices and patients. Noting that representatives from assorted interest groups were "pretty hot under the collar" about the cesarean rate, Marieskind sought facts, not anecdotal evidence or emotional claims. She devoted the bulk of the HEW report to a systematic examination of the factors contributing to the rise. While most physicians she interviewed cited their fear of a lawsuit as the reason for their growing propensity to perform a cesarean, she could find little basis for their claim. Only a tiny minority of the doctors she interviewed had been sued or knew anyone who had been sued. She found instead that more significant contributors to the increase were American physicians' unwillingness to allow vaginal births after a previous cesarean, changes in the training of obstetric residents, the unsubstantiated conviction that cesarean section saw outcomes that were superior to vaginal birth, a willingness to accept vague justifications for cesareans, and a declining fertility rate that amplified the notion "every baby counts." She also noted that obstetricians had begun to look to cesarean section as a solution for every problem they encountered during labor, even as they dismissed the notions that vaginal birth benefited neonates and posed fewer risks to mothers. She reported that obstetricians repeatedly asked her during interviews, "What's so great about delivering from below, anyway?"[5]

The year that HEW issued its findings, the Comptroller General's office sent a report to the US Congress describing the consequences for the nation of contemporary obstetric practices. While the Comptroller General's office was unable to draw any specific conclusions about the effects of a high cesarean rate—too few studies on the subject had been conducted—the report's authors urged the government to do "more to help resolve the controversy over OB practices." The American College of Obstetricians and Gynecologists (ACOG) responded on behalf of its members, insisting that the government should not be in the business of telling physicians how to practice medicine.[6]

Two years later, the NIH issued a report akin to the HEW's, concluding that there was no relationship between the increase in cesarean sections and recent improvements in maternal and neonatal outcomes. To the contrary, the report argued, if the surge in cesareans ebbed, maternal and neonatal outcomes would continue to improve. Authors of the report cited a host of contributors to the burgeoning cesarean rate that had nothing to do with medical need—the ease of cesarean surgery versus the challenge of forceps; the new concept of "defensive medicine"; the longtime tenet, "once a cesarean, always a cesarean," now unwarranted thanks to the low transverse cut; assorted financial incentives; and the effects of electronic fetal monitoring (EFM). The NIH advised that obstetricians address dystocia—the number-one reason doctors gave for performing a cesarean in the 1970s—with benign treatments such as hydration, ambulation, and rest rather than a cesarean section.[7]

By the early 1980s, on the heels of the government reports, grassroots organizations calling for fewer cesarean births were increasingly visible and vocal. The Cesarean Prevention Movement vividly described women's assorted reactions to their surgeries. The "Cesarean Patient" was tired, in pain, and foggy from Demerol. The "Cesarean Mourner" had never made peace with not having a vaginal birth. The "Cesarean Victim" suspected her surgery had been unnecessary. The "Cesarean Learner" was now empowered to seek a vaginal birth the next time around. The "Cesarean Surrender" had given up the fight. The "Cesarean Gratitude" was thankful for the surgery that had saved her and her baby. The "Cesarean

Activist" was determined that no woman ever have unnecessary surgery again. The "Cesarean Phoenix" rose "victorious from bitter ashes! . . . extend[ing] the same welcoming acceptance to the spectrum of birth feelings expressed by other women . . . return[ing] to the supportive sources which first offered help to us." In short, obstetricians had good reason to feel pressured—criticism came from not only the US government but daily interactions with patients, from which there was no escape.[8]

Pedaling and Backpedaling on Vaginal Birth after Cesarean

Both the HEW and the NIH had cited, as one of many reasons for the rising cesarean rate, the unwillingness of American obstetricians to attend a vaginal birth after a woman had given birth previously by cesarean. In Europe, obstetricians had been overseeing VBACs for more than 70 years, ever since a German obstetrician developed the low cervical cesarean incision in 1907. That cut, made at the bottom of the uterus in a horizontal line, created stronger scar tissue than the classic cut preferred by American physicians. Yet the classic cut, a vertical line beginning at the umbilicus and ending at the bottom of the uterus that produced a scar prone to rupture in subsequent labors, was the very technique that prompted Edwin Cragin to issue his dire "once a cesarean, always a cesarean" admonition. Nevertheless, even as VBACs became common in Europe, American obstetric textbooks continued to describe the "classical cesarean section" as preferable, dismissing the European innovation as "slightly more difficult" to perform.[9]

VBACs thus remained unthinkable in the United States. Obstetricians were so wedded to Cragin's dictum that a physician who began medical school in 1960 recalled a woman who entered the hospital with her cervix fully dilated and her baby's head crowning. A trouble-free birth appeared imminent. But her first birth had been by cesarean. So "obstetricians in the back came in and performed a[nother] cesarean." He characterized the state of mind that prompted the woman's unnecessary second surgery as unbendingly, "Once a cesarean, always a cesarean, by God!" Even in the early 1980s, as the low transverse cesarean became more common in the United States, a previous cesarean remained a contraindication to vaginal birth.[10]

Determined, edified patients eventually pushed American physicians to perform VBACs. Nancy Wainer Cohen, coauthor of the 1983 book *Silent Knife: Cesarean Prevention and Vaginal Birth After Cesarean (VBAC)*, was one of the earliest leaders of the VBAC movement. When Cohen was pregnant in 1974 with her second child after giving birth to her first by cesarean, she and her husband searched for

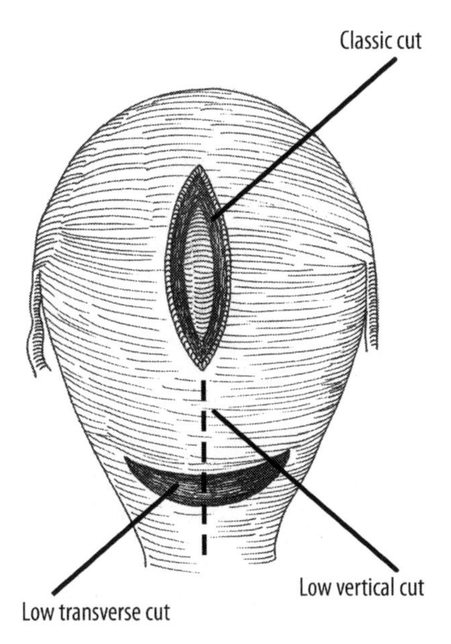

The two types of cesarean section incisions: classic and low transverse. The scar resulting from the classic incision is prone to rupture; the scar resulting from the low transverse incision is stronger and, today, is performed almost exclusively.
Illustration by Maryam Khaleghi Yazdi, adapted from Hacker and Moore, *Essentials of Obstetrics and Gynecology*, 355.

a doctor who would allow her to give birth vaginally. The physicians they consulted, however, described the request as "outrageous, irresponsible, unthinkable!" The Cohens remained resolute, however, and, ultimately, Cohen had a vaginal birth, although not exactly in the manner she had envisioned. "Lots of medical and technical interference (which we felt helpless to refuse)" undermined her triumph. When she was pregnant with her third child, she eschewed hospitals and obstetricians altogether in favor of a home birth attended by midwives.[11]

Cohen began to conduct "VBAC Workshops" for interested mothers and received hundreds of appreciative notes from her students after their VBACs. Many of those women, like Cohen embittered by their experience in the hospital, opted for home births. "A VBAC at home!" one mother wrote in 1984. A 1985 birth announcement read, "After a previous c-section for CPD [cephalo-pelvic disproportion] & a Hospital VBAC, our Home [double underscored] is where she made her first appearance. . . . And Daddy was there to 'catch' her!" Another mother who had a home birth in 1985 celebrated the event and its aftermath while simultaneously ridiculing pelvimetry: "Midwives did wonderful peri massage and hot compress to help me not to tear too much. I have notified the Dr. who turned me down for homebirth backup that my 9 cm diagonal conjugate pelvis—his opinion—had a 9 lb baby with a 14 inch head." Mothers who had their VBACs in the hospital felt equally empowered by Cohen's training and encouragement: "Without the proper education it would have been difficult to have a VBAC delivery. We're still on a high and we have the most wonderful memories of [our daughter's] birth. You do wonderful work and we hope you'll continue to educate the public." Years before "VBAC" became a well-recognized acronym, Cohen spread word that she was willing to speak anywhere in the country on "Vaginal Births Following Cesareans" as well as "Preventing Emotional Sequellae of Cesarean Childbirth."[12]

Before Cohen began her crusade, women seeking VBACs had difficulty finding any assistance, even from cesarean support groups. "The people I've talked to have left me feeling I should just resign myself to future cesareans, that a vaginal delivery is a nice idea, but not a very likely reality," wrote one disillusioned mother who had sought help from such a group. She described her first birth bitterly: "The magic lump in my tummy was suddenly a disease that must be cured at all cost and with great speed, and my baby was an incidental by-product, like a tooth handed back after it's been pulled for causing a toothache." She was determined to avoid a similar experience at her next birth. Another mother wrote of her quest for a VBAC, "The doctors and general public in this area have been brainwashed. . . . They all say it is dangerous to allow a trial labor!" Another mother noted, "I am your basic 'Once a cesarean—*don't want* to always be a cesarean.' "[13]

As more American women who had given birth by cesarean surgery sought vaginal births, American obstetricians learned what their European counterparts had long observed—that the low transverse cut had advantages over the classic cut that included less blood loss, easier repair, fewer surgical adhesions, and, key to VBAC safety, significantly diminished risk of uterine rupture in subsequent labors. Yet even as the low transverse cut became the routine in the United States, a series of contradictory recommendations issued by the ACOG ensured that medical enthusiasm for VBACs would be erratic. Initially, the ACOG advisories lauded VBACs, and the VBAC rate increased from 3 percent of all post-cesarean births in 1980 to 27.5 percent in 1995. Then, the organization issued a series of caveats about the procedure, and the VBAC rate plummeted.[14]

ACOG's first VBAC guideline, issued in 1982 as the cesarean rate approached 20 percent, advised that uterine rupture after a cesarean was "rarely catastrophic," thanks to a number of innovations: the low transverse cut, the fetal monitor, 24-hour blood banks, and an "immediately available" physician capable of performing a cesarean in an emergency. Six years later, after the cesarean rate reached 24 percent, another ACOG pronouncement was even more encouraging—data indicated that the maternal and perinatal death rates after a VBAC were lower than after a repeat cesarean. ACOG suggested that obstetricians "counsel and encourage" mothers to attempt VBACs—provided the hospital where they planned to give birth had the resources to perform an emergency cesarean within 30 minutes.[15]

That advisory had tangible effects. For the first time since the cesarean section rate had begun its precipitous increase in the late 1960s, the rate decreased. Enthusiasm for VBACs among doctors became so common that an obstetrician who began her residency in 1991 recalled, "we were very pro-VBAC. . . . In fact, even people who didn't want to VBAC were not allowed to schedule a cesarean. They had to wait until they were in labor and then come in. . . . It was thought to be the best way to go." The policy did not always work out well. "We had . . . a term," she recalled, " 'the reluctant VBAC' . . . and it was horrible."[16]

Another ACOG statement in 1994 inspired doctors to press women even more vigorously to have VBACs. Not only were mothers still to be counseled and encouraged to undergo a trial of labor, now an obstetrician simply had to be "readily" (rather than "immediately") available to perform a cesarean in an emergency. And the 30-minute constraint had vanished. A member of the ACOG committee that authored the guideline explained the reasoning behind the rewording. "Whenever you lay a time down—30 minutes," you invariably encounter trouble. If a physician arrived to perform an emergency cesarean "in 32 minutes [and then something untoward occurred] . . . you can't defend it. So, I remember we specifically wrote 'a reasonable period of time' " in lieu of a specific amount of time. In 1995, the ACOG championed VBACs with its strongest wording yet: repeat cesareans should not be performed routinely, only for specific indications. Between 1988 and 1997 the cesarean rate declined 20 percent.[17]

ACOG began backpedaling on its pro-VBAC stance in 1998. In yet another recommendation, American obstetricians' premiere professional organization noted that most studies of VBAC safety had been conducted at either university hospitals or tertiary care centers; outcomes at community hospitals were not well documented. Although the ACOG still recommended that "most women" be offered a trial of labor after one previous cesarean, the organization now advised "global mandates for a trial of labor . . . are inappropriate." The following year, in response to a study highlighting the "small but significant" chance of uterine rupture during labor after a previous cesarean, even after use of the low transverse

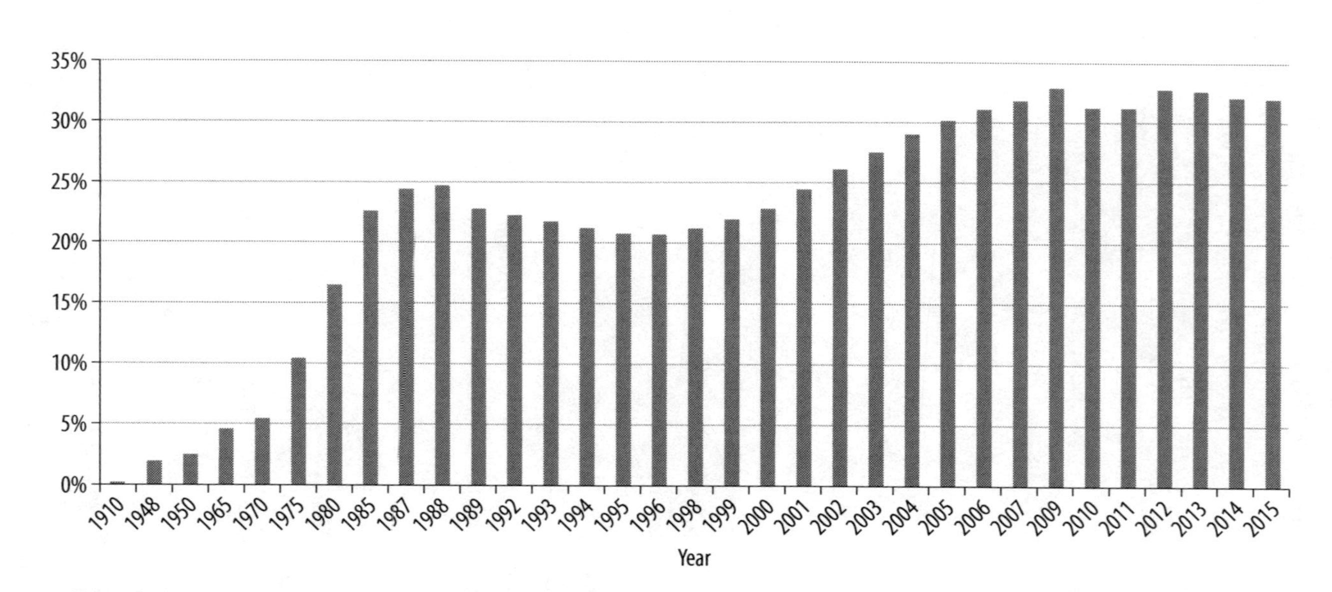

Effect of VBAC rate on cesarean rate. The changing guidelines for VBAC issued by the American College of Obstetricians and Gynecologists between 1988 and 2004 affected the cesarean rate. In 1988, when ACOG first suggested that obstetricians "counsel and encourage" mothers to have VBACs, the cesarean rate began to decrease as the VBAC rate increased. When the organization began to backpedal on that advice in 1999, the cesarean rate started to go back up and continued to increase as the VBAC rate eventually returned to mid-1980s levels.

cut, and an increase in lawsuits against obstetricians as a result, a single word change in yet another ACOG bulletin reversed the progress toward normalizing VBACs. Rather than be "readily" available to perform a cesarean, ACOG recommended that a physician be "immediately" available when mothers attempted a VBAC—"because uterine rupture may be catastrophic." The single word change conveyed two messages: cesareans were safer than VBACs, and VBACs posed imminent danger no matter the surgical technique used previously.[18]

When a physician's professional association issues a professional standard, doctors who do not adhere to it do so at their own peril—not observing the guideline increases their liability in the event of an adverse outcome. ACOG's 1999 ruling consequently prompted rural and small urban hospitals to severely limit or outright forbid VBACs. The organization reiterated its immediately available (as opposed to readily available) position in 2004. The VBAC rate plummeted to 8.5 percent in 2006 after reaching a high of 28 percent in 1996. By 2009, the overall cesarean rate in the United States was nearing 33 percent.[19]

The American Academy of Family Physicians (AAFP), unhappy with ACOG's 1999 and 2004 positions, issued their own guidelines in 2005, "since there is no evidence that these additional resources [obstetricians immediately available to perform a cesarean] result in improved outcomes." The NIH eventually sided with the AAFP, calling for a collaborative effort between the ACOG and the American Society of Anesthesiologists to alleviate "or even eliminate" barriers to VBACs. ACOG nevertheless remained steadfast, reiterating in 2010 that "a trial of labor after a previous cesarean delivery should be undertaken [only] at facilities capable of emergency deliveries . . . with staff immediately available to provide emergency care."[20]

The NIH position did nudge the ACOG to more fully explain their position, however. Later in 2010, the organization issued a glossy brochure clarifying that the years of assorted guidelines had been intended only to assure the safest possible births, "not to restrict women's access to VBAC." Some physicians considered the organization's explicit support of the universal availability of VBACs long overdue. As one maternal-fetal medicine specialist at Ohio State University Medical Center observed, "How can a hospital say it can handle an emergency c-section due to fetal distress," as all hospitals with maternity floors must, "yet not be able to do a VBAC?" If a hospital was not equipped to oversee a VBAC, he implied, that hospital should not be delivering babies at all.[21]

Despite ACOG's attempt to backpedal its backpedaling, the VBAC rate in the United States did not recover. More than three decades of equivocations had

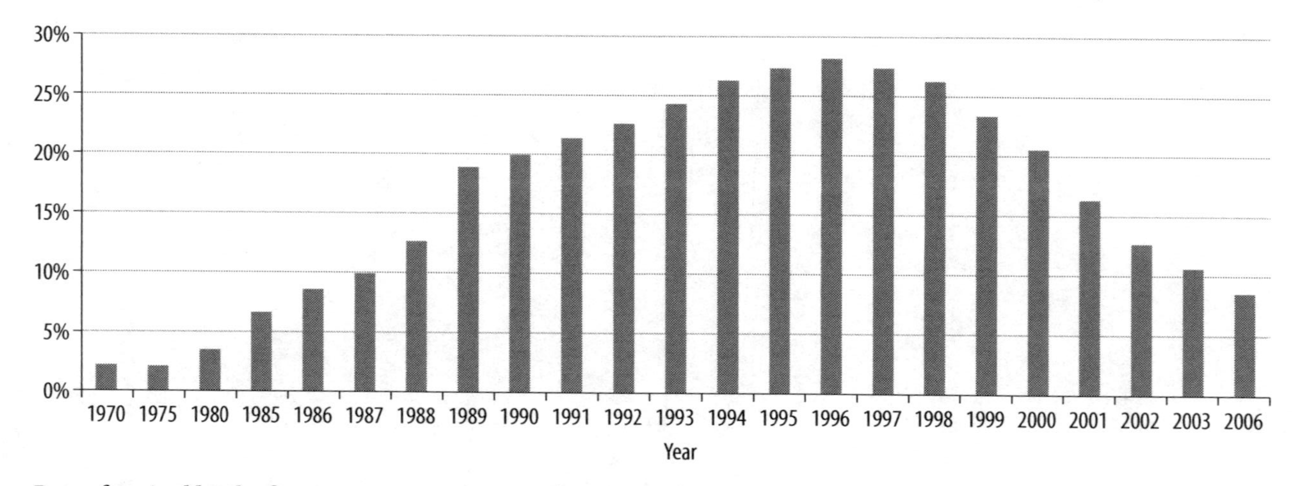

Rate of vaginal birth after cesarean, 1970–2006. The VBAC rate in the United States has risen and fallen over the years, depending on the latest ACOG guidelines. Although ACOG stated in 2010 that the years of assorted guidelines were intended only to assure the safest possible births, "not to restrict women's access to VBAC," the VBAC rate has not recovered since 1999, when ACOG first recommended that obstetricians be "immediately," rather than "readily," available to perform a cesarean when a woman is laboring with a cesarean scar on her uterus. At least one obstetrician has suggested that the recommendation made no sense: if a hospital was not capable of performing an emergency cesarean whenever necessary, the hospital should not be allowing births of any type.

Sources: American College of Obstetricians and Gynecologists Resource Center, 2004: NVSR 54(8), table E; 2003: NVSR 54(2), table 39; 2002: NVSR 52(10), table 39; 2001: NVSR 51(2), table 39; 2000: NVSR 50(5), table 39; 1999: NVSR 49(1), table 39; 1998: NVSR 48(3), table 39; 1997: NVSR 47(18), table 39; 1996 MVSR 46(11 Supp), table 39; 1995: MVSR 45(11 Supp), table 39; 1970–1985: MMWR 42(15), table 1; Osterman and Martin, "Trends in Low-Risk Cesarean Delivery"; "Decline in Rate of Vaginal Birth after Cesarean Tied to Restrictive Policies."

reinvigorated American obstetricians' qualms about the procedure. One obstetrician, who graduated from medical school in 1988, when VBACs were being "encouraged," described the change in attitude she had witnessed during her career. When she was a resident, she and her cohorts had grown quite comfortable with VBACs. In contrast, the residents she supervised in 2006 exhibited palpable anxiety during the procedure. They hovered nervously around women, behaving, she said, "like the patient is about to blow up."[22]

Forgetting the recent past, when obstetricians had enthusiastically touted VBACs, was understandable—the medical and public perceptions of risk and VBAC had shifted yet again. In 2001, newspapers reported that when labor was chemically induced, VBACs posed a much higher risk of uterine rupture when compared with women undergoing a second cesarean than previously thought—15 times higher in women if their labor was induced with a prostaglandin and 5 times higher in women given other hormones for induction. The alarming news affected obstetricians financially. By the end of the first decade of the twenty-first century, doctors who attended VBACs were paying higher malpractice premiums than physicians who did not.[23]

Yet the actual numbers revealed by VBAC studies were not nearly as alarming as newspaper headlines indicated; unfortunately, reporters rarely explain the nuances of statistics to the public. Women with a low transverse scar undergoing *spontaneous* labor, that is, forgoing dangerous prostaglandins and other methods of induction, had a 99.5 percent chance of not suffering a uterine rupture; women undergoing a repeat cesarean had a 99.8 percent chance of not suffering a deadly complication from the surgery. These statistics can be interpreted in two ways. Women undergoing a VBAC have a 166 percent greater chance of suffering a uterine rupture than women undergoing a repeat cesarean have of suffering a deadly complication. But the two numbers—0.5 percent in the case of VBAC and 0.2 percent in the case of repeat cesarean—are both such miniscule figures that the difference between them is not statistically significant. In other words, the odds of experiencing a uterine rupture during a VBAC or death following a second cesarean are virtually identical. Nevertheless, perception of risk has proven to be as effective a driver—of obstetricians' decisions, patients' choices, malpractice rates, and lawsuits—as actual risk.[24]

Viewing Pregnant Women as Litigants-to-Be

ACOG's many, at times contradictory, advisories contributed to this "mixed-up perception of risk." In the late 1990s, pro-VBAC activists reported that some physicians were insisting that patients seeking a VBAC sign a "VBAC Consent Form" that informed patients of risks that included fetal death and brain damage. Activists protested, "Where is the discussion of VBAC *safety*? Why are the *risks* of major abdominal surgery not itemized?"[25]

The "VBAC Consent Form," and its implied message warning women away from VBACs, was a sign of the times. Increasingly, obstetricians worried about risks not only to laboring women but also to themselves. When Helen Marieskind interviewed obstetricians for the HEW's 1979 report, most cited malpractice threats as the primary reason for the increase in cesareans. Their fear of liability was not unreasonable, although they should not have linked their concern to cesareans. The National Association of Insurance Commissioners (NAIC) estimated in 1979 that an obstetrician/gynecologist faced ten times the risk of being sued compared to physicians in other specialties. Yet when the NAIC issued that estimate, fewer than 10 percent of the claims against obstetrician/gynecologists were related, even tangentially, to cesarean birth. Marieskind observed similarly that, even as the cesarean rate rose, there had been only "one or two really whopping suits" in the entire country linked to cesarean section. And those few suits stemmed from bad maternal outcomes *as a result of the surgery*, not due to a damaged infant who might have been saved by the surgery. In the medical malpractice arena of the 1960s and 1970s, patients and their attorneys identified cesareans as problems, not solutions.[26]

Nevertheless, while the obstetricians interviewed by Marieskind mistakenly linked cesareans with their ability to thwart a lawsuit, their more general concerns about malpractice threats had a basis. The medical community had recently weathered its first malpractice "crisis point." There have been three such crises in US history, each marked by a rapid, large increase in either award size, malpractice premiums, or both, usually due to insurers' investment losses. The first crisis occurred in 1975, five years after the cesarean rate began its rise but several years before Marieskind conducted her interviews; the second occurred in the mid-1980s; and the most recent happened at the start of the twenty-first century. And although at and shortly after the crisis points all physicians' malpractice premiums increased considerably, obstetrician-gynecologists' increased the most. In a single year (1975, the first crisis point), malpractice insurance rates for obstetrician/gynecologists working in California, as just one example, quadrupled. Yet even then, most suits brought against obstetrician/gynecologists were for gynecologic, not obstetric, errors.[27]

Perception of risk, however, does not have a rational basis. While malpractice suits brought against obstetricians for failure to perform a timely cesarean had nothing to do with the initial, precipitous rise in the cesarean rate—because those suits did not exist—the introduction of the electronic fetal monitor in the late 1960s played no small part in forging the notion that there was a relationship between a diagnosis of fetal distress and obstetricians' obligation to perform a timely cesarean. Before EFM, malpractice suits against obstetricians for any reason were rare simply because a would-be litigant was seldom able to provide concrete proof of negligence. While the use of fetal stethoscopes during labor had allowed doctors to assess fetal well-being periodically, physicians' memories and handwritten notes were the only record of the intermittent evaluations. EFM, on the other hand, seemed to provide tangible, objective documentation of the nuances of entire labors.[28]

Using fetal monitor strips as seemingly incontrovertible evidence, medical malpractice claims against obstetricians became more numerous and lucrative. One obstetrician trained in the 1970s "still grieve[s]" the litigious climate spawned by electronic monitoring. After the monitor, she observed, a lawyer could point to a squiggle on a printout and claim, "'Well, that's where the baby was damaged.' How do you disprove that?" Lawyers began to tell juries: if only the obstetrician-defendant had performed a timely cesarean section in reaction to the message provided by the monitor, lifelong damage would have been prevented, and there would be no court case. As one attorney points out, EFM is a "no-win situation" for obstetricians. "Without EFM you're automatically liable for a bad result. With it, you provide instant replay for juries and evidence of a missed opportunity to save a damaged child," however debatable the reliability of that instant replay may be. He condemns the ACOG for not speaking out more firmly in favor of the fetal stethoscope and against EFM.[29]

Before pursuing any political ambitions, John Edwards—who eventually became a US senator from North Carolina and a one-time presidential and vice-presidential candidate—pioneered the use of EFM in litigation against obstetricians in the 1980s. Edwards was instrumental in inventing the claim that a physician's failure to recognize fetal hypoxia during labor, as indicated by a fetal monitor, caused cerebral palsy and other forms of neurological damage. Admirers cast Edwards as the champion of severely disabled children. The *Boston Globe* described his efforts as going "beyond a recitation of his case to a heart-wrenching plea to jurors to listen to the unspoken voices of injured children." He argued cases by pretending to be the fetus in the womb begging to be let out before it was too late. With a severely disabled child—usually due to cerebral palsy—sitting at the prosecution table, juries proved sympathetic. Edwards amassed a $38 million personal fortune, won at least $205 million for his clients, and almost single-handedly created the concept of failure to perform a cesarean as a valid medical malpractice claim. Lawyers in communities around the country mimicked Edwards's success. A jury awarded $35.6 million to one Brooklyn girl whose cerebral palsy affected her speech and ability to walk; her lawyer had charged that her physician failed "to deliver her at birth by cesarean section . . . despite obvious warning signs." Another attorney who won a $29 million settlement for a "brain-damaged and wheelchair-bound" Bronx teen blamed obstetric residents working without supervision. Although the boy was eventually born by an emergency cesarean, his lawyer complained, "It was a situation where they said 'We can wait, we can wait,' and then they waited too long."[30]

Yet most, if not all, of these cases were without merit. Cerebral palsy occurs almost exclusively during fetal development, or because of extreme prematurity, rather than as the result of an event occurring during a full-term birth. That is why, despite an almost sevenfold increase in cesarean sections since the advent of the near-universal use of the electronic fetal monitor, the incidence of cerebral palsy, at 1 in 500 births, has remained unchanged. Nevertheless, by the mid-1990s, 60 percent of malpractice premiums paid by obstetricians went to cover allegations of birth-related cerebral palsy caused by failure to perform a cesarean. Performing cesarean sections became one of the primary strategies used by obstetricians to immunize themselves against lawsuits. Researchers began to cite obstetricians' "siege mentality" as the reason that lowering the cesarean rate had become such a challenge.[31]

Damage awards became so high that, increasingly, hospitals refused to offer staff positions to obstetricians who carried less than $1 million worth of malpractice coverage. By the late 1980s, physicians who delivered babies, whether they were obstetricians or family physicians, were paying higher malpractice premiums than almost any other type of doctor. On average nationwide, obstetricians were paying $30,000 a year for insurance, and in New York, California, and Florida, premiums were double that. No one believed rates could go much higher until the third malpractice crisis point, in the early twenty-first century, when obstetricians' premiums skyrocketed in some states to $200,000 annually. The ACOG president in 2002 and 2003 complained that premiums were "well over $100,000 a year before you [even] deliver your first baby" and warned, "it's going to destroy our specialty, because we're the number-one target; there are two patients in every encounter, mom and baby."[32]

An obstetrician who began practicing in the early 1950s recalled that he and his original cohort never worried about lawsuits. "Everybody I knew had $10,000 malpractice insurance. I knew essentially nobody that was sued, except who really deserved it." An obstetrician who practiced in Illinois until his retirement in 2008 similarly remembered that when he began to practice medicine 40 years earlier, his premiums had been negligible—his first annual policy cost $37. In contrast, just before his retirement, his premium had ballooned to a "crazy" $160,000. Of necessity, obstetricians began to view pregnant women as litigants-to-be, at least as much as mothers-to-be. One obstetrician advised the residents he supervised that even if a baby was "'less than perfect,' if a Caesarean had been done they were 'covered.'"[33]

Before the introduction of antibiotics after World War II, doctors and the public alike viewed medicine as fallible. Bad things happened. Undesirable outcomes were unfortunate but often unavoidable. A retired obstetrician recalled of his training, "you learn[ed] Mother Nature . . . presents you with problems that you really can't do too much about." By the time he retired, though, malpractice settlements implied that obstetricians had the power to ensure good outcomes. Mortimer Rosen, director of obstetrics and gynecology at Columbia-Presbyterian Medical Center in New York City in the late 1980s, testified as an "expert witness" during many malpractice cases. He noted, "it's become apparent to me that death and damage are no longer viewed simply as tragedies, but as tragic consequences of a mistake made somewhere by someone." A certified nurse-midwife agreed: "For the trend now seems to be that if the perinatal team fails to provide perfection, it may be compelled to pay—financially and emotionally."[34]

Obstetricians lived with the stress daily. One explained, "The threat of a lawsuit, the threat of a damaged infant. . . . It's always there. . . . It's not objective. . . . This is a baby . . . and you want, just as much as the patient wants to have a baby that is a Harvard-graduate-slash-tennis-player, you want to give them that baby." Thus, she observed, "the default becomes a c-section." And just one lawsuit, whether experienced personally or vicariously, could change a doctor's behavior. As another obstetrician explained, "For a physician to be sued is very damaging to their functioning. It is hard with the next patient [who] . . . has anything on the [monitor] tracing. . . . It's very hard . . . to overcome that."[35]

If obstetricians were nervous before John Edwards launched his litigation strategy in the mid-1980s, Edwards's success in the courtroom caused anxiety to proliferate, as if by contagious infection. "There is no question," an obstetrician observed, "it's had a steady incremental effect on how conservative obstetricians are in their practices." And while "conservative" in earlier decades meant employing every trick to avoid a cesarean, by the late 1980s "conservative" meant performing a cesarean in the face of even the slightest doubt about the trajectory of a birth. One obstetric department chair told his doctors, "I would never criticize you for doing a c-section too soon," adding, "I'd be happy if our c-section rate is 65–70 percent." His hospital was self-insured; consequently, he viewed cesareans as a prophylactic measure, a means of immunizing doctors and their hospitals against lawsuits.[36]

More Cesareans, More Money

Indeed, concern over hospitals' and obstetricians' incomes helped to promote cesareans. In 1963, at the tail end of the baby boom, the ratio of births to obstetricians was 261 to 1. Twelve years later, after births decreased and the number of obstetricians increased, the ratio had fallen to 145 to 1. Yet obstetrician-gynecologists were earning more money than ever before. "It seems to me," said one public health physician at the University of North Carolina in 1980, "that in order for those obstetricians to maintain that sort of livelihood, they are forced to resort to more expensive and elaborate technologies, of which, I think, Caesarean section is one." Later studies seemed to corroborate that supposition. The states with the largest declines in fertility were seeing the largest increases in cesarean delivery, although researchers could not prove a causal effect—only that low fertility was correlated with a high cesarean rate.[37]

Like the burgeoning malpractice claims that spurred the cesarean rate, the rise in private, employer-based, insurance coverage of maternity care, which was virtually nonexistent before the late 1970s, also contributed to the increase. If Americans had health insurance at all as the cesarean rate tripled through the 1960s and most of the 1970s, coverage was usually provided by Blue Cross / Blue Shield through employers. These plans seldom covered maternity care, however. Before the late 1970s, health insurance companies, including "the Blues," deemed pregnancy a voluntary condition and excluded it from coverage. The few plans that did cover prenatal care and childbirth covered only a small portion of the cost. And in the highly unlikely event a policy did fully cover maternity costs, exemptions were common: costs were not covered until ten months after the policy became active, for example, and/or the policy did not cover the newborn during the first

10 days of life. Maternity coverage of any sort was such a rarity that an ACOG "statement of policy" issued in 1976 called for insurers to provide maternity care "on the same basis as other medical and surgical procedures." Not until 1978, though, as the cesarean rate approached 15 percent, did the US Congress pass the Pregnancy Discrimination Act, mandating that pregnancy be treated as a medical condition covered by insurers no differently than other medical conditions.[38]

Health economists have confirmed that hospitals' and physicians' incomes are part of the cultural stew promoting cesareans. Obstetricians working at for-profit hospitals perform cesareans at a rate 1.41 times higher than obstetricians delivering babies at nonprofit hospitals, regardless of women's risk factors. Of all forms of health insurance, private insurance offers the largest reimbursement for a cesarean, and, since the advent of Medicaid in 1965, there has been a noticeably higher rate of cesareans among privately insured women than among women insured by Medicaid. The hefty reimbursement differential between Medicaid and private insurance is the likely cause. In 2010, a cesarean cost Medicaid an additional $4,459 per birth; it cost private insurers an additional $9,537 per birth.[39]

The history of Medicaid payments alone demonstrates a relationship between cesareans and reimbursement rates. Whenever Medicaid has raised physicians' payment for cesareans, the cesarean rate among women covered by Medicaid has increased—but only among women whose doctors did not earn a predetermined salary as employees of an HMO. A 10 percent increase in cesarean payments, no matter the source, has been associated consistently with a 1.5 percent increase in the cesarean section rate. In short, the higher the financial reward, the more likely physicians have been to perform a cesarean. While in the nineteenth century, impoverished women and women of color gave birth by cesarean in inordinate numbers, in the late twentieth and early twenty-first centuries women of means, or at least women with superior insurance coverage, have experienced the highest cesarean rates. The National Center for Health Statistics reported that even within the same hospital, privately insured patients see substantially higher rates of cesarean delivery than under- or uninsured women, despite identical diagnoses.[40]

In the 1980s, birth reform activists pounced on these sorts of findings, citing doctors' "greed for money" as their motivation for performing cesareans. In referencing an American Medical Association finding in 1985 that cesarean sections put an additional $175 million in obstetricians' pockets and $1.1 billion in hospitals' coffers annually, a syndicated columnist editorialized: "The new sound of joy heard in delivery rooms is not 'It's a boy' or 'It's a girl,' but 'It's a bonanza!'" Yet this sort of financial reward was hardly unique to obstetricians. It was, and continues to be, a problem across the American medical landscape. Most American physicians are embedded in a fee-for-service system that allows them to charge for each office visit and every individual service performed during that visit, creating a built-in incentive to opt for more expensive, and simply more, procedures and tests.[41]

Indirect financial considerations have similarly stoked the cesarean rate. The more cesareans they could schedule, the more confidently obstetrician/gynecologists could arrange the larger, and even more lucrative, portion of their practice—routine gynecological appointments and gynecological surgeries. The decrease in hospital-based midwives likewise contributed, directly and indirectly, to the increase in cesarean surgeries. One obstetrician attributed the tricks she learned to avoid a cesarean to the midwives who worked at the hospital where she had trained as a resident in the early 1990s. "We loved our midwives," she said. "We would page them when we were in labor and delivery saying, 'This patient's xyz is happening. What is the thing you guys do to make the baby turn?'" Several years after she completed her residency, though, the hospital shuttered its midwifery service. The midwives spent a good deal more time with their patients compared to the hospital's obstetricians, seeing only six or seven patients per day versus obstetricians' 15 patients in half a day. As malpractice premiums soared to $200,000 per practitioner—for midwife and obstetrician alike—the hospital's administrators decided the low revenue generated by midwives no longer justified their malpractice costs. The obstetrician who had learned so much from midwives thought their worth should have been calculated in more than just dollars. "We're always nervous that bad things are about to happen," she said of obstetricians, "but the midwives are very hands off." She was sad for the current coterie of obstetric residents in her hospital, "because they don't get that kind of thing anymore. That there's another way . . . a way to approach labor as a natural life event." Another obstetrician, who did her residency at a hospital with "a lot of volume and a lot of uninsured . . . and also the very complex cases," similarly vouched for the value of midwives. "As students, if you wanted to get in a quote unquote 'normal' delivery, then you knew your money was with the midwives." With midwives vanishing from hospital maternity floors due to liability costs, an increasing number of obstetric residents found their perspective and training narrowed, further notching up the cesarean rate.[42]

"The More You Do Something, the Better You Get at It"

Other circumstances diminished doctors' skills as well. Beginning with the end of the baby boom and then snowballing, obstetric residents did not have the same opportunities to acquire the skills that had allowed their progenitors to avoid cesarean surgery. One obstetrician, who completed his residency in 1969, recalled that as a resident he delivered at least 20 to 30 babies each month. Now, he said, the average obstetrician delivered four or five infants each month. "When I was a resident," he explained, "we had three residents a year [at my hospital], now there are ten. There are the same number of deliveries . . . divided among ten residents that were divided among three. . . . The more you do something, the better you get at it." The abundant opportunities to hone skills that he and his cohorts enjoyed had simply disappeared.[43]

By the 1990s, doctors' skill levels were a reliable predictor of the chance their patients would have a cesarean birth. Pregnant at age 44, eight years after her first child had been born, Barbara told her longtime obstetrician she wanted neither epidural nor c-section. After years of treatments for secondary infertility, she explained, "I've had enough surgeries." Adhering to her wishes, Barbara's experienced doctor managed to turn her baby, who was positioned sideways, to the cephalic position during labor and hold him there for 45 minutes to ensure he did not return to the unfavorable position. Although the baby's heart rate slowed "precipitously" at one point, the physician did not rush to perform a cesarean. Barbara had a vaginal birth.[44]

In contrast, while older obstetricians had abundant opportunities during their training to treat every conceivable complication of a vaginal birth, the one procedure that more recently trained obstetricians are especially comfortable performing is a cesarean section. A second-year obstetric resident noted in 2013 that most of the 350 births she and her cohorts had attended thus far were cesarean deliveries. She was more at ease performing a cesarean—"probably the skill that we get the most experience in"—than attending a vaginal birth. She and other residents joked among themselves, "we could do a c-section on a desert island."[45]

The 1979 HEW report recognized that many training opportunities had indeed vanished. Obstetric residents no longer learned how to use a fetal stethoscope. They used the electronic fetal monitor instead. Nor did they learn how to apply forceps. One obstetrician recalled that when she and her cohorts were residents, they looked for any opportunity to use forceps to perfect their skill. "Whether it was right or wrong, when we came in on the shift, we would sort of look and see which patient was going to be a good candidate . . . never at the risk of the patient, but we really tried to do forceps deliveries, so that we could all learn. And the attendings encouraged that." Now, she observed, "we're kind of a dying breed." And, as another obstetrician noted, the relationship between lack of skill with forceps and an increase in cesareans was obvious: "When they [forceps] went away, the cesarean rate went up even more."[46]

Obstetricians' malpractice fears and the reduction in their skills were interrelated. Applying forceps, for example, had always been a far more difficult skill to teach, learn, and execute than performing a cesarean section. A physician who completed her residency in 1974 fully trained in the use of forceps described the intricacies of using the instrument. Obstetricians had to constantly weigh many factors: "the position of the baby, how far it's descended, how long the labor's gone on, the status of the baby by monitoring." She learned to "think through those issues . . . you have to know how hard to pull, or how hard not to pull. All those things are part of the training experience of operative vaginal delivery." Another obstetrician noted that, because the adept use of forceps was so hard to learn, as cesarean surgery became safer, forceps were classified as another "liability thing." Even when she wanted to learn how to apply forceps as a resident, her mentors told her, "Go bleep yourself, we are not doing that!"[47]

Today's alternatives to forceps dismay the obstetricians trained in the instrument's use. In describing the vacuum extractor, one sniffed, "It is used by people who haven't developed the skills with forceps. The timid and the poorly trained use vacuum. The well-trained use forceps." Another obstetrician agreed. "Those of us who are well trained in the use of forceps kind of stick our nose up at vacuum and call it 'housework.'" Certainly, this sort of attitude is, in part, an example of a generational smugness seen often not only in medicine but in daily life. This tendency was perhaps most effectively satirized by the "Grouchy Old Man" in the late 1980s and early 1990s, who railed on *Saturday Night Live*, the popular late-night comedy show on NBC, against every newfangled thing he had not grown up with, from seat belts to hair dryers. But in medicine, physicians' skills, and the choices they make based on those skills, have particularly high stakes.[48]

Another obstetrician noted that the absence of forceps training was the "same thing, same thing" for breech births. Rather than learn how to deliver a singleton breech as a resident, she learned only how to deliver a second twin in the breech position. Other hospitals forbade residents to learn even that. One obstetrician, who delivered "plenty" of second twins in the breech position during her residency, became "very comfortable with it." Then, in 2001, after starting a job at another hospital, she encountered a different attitude. She had just delivered one twin in the cephalic position and was about to deliver the second twin in the breech position when "a more senior attending" intervened. He berated her: "Are you crazy? . . . You've got to do a c-section. This baby is coming down breech!"[49]

After studies in the 1990s found that fetuses in the breech position faced more risks when born vaginally, ACOG responded with, in the words of one obstetrician, "a very damaging position statement saying the safest way to deliver breech is by c-section. And when that came out, the day it came out, we all said, 'there goes vaginal breech.'" Even in academic medical centers where older faculty could teach the skills needed to successfully execute breech deliveries, the practice has been discouraged. At least one retired obstetrician did not mourn the development, though. "We delivered breeches of any sort . . . and really sweated through a lot," he recalled. He pointed to his white hair. "That's how I got some of these."[50]

Although ACOG softened its position on vaginal breech deliveries in 2006, the edict that "planned vaginal delivery of a term singleton breech fetus may be reasonable" did little to increase vaginal breech births. For years, few residents had been sufficiently trained; in 1999, 84.5 percent of mothers in labor with a breech presentation were delivered by cesarean section. The 2006 *ACOG Committee Opinion* acknowledged the problem: most obstetricians would continue to opt for a cesarean "because of the diminishing expertise in vaginal breech delivery," a capability that ACOG's earlier ruling had further weakened. Some older obstetricians view the deskilling of their more recently trained colleagues as potentially harmful to patients. One physician who started her obstetric residency in 1982 noted, "If you've never had a vaginal breech, and one comes in, you know, sticking out of the vagina, you're gonna be in trouble."[51]

Rather than learning how to apply forceps or deliver babies in the breech position, residents trained in other, newer skills—how to interpret fetal monitor printouts, how to perform fetal scalp blood sampling, and how to use an ultrasound machine. And those diagnostic tools, in turn, further limited training opportunities. The placement of EFM straps, for example, rendered the "competent abdominal examination" not only impossible to perform but seemingly irrelevant—the monitor already provided the data. Ultrasound equipment, and its ability to relay information to the physician about the condition and position of the fetus, likewise made external palpation seem largely unnecessary. The admonition issued by J. Robert Willson, ACOG's president in 1981, that as residents learned "to rely more and more on fetal monitors" they were "learn[ing] less and less about labor," had come to fruition.[52]

"I Felt I Had No Choice"

The diminished skill of obstetricians limited their patients' choices. One woman, pregnant in the early 1980s, did not learn that her baby was in the breech position until she "entered the hospital, full term, with my membranes ruptured. I was immediately informed that my birth would have to be by cesarean, that the risks of injury and asphyxia were too great for a vaginal birth." She wondered why no factors, other than the fetus's breech position, were being considered—her pelvic size, her baby's weight, or the type of breech, either frank or footling. As a nurse practitioner, she knew breech babies could be delivered vaginally. She had "even assisted a woman with a precipitous vaginal breech birth. The baby had an Apgar of 8!" But, she said, "I felt I had no choice." No doctor present when she entered the hospital knew how to assist a vaginal breech birth. "I came away from my first birth with so much anger!" She had learned firsthand that women now had to set their expectations for birth based on their physicians' limited skills, and some women found this frightening. "I would appreciate your literature on drug free births," one woman wrote to a feminist health reform organization in the late 1980s. "My last birth was very hard with an epidural. . . . I was very lucky not to have a c-section." Pregnant with her second child, she hoped to once again avoid a cesarean but was not sure she could. "I'm due again 20th Feb with a new doctor 29 years of age. . . . I'm very scared of a c-section because of this doctor's inexperience."[53]

One mother of three children had three very different birth experiences, each shaped by the skill level of her physician. During her first birth in 1998, she "was ultrasounded to death," although she blamed herself. "I was really being conventional over the birth." A week after her due date, her doctor insisted on inducing labor. "They are so fanatical about 'if things are late.'" The moment she felt pain she asked for an epidural. When the doctor instructed her to push, she did, ending up with a "terrible" fourth-degree tear. But she treated it philosophically, telling the nurse, "well at least it is not a fifth" degree tear. "And they were, like, 'there is no fifth!'"[54]

When she was 40 weeks pregnant with her second baby, her new obstetrician suggested induction because, he explained, the baby was getting too large—over 9 pounds. Only after the baby was born did she learn the baby's actual weight—7 pounds 12 ounces—but the fourth-degree tear during her first birth had frightened her. She did not want to risk another, so she consented to the induction. But the birth did not go well. The epidural numbed her to a far greater degree than during her first birth. She began shaking. She was making no progress. After 24 hours, the doctor suggested "very casually, 'how about a c-section? Then we don't have to worry about the tear.'" He had exploited her worst fear, and she was exhausted. "I wanted it done with. And so he did kinda talk me into it. And I wasn't really against it . . . it all made sense at the time. When you are in the fog, it all makes sense."[55]

Her third birth, attended by the most skilled of her three obstetricians, was her favorite "because I had finally learned!" She saw an older obstetrician who was "the master of the VBAC." The baby was "sunny side up," in the occiput posterior position, but her physician was unruffled. He knew exactly what to do. "He literally took his hand and turned it and we were done. . . . It took one second to turn that baby." That upset her only because her second baby had been in the same position, and that was the reason given by her previous obstetrician for her stalled labor and the need for a cesarean section. He never attempted to turn her baby or even suggested the maneuver to her as a possible solution.[56]

April, who also gave birth to three children in the early twenty-first century, had a similar experience with her three birth attendants—each displayed differing skill sets. Her first son was born vaginally at a birth center in California without even a fetal monitor in the room. A midwife oversaw the birth. When she gave birth to her second son, she was living in rural Ohio. With no birth center in the area, and given her discomfort with home birth and the fact that her health insurance would not cover "the midwife route," her only option was an obstetrician-attended, hospital birth. Despite the venue, she wanted her second birth to be similar to her first.[57]

When she arrived at the hospital, she declined an IV. An obstetrician exhorted, "At least let us put the port in." But April was steadfast. She told the doctor, "This is not a matter of life and death and I don't want you filling me full of water that I'm going to have to pee out at some point. No." In another feisty move, she refused fetal monitoring. "Frankly," she said later, "I didn't care whether I was being a difficult patient or not. It was my birth." Toward the end of second-stage labor, her son suffered a dangerous complication—shoulder dystocia. "His shoulders, . . . just a centimeter wider than his head," became stuck after his head left the birth canal. Her well-trained obstetrician responded adeptly. She "popped his collar bone with her thumb and slid him out." The baby's collarbone eventually "healed perfectly."[58]

April wanted more children, and she assumed her third birth, like the first two, would be vaginal. "My sister gave birth to a 10-pound baby. . . . I really wasn't worried about needing a c-section." During her third pregnancy, however, she had an obstetrician only six years out of her residency. The shoulder dystocia suffered by April's second baby made her nervous. She urged April to opt for a planned cesarean. The young physician explained, "I do not feel confident enough to guarantee you that I can do what [April's previous obstetrician] did if the baby gets stuck. . . . I don't have the skill to deliver this baby." She warned April that if she refused a planned cesarean, she would "likely" end up needing an emergency cesarean "which is much more traumatic and difficult in the recovery than if we just did an optional c-section without you going into labor." The obstetrician also warned April that if she insisted on a vaginal birth, she risked permanently paralyzing her baby's arm if he, too, had shoulder dystocia. There would be no obstetrician present capable of handling the emergency.[59]

The obstetrician's final admonition swayed April. "That was the thing for me. It wasn't about what happened to my body; I was prepared to take the risks with my body. I was not, however, prepared to take risks for the baby." April agreed to a planned cesarean. The surgery took place the next morning. "That's where they get you," she said later. "Because of course you're going to do whatever you need to do to have a healthy baby. . . . When your OB says to you, 'I can't guarantee you that I can do that, that I can save your baby from a lifetime of disability,' what choice are you going to make?"[60]

April suffered in the immediate aftermath of the cesarean. She was allergic to the morphine doctors gave her to control her pain, and she vomited for 13 straight hours. "I was trying to breastfeed, you know, so I've got [my baby] in one arm and a friend of mine holding the little puke bucket in the other and it was literally 13 hours." One nurse scolded her, " 'You know you aren't supposed to eat or drink anything the night before the surgery.' I was like, 'Lady! I did not! I did not! Just hold the bucket.' " And her allergic reaction to the morphine was not her only postpartum complication. "I was purple as an eggplant from navel to the tip of my pubic bone because they had to pull a lot" when the baby became "partially engaged" in the birth canal "so they had to disengage him and then flip and pull to get the head out." For weeks after the birth she could not lift her feet to get into a car—a cesarean surgical incision goes through muscles as well as flesh. "You don't realize what all of those muscles, how many . . . movements they are tied to. I could not pull myself into my own bed. . . . And they don't tell you that stuff. They don't tell you how serious a c-section is in terms of major surgery."[61]

She remained bitter about her experience. "I popped out one, I popped out two, and I'm . . . pretty sure I could have popped out baby number three . . . had I been given the chance." Yet her young obstetrician's limited skills narrowed her options.[62]

Unexpected Consequences of More Female Obstetricians

During April's prenatal appointments with the young obstetrician who delivered her third baby, she learned that her new doctor "had an extremely painful, horrible first birthing experience." And, "in order to save women from that kind of pain," she sometimes recommended a cesarean. "So I knew from the get-go that her own birthing experience had significantly influenced the way that she . . . approached any kind of difficult case."[63]

April had identified one of the many paradoxes of modern American obstetrics. In the 1970s, when birth reform activists were at their influential height, they argued that the male physicians who dominated obstetrics were singularly responsible for subjugating women by foisting on them a technocratic approach to birth. Feminist activists did not mince words. Male obstetricians were the problem: "man . . . institutionalized birth in the hospital. Man placed woman on her back in labor, then devised metal tools to pull her baby out, then knocked her senseless with anesthesia." Male doctors orchestrated "carefully timed and controlled" deliveries, not for the benefit of his patient or her baby, but for his own convenience, "when he is on the spot and ready." Activists charged that "the male obstetrician" was uniquely capable of condescension and chauvinism: he "comforts woman by advising her to leave everything to him, to simply place herself in his hands and abide by the procedures of his institution, the hospital." If only female obstetricians replaced male obstetricians, reformers imagined, unwanted medical interventions would vanish, and birth would become the humane, "natural" experience it was meant to be. Doctors who were women would protect other women from the routine, largely unnecessary, uncomfortable treatments that had become so common.[64]

Over the next four decades, feminist activists got their wish. Female physicians came to dominate obstetrics. By 1990, 20.9 percent of all ACOG members (13 percent of fellows and 44 percent of junior fellows) were female. Ten years later, 36 percent of all ACOG members (29 percent of fellows and 64 percent of junior fellows) were women; in 2015, more than half of ACOG members were women. Just under half were fellows, while a whopping 82 percent of junior fellows were women. Overall, female junior fellows overtook males in 1994; female members of ACOG surpassed males in 2011.[65]

Yet women taking over the specialty did not have the effect feminist activists had predicted. Quite the contrary: as women became obstetricians in ever-growing numbers, the cesarean rate and other interventions, such as planned induction and epidural anesthesia, increased. Female obstetricians not only displayed the same affinity for medical interventions as their male counterparts, they also spoke to patients with a dual authority—as trained physicians and as women who either had experienced birth or might in the future. As such, they could be even more directive than their male counterparts.

Female obstetricians, like all conscientious physicians, tend to want for their patients what they want for themselves. One Chicago obstetrician regularly reminded her patients that during her own first birth she "could not go without an epidural past one centimeter." To save her patients from the pain she had experienced, she "strongly pushed" them to ask for epidural anesthesia early in labor. Another obstetrician gave birth vaginally via forceps to four large babies between 1983 and 1990—her first child weighed 11 pounds. And she, too, would conjure her personal experience when advising patients. She regularly told them that "the complications of delivering a large baby" dogged her "years later . . . things like bladder prolapse, surgery, hysterectomy." She used her own experience "to tell patients the good sides of a c-section," advising some, "if you have the c-section, you won't have to deal with these consequences." Another obstetrician who had three cesareans—the first for failure to progress, the second after a failed VBAC, and the third by a planned cesarean—admitted that when advising patients, "You do bring your own past experiences into it." Although she told patients that she never regretted attempting the VBAC that ultimately failed, she also explained to them that her easiest cesarean was the planned one, "to just know what you're going to do and go in and do it in terms of planning your day." She also comforted patients facing an imminent cesarean with the observation, "I have a scar on my abdomen [but] I don't have one on my perineum. So, I can live with that."[66]

Female obstetricians influence not only their patients but also the residents they supervise. One obstetrician described a colleague who gave birth to her first child by elective cesarean section. "She never labored. She just wanted a section." After the birth, the new mother instructed the residents whom she oversaw to offer elective cesareans to each pregnant woman they examined. Another obstetrician described a colleague who likewise had an elective cesarean. Her choice, the obstetrician observed, telegraphed to her residents a strong position favoring cesareans that were not medically necessary.[67]

The few studies conducted on the attitude of female physicians toward their own births indicate that a greater percentage of female obstetrician/gynecologists, urogynecologists, and maternal-fetal medicine specialists than the population at large prefer for themselves an elective cesarean rather than a low-risk vaginal birth. In one study, 17 percent of female obstetricians chose a cesarean section for themselves in the absence of any medical reason. In later studies, they showed an even greater preference for elective cesarean—21 and 31 percent in successive studies. Researchers described female obstetricians as exhibiting a "liberal attitude" toward cesarean sections in general and warned that, given their dominance in the field, their views could counter efforts to reduce the cesarean section rate. Another study found a positive relationship between a physician's personal preference for cesarean surgery and the percentage of her patients who delivered abdominally.[68]

The generational divide between obstetricians is often evident when they discuss the course their specialty has taken. While very recently trained obstetricians tend to describe the cesarean section rate with resignation, their more experienced colleagues do not. An obstetrician who started her residency in 1992 had three cesarean births due to "a size issue," which she characterized as "a big fat bummer." But she described one colleague—they had been residents together—who "came to see us for prenatal care. . . . And she said, 'I'm only going to have this one baby. Let's just do a c-section.' So, we did." An older obstetrician, who started her residency in 1973, cannot abide this. "It's their own biases," she said of her younger colleagues. "Some of them even have . . . I can hardly say the words . . . elective primary cesarean deliveries." Of the upsurge in cesareans in general she said, "When you have a hammer, you look for a nail, and I think having the person taking care of a patient who can also do the cesarean sometimes influences" the course of the birth. She had seen this often enough that when she gave birth to her own children, one in the late 1970s and the other in the early 1980s, she opted both times for a midwife rather than an obstetrician. "That was back at a time when the cesarean delivery rate was doubling every few years. And I thought my only chance for a normal birth was to use a midwife." She chose the nurse-midwife who was part of her maternal fetal medicine practice group: "And she obviously had an astoundingly high vaginal birth rate, and I picked her."[69]

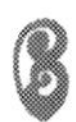

J. Robert Willson—who would eventually hold a host of leadership positions in the obstetric world, including president of the American College of Obstetricians and Gynecologists and director of the American Board of Obstetrics and Gynecology—chided colleagues in 1953, as baby boom birth protocols were being put in place, that maternal mortality had been reduced over the decades by eliminating medical procedures that increased the possibility of infection, not by performing more procedures. Yet today, obstetricians view not intervening as the risk. As one obstetrician explained, if she allowed a vaginal birth "and I turn out to be wrong, then the outcome is much more devastating for the family, than if I say, 'you need a cesarean section,' and it turns out the baby's gases are fine." Antibiotics and blood banking, the assorted diagnostic tools introduced in the 1950s and 1960s, particularly the electronic fetal monitor, and the many changes in medical culture since the late 1960s colluded to amplify obstetricians' inclination, not just to intervene during childbirth but to intervene with what traditionally had been the most extreme intervention—cesarean section.[70]

Electronic fetal monitoring had already convinced obstetricians that fetal distress occurred far more frequently than they ever suspected. Then came ACOG's conflicting professional recommendations governing VBACs; varied health insurance reimbursement rates for vaginal versus cesarean births; soaring malpractice premiums; the increase in lawsuits against obstetricians for dubious claims, most notably that failure to perform a timely cesarean caused cerebral palsy; medical training focused increasingly on medical technologies and surgical birth and decreasingly on methods to ensure safe vaginal birth; and the unique perspective of female obstetricians. Individually, but especially in the aggregate, these factors encouraged ever more cesarean births. Obstetric texts reinforced the trend. The authors of the 1980 edition of *Williams Obstetrics* noted, "In modern obstetric practice, there are virtually no contraindications to cesarean section." Sprinkled throughout the same book's thousand-plus pages were the many contraindications to vaginal birth in "recognition of [fetal] impairment, actual or suspected . . . if . . . vaginal delivery were attempted." The onus of risk was now squarely on vaginal birth.[71]

Yet medical practice has never been cut and dried—not in J. Whitridge Williams's and Joseph DeLee's day, and not in the twenty-first century. Despite the normalization of cesarean section, most doctors recognize the procedure carries all the attendant risks of any major abdominal surgery. And this weighs on them. "I remember last week I did a c-section on a woman who was having her second baby," recalled one physician, "and she had pushed for a fairly good while and just wasn't coming down. . . . The baby was posterior and I tried to rotate her and so I offered her the c-section and she accepted it." The obstetrician still wondered, though, "Could we just have waited?" But she had other considerations when she offered the surgery to the laboring mother. As Robert Harris discovered more than a century earlier, cesareans are safer when performed earlier in labor. "Had she labored another hour and the baby got further in the pelvis and we still couldn't get the baby [out] . . . now it's going to be a terribly difficult c-section. She's much more likely to get an infection. You are much more likely to tear down into the vagina and have a difficult repair and recovery. The baby is going to be more stressed."[72]

For any obstetrician, the memory of a devastating outcome, however rare, lingers in a way that the many good outcomes do not. One obstetrician will never forget the fetus who appeared to be fine throughout labor—"I thought I was reading the [EFM] strip right"—but the baby was stillborn "and never took a breath and it was life altering . . . devastating." Consequently, obstetricians continually second-guess themselves: "you look back at that and say 'at what point should I have or could I have?'" Despite her excitement witnessing "that rare birth that happened without any intervention," another obstetrician described the more influential "fear around the birth process" that festers "both for obstetricians and for trainees in obstetrics . . . because you are privy to the stories about the negative things . . . and that sometimes overrides that sense that this is something that's natural." A momentary lapse in judgment can have any one of a number of devastating consequences—the loss of a young woman's uterus, a disabled child, a stillborn baby, a dead mother. And the fear of any one of those consequences pushes obstetricians toward the procedure that they currently identify with diminished risk—a cesarean section.[73]

Professionally speaking, obstetricians tend to be conservative by nature. That is why physicians practicing in the nineteenth through the mid-twentieth centuries avoided cesareans; the surgery posed manifold risks. An obstetrician who began to practice in 1952 listed those risks: "In the first place you have a major anesthetic. I don't care if it's a spinal, an epidural, or a general . . . [and] you have the potential of an incision that's going to get infected and not heal . . . and just because you do a cesarean section doesn't mean you're not going to harm the baby. . . . And when you add them all up there is a higher morbidity with a major operation than with not." Today, physicians take a similar inventory and come to the opposite conclusion. As a young obstetrician noted, "I have a partner who says that, 'No baby ever died from a c-section. I've never felt bad about doing a c-section.'" With the growth in surgical safety, the default for a difficult birth became cesarean surgery, enhancing the belief that cesarean section offered better outcomes than vaginal birth.[74]

For mothers, the increase in cesarean surgeries transformed how they would anticipate, and ultimately experience, birth. As their physicians framed vaginal birth as dangerous, mothers' choices narrowed. Having been told their infant faced serious risk if they chose vaginal birth, many had no option but to consent to a cesarean. And as the surgery normalized, more mothers anticipated that their birth would quite likely end in cesarean section out of necessity. What had generated consternation in one generation of mothers was about to be largely accepted by the next.

Chapter Seven

Giving Birth in a Culture of Risk

Consequences for Mothers

Mothers' anticipation and experience of birth have often conflicted with obstetricians' approach to and medical understanding of birth. This clash became especially obvious in the 1970s and 1980s, when feminist activists condemned as unnecessary, demeaning, and even harmful, many treatments that obstetricians had long touted as beneficial. Although mothers and doctors attempted to respond to each other's positions, they often talked past one another. The largely white, female, college-educated activists who challenged the nation's largely white, male obstetricians never fully appreciated the array of pressures that obstetricians contended with. Nor did most obstetricians fully grasp the legitimacy of mothers' complaints about inhumane treatment. This rift between women and the physicians specializing in women's medicine has had broad, persistent consequences.[1]

Generation Gaps

While neither all physicians nor all mothers have ever approached childbirth in a monolithic way, specific views have predominated in each generation. The women who gave birth to the baby boomers in the 1940s, 1950s, and 1960s sought and received medical care in an era of physician paternalism—a form of control that was particularly pronounced in obstetrics and gynecology. Doctors were the experts. They made the medical decisions. Who was the patient to question them? One mother who gave birth to her first child in 1949 and her second in 1952 exemplified that tradition. She recalled of her pregnancies and births: "The doctor was in command. . . . The doctor was God. And when the doctor told you this is how it's going to be, you didn't worry. You let the doctor worry."[2]

The baby boomers, the daughters of these women, matured in a different world. Most were still in school in the 1960s and 1970s, as the women's rights movement came to the fore. That movement helped shape their views and aspirations. Rather than accede to doctors' instructions and hospital routines during birth, as their mothers had, they questioned everything. One woman wrote of her impending birth, "I am enraged about having my baby in a hospital! The doctor said *I must* be on my back in stirrups, *I must* have a pubic shave, and *I must* have an enema. . . . I ask, who is having this baby?" Criticism of women's medicine became the overriding narrative among health reformers in the 1970s, challenging the authority of male physicians and driving change.[3]

The next generation of American women took the successes of the women's movement for granted. They had grown up in a world where federal law mandated gender equity, where women working outside the home was the norm, and where schools, from the primary grades through higher education, nurtured women's academic and athletic talents. Yet the legal mandate that women must receive the same treatment as men in public life did not necessarily result in equal treatment for women. Women carry and grow fetuses. They give birth. They lactate. In the absence of social supports formulated to respond to those realities, such as the paid maternity leave and government-subsidized daycare enjoyed by working women in almost every other industrialized country, American working women found themselves at a disadvantage to working men. Same treatment did not translate to equal treatment. Without accommodations for women's special abilities, the change wrought by the women's movement made life more, rather than less, difficult for the growing number of women who were new mothers and also working outside the home.[4]

Given their milieu, this latest generation has approached childbirth not as the empowering activity so many of their mothers celebrated but as one more draining task in an already too-busy life. As one young woman chided, "In a world where women are constantly proving their worth—in the office, on the playing field, at home—unmedicated childbirth need not be singled out as 'proof' of one's strength." These women tended to ridicule the natural births that so many of their mothers found inspiring. If medicine could tame the intensity of labor, then why not embrace the treatments? If an intravenous Pitocin drip provided the means to schedule a birth that would otherwise interfere with work commitments and the care of other children, why not use it to mitigate the disruption? If epidurals allowed mothers to sleep, read, converse normally, and watch television during labor, why not opt for the relief? One woman who gave birth to her first child at age 29 in 1993, was appalled, not emboldened, by what she learned in her Lamaze class. "I was just so angry at what was coming. . . . I kept saying 'I am on a rollercoaster headed toward a cement wall and I cannot get off.' " She declared the classes ludicrous. "I thought they were froufrou-y and stupid. I went in saying, 'if it hurts, I am going to make sure I take drugs and I am not going to start the breathing.' "[5]

These three generations of American women tended to view cesarean sections as differently as they viewed childbirth in general. The rare woman who gave birth by cesarean in the decades just before and after World War II usually viewed the surgery as a life-saving necessity. And generally, as in Jackie Kennedy's births, it was. Much like their mothers, the women who came of reproductive age in the 1970s rarely anticipated the possibility of a cesarean section; unlike their mothers, when they did have one—increasingly likely as the section rate surged through the 1970s and 1980s—they tended to react with anger. One mother, who gave birth to her first baby by cesarean in 1971, said years later that she wished she had been privy to what she termed "the '80s knowledge," a byproduct of the women's health reform movement, before the birth. She was sure that her surgery had been unnecessary and that doctors had "denied [her] something very, very important," yet at the time she did not have the information to challenge their authority. Since the end of the twentieth century, yet another generation has exhibited a third point of view, seeing more positives in their surgeries than negatives. "I birthed him," said one mother who had a cesarean in the early twenty-first century. "I know others would disagree, but I fought and struggled and went to the mat to see my baby at his birth. And I did it. And in a lot of ways that empowers me to think about trying birth again."[6]

Despite their contradictory views, the baby boomers, and later their adult daughters, both determinedly sought control during childbirth. The boomers sought control by rejecting medical treatments and their daughters by doing the opposite—embracing medicine. The woman disgusted by her Lamaze class in 1993 viewed "natural" childbirth as the epitome of a lack of control: "Here I was almost this 30-year-old woman, in control of my life, and, as I saw it, there was no control in that scenario."[7]

The chair of the Department of Obstetrics and Gynecology at Sloane Hospital for Women in New York City confirmed in the late 1980s that women were making this type of assessment about spontaneous vaginal birth. "Patients have been very demanding in saying, 'If there's absolutely *any* question of risk, I want you to do a cesarean.'" His statement implied that cesarean birth conferred control by thwarting all risk. The message was a powerful one, embraced by a growing number of young women. One woman had long been frightened by the fate of a friend's brother, who had been deprived of oxygen during birth, leaving him "incapable of movement or speech, and dependent on full-time care." She was certain that "injury by the birth itself" was easily avoided—by having a cesarean section. "That didn't strike me as cowardly or selfish" to choose a cesarean, she said. "It struck me as good parenting." Yet another mother affirmed this view in extolling her planned cesarean: "The certainty—knowing how it's going to go—is a good thing. With labor, you have absolutely no control—you don't know when it's going to happen; you don't know how it's going to go." To some, in contrast to methodical abdominal surgery, vaginal birth was beginning to appear unnecessarily, and dangerously, uncontrollable.[8]

Mothers Ask Why

Cesarean section was an unusual event in the early 1970s—so rare that women were often confused when they found themselves in a surgical suite during labor with an obstetrician poised to operate. Their mothers had almost certainly given birth vaginally. Their friends were unlikely to have given birth by cesarean. Making their cesarean surgeries even more unpleasant, the nascent birth reform movement had not yet succeeded in altering obstetricians' bedside manners—doctors were still overtly paternalistic when interacting with pregnant patients.

Theresa's story was thus not unusual for the era. She gave birth to her first baby by cesarean at age 20 in 1971 due to a diagnosis of "fetal distress." She was wholly unprepared for the surgery—doctors told her husband she needed a cesarean but never even mentioned the surgery to her until after they had wheeled her into a surgical suite and she asked why she was there. Despite the diagnosis of fetal distress, her son was born with an initial Apgar score of 9. Theresa did not feel then, nor does she believe now, that the cesarean was necessary. Eighteen months later, she bore her second son. Vaginal birth after cesarean (VBAC) would not be on the American medical radar for another decade; her physician never mentioned the possibility of a vaginal birth. Quite the contrary: early in her pregnancy he informed her that he would perform another cesarean and that she had no choice in the matter. "Once a c-section, always a c-section," he told her.[9]

Not until she gave birth to her third child almost five years later, after the messages of birth reform advocates had permeated newspapers and magazines, did Theresa question her previous obstetrician's declaration. Like other pregnant women moved by the urgings of feminist activists, she bypassed her physicians in a search for information and learned that in England women rarely had repeat cesareans. VBAC was the norm. She tried to tell her latest obstetrician about her discovery. But, she recalled, "He was not going to hear it." Instead, he responded with a non sequitur: "You have had three abortions. What do you care?" Theresa was certain that mentioning her abortions was his way of "shutting me up." Unable to switch providers because her health plan required her to give birth at a specific hospital with a specific group of obstetricians, she felt stripped of all options.[10]

Her third cesarean was a nightmare. Seconds after the anesthesiologist administered spinal anesthesia, Theresa was unable to breathe. Another doctor tried to assure her, "you might not think that you're breathing. Try a little harder." She still could not breathe. The anesthesiologist administered general anesthesia. When Theresa regained consciousness, she was on a respirator, unable to speak, with a terrible spinal headache. She learned later that the anesthesiologist had injected the spinal anesthetic too high on her spinal column. "He'd frozen my diaphragm."[11]

During her first two surgeries, regional anesthesia had allowed her to see her babies immediately after their births. "That is different," she explained, "than just being told four hours later when you wake up" that you have had a baby. To make matters worse, while she was unconscious no one mentioned her inability to breathe in the operating room to her husband. While he waited for her to wake up, he called family and friends to share the happy news that he and Theresa had a daughter. Learning about the phone calls compounded Theresa's fury about the third cesarean and the general anesthesia: "Everybody in the world knew I had a baby girl before I knew I had a baby girl!" The memory summoned her old anger: "THAT REALLY PISSED ME OFF!" She was "in pain and misery" when the anesthesiologist entered her room. "Well, it happens to the best of us," he told her. Her head still pounding, Theresa responded to his unapologetic apology with an irate rejoinder: "You think you're the best?"[12]

Theresa and her now-grown children still suffer from side effects of the births. Her sons have asthma and allergies, conditions she attributes to the cesareans; contemporary studies support her suspicion. Theresa herself has suffered from surgical adhesions—a common side effect of multiple abdominal surgeries—that have caused her a good deal of pain. Although the phrase "natural childbirth" was not part of her vocabulary when she gave birth to her first child in 1971, she had always harbored one basic assumption about birth before her first cesarean. "I assumed it was kind of a natural process. I mean, that was what I felt from my mother."[13]

Mothers Condemn Cesareans

Another mother, who also received general anesthesia during her cesarean, awakened after the surgery, like Theresa, to learn she had a baby girl. "I said to myself 'I really don't give a hoot. I could care less if the baby lives or dies.' " Six weeks later, suffering from postpartum depression, she saw a psychiatrist. She told him she did not want her daughter. "But," she said later, "I also had a feeling that I didn't *have* my daughter either."[14]

Nancy Wainer Cohen described her devastation after her first birth, by cesarean, in 1972. Searching for a way to heal psychologically, she asked the instructors of her childbirth education class if they knew other women who had undergone a similar experience. The instructors invited her to submit her query to their newsletter. Although they only distributed the newsletter locally, women apparently shared it with others. Stories came in from all over the country. "The responses," Cohen wrote, "never stopped." One mother described her cesarean as akin to "being raped. I couldn't do anything but wait until it was over." Cohen had struck a nerve.[15]

In 1973, she cofounded Cesareans/Support, Education, and Concern—C/SEC. The women who flocked to the organization blamed the routine accoutrements of a hospital birth—the IV, the artificially ruptured membranes, the Pitocin drip, the electronic fetal monitor, the epidural, and the medical impatience that accompanied each procedure—for their cesarean sections, echoing the traditional objections of birth reformers in general. C/SEC had two purposes: to lower the cesarean rate and to "humanize" the cesarean experience by sponsoring support groups for mothers distressed by their surgeries. C/SEC's work influenced even the women who had not been traumatized by their surgical births. "The more I learned," wrote one woman after her second birth in the late 1970s, "the more I came to realize that there was far more risk involved in submitting myself to major abdominal surgery than there was in attempting a vaginal delivery." She had not resented her cesarean until experiencing a VBAC. "ROUTINE REPEAT CESAREANS," she wrote, "ARE AN OUTRAGE." Mainstream newspapers, women's magazines, and the black press helped to alert their readers to the high cesarean rate and its dangers. *Jet* magazine reported in 1984 that, despite the rising numbers, cesareans were "considered unnecessary in most cases."[16]

Determined to assert control in subsequent births, many of the unhappy mothers who sought help from grassroots organizations like C/SEC determinedly sought a VBAC. One mother ecstatically reported giving birth to her fourth child "in the warmth and privacy of [my] own home . . . totally free of medical intervention." She offered an indignant description of her first birth, the one that set her on a path of two more c-sections before the home birth: "cesarean because of 'failure to progress because of possible CPD' [cephalo-pelvic disproportion] which was actually premature rupture of membranes with no labor and impatient obstetrician." Another mother wrote of her VBAC, "I am *so* happy. *So* content, & so grateful. My body has healed so fast—our family is so peaceful and my marriage is not suffering any of the effects of the 'knife.' I am *whole*."[17]

The women who defiantly orchestrated VBACs sought to become role models, not only for other women but for obstetricians as well. A California woman who experienced "a traumatic cesarean" in 1973 did not give birth again until 1983. Determined to "NOT be a victim again," she retained a midwife. She attended childbirth preparation classes. During her third month of pregnancy, she began to lobby for use of the "Alternative Birth Room" at her local hospital—"one of the most rigid, conservative, monolithic medical establishments in Calif." When the hospital's head of obstetrics warned her about uterine rupture, she told him she was willing to risk the 0.5 percent chance. Ultimately, with the backing of her personal physician, she received "a reticent OK" from the hospital's obstetric chief to use the birth room.[18]

During labor, she continued to defy hospital protocol. She sipped white grape juice after nurses told her she could not have anything to drink. She labored in unconventional positions—standing, kneeling on the floor, sitting on the toilet—"everywhere but lying down on the bed." After her cervix remained at six centimeters dilation for four and a half hours, "the head of obstetrics threw a fit in the hallway, insisting that my labor was arrested and I should be sectioned. He even had a gurney in the hall ready to take me away." Someone called in a psychiatrist to lecture her on "why I should not look at another c/section as a defeat." As the psychiatrist upbraided her, she had the urge to push. When the baby's head began to crown, a hospital nurse could not believe what she was witnessing. She marveled, "I've never seen anyone do that without an episiotomy first!"[19]

Even as cesarean birth normalized, the International Cesarean Awareness Network (ICAN) continued to collect and publish women's upsetting stories in the early twenty-first century. "That first night, I drop my baby. I can't take care of her—can't even hold her. Can't be grateful. Can't feel joy. All I feel is pain and tiredness and frustration at not being able to start being a mother." Another woman described the string of medical interventions she endured before her birth ended in abdominal surgery. She had "reluctantly agreed to an induction." Twenty-four hours later, doctors declared the induction a failure and sent her home. When her water broke two days later, she headed back "to the hospital in rush-hour traffic for an hour, and labored for 12 hours, eight hours spent at eight to nine centimeters with an epidural that didn't work and Pitocin that worked too well." She concluded angrily, "I GOT CUT OPEN ANYWAY."[20]

Mothers Blame Themselves

Yet mothers' feelings about their cesareans were certainly not uniform. Some were angered by an experience they considered unnecessary and demeaning, while others were satisfied with their births. And even dissatisfaction did not necessarily drive a woman to seek a different type of birth with her next pregnancy. To the contrary, a negative experience could prompt fatalism—a mother resigned to put herself in her doctors' hands the second time around.

Mary's responses to her two births demonstrate all of those conflicting reactions. Before and during her first pregnancy, she looked forward to a "natural" birth. Mary did not fear an unmedicated labor. She feared the opposite—"intervention by hospital personnel." Her first birth, in 1990 when she was 36, validated her trepidation. She found doctors' and nurses' "treatment and handling" of her so upsetting that, at her six-week postpartum checkup, she complained to her obstetrician. Her "main bitch" was that nurses and doctors had disregarded her persistent request to be taken off the fetal monitor. She told her physician that there had been no need for continual monitoring; her baby "at no time showed any signs of suffering from the effects of my labor."[21]

That was not Mary's first clash with her obstetrician. During her pregnancy, after her due date came and went, the doctor told her to make an appointment with the hospital for labor induction. Mary declined. When he said she had no choice, she fought back tears. She saw "no need to play with nature." She was thus delighted when she began to labor spontaneously two days before the scheduled doctor-mandated induction.[22]

During the 30-minute ride to the hospital, Mary noticed that the contractions that had been gathering strength at home had slowed. Then, as she and her husband, Michael, walked across the hospital parking lot, the contractions regained their strength. Shortly after the birth, Mary observed in a letter to a friend: "In retrospect, this as well as the later events" seemed to demonstrate that "being up and moving around . . . increase[d] the frequency and intensity of the contractions whereas inactivity . . . slow[ed] them down."[23]

Her hospital experience began well enough. The paperwork Mary had completed in anticipation of her scheduled, and now unnecessary, induction was waiting for her at the registration desk when she and Michael arrived. As she settled into her room, a nurse hooked her up to a fetal monitor "and confirmed that our baby's . . . heartbeat was constant and strong." But after a physician performed an internal exam, Mary was discouraged to learn she was only two centimeters dilated. The news did proffer a benefit, though. Because she was still so early in labor, the nurse took Mary off the monitor, releasing her to wander the hospital corridors, albeit with strict instructions to return to the room by the time Mary's doctor was expected to begin his rounds.[24]

Mary and Michael enjoyed an ambling tour of the maternity floor. "I was still very loquacious, keeping a light banter with defenseless" Michael. As they walked, her contractions intensified. She wondered why she did not see other couples strolling the corridors. At the appointed time, they returned to her room for another monitor check. After nurses confirmed that her baby was doing well, she expected to be released for another walk. Instead, she remained attached to the monitor while two nurses and, eventually, "an insolent intern" performed periodic internal exams to assess her progress.[25]

Mary was miserable. Staying in bed during labor "seemed like unnecessary torture. . . . [The] forced immobility . . . made the pains even worse." When the intern returned for another examination, he warned her that if her cervix had not dilated any farther since the last exam, he would break her bag of water. At that point in her labor, Mary would brook no threats. "With a crochet hook looking device poised to enter my vagina, I told him he would do nothing of the kind, & furthermore . . . I wanted to get out of bed & move around." The intern was "truly shocked" by Mary's resistance. He left the room to report her impertinence to her doctor. When her doctor arrived, he explained to Mary that her cervix had been dilated five centimeters for a number of hours and that breaking her amniotic sac would ensure that her labor progressed more rapidly. A nurse chimed in to report another problem—she was having trouble "getting a solid [monitor] reading on the fetus," a possible sign of fetal distress. The nurse informed Mary she could not resume her walk "until a good, steady fetal reading was obtained." Mary's doctor pierced her amniotic sac. But rather than strengthening as the doctor had predicted, her contractions subsided and did not regain their prior power and frequency until 30 minutes later.[26]

That sort of ebb and flow of uterine contractions had become familiar to Mary. As she wrote a month later to her friend, "the same slowdown had occurred each time they strapped me into the monitors trapping me in the bed. . . . As soon as there was medical intervention, the contractions tapered off in reaction to it—an opposite response to what the doctors wished to achieve." When her doctor checked again, only to find that cervical dilation still remained static, he announced Mary must have an intravenous Pitocin drip. She was not happy with that plan. During her pregnancy, she had read about the sudden, powerful contractions caused by the synthetic hormone. "I was afraid of losing control."[27]

At that point, however, she was starting to blame herself, rather than doctors, medical interventions, or hospital rules, for her predicament. "My body was not cooperating and not responding as I had expected it to." At 2 p.m., the doctor started the Pitocin drip. As Mary had feared, her physical reaction was strong. "The contractions began to creep up on me with a vengeance. . . . They came right up my spine, centering their fury at the small of my back, radiating out to the top of my uterus, then receding after a prolonged plateau period." Michael became essential to her well-being—"his calming voice" helped her maintain focus. "I managed to get through 4 hours of heavy contractions with his encouragement, without taking any sedatives or painkillers."[28]

Mary continued to blame herself. "I suppose if I had not been so anxious to have a 'natural' delivery, the measures taken by the doctors might not have had so much bearing on the contractions." She imagined her "old uterus" was the likely source of her lack of progress: "my doctor did say it might indeed be due to my age that I didn't dilate—old, unused muscle that didn't know how to do it?" At 5 p.m., a doctor informed her that she was still only five centimeters dilated. Now Mary's obstetrician told her he was worried that when her cervix did "finally" dilate fully, she would be too exhausted to push. "Everything I had hoped would not happen to me . . . was happening. I felt broken. But here I was in the middle of this mess & there was no out."[29]

To enhance their ability to monitor the fetal heartbeat, nurses ran an electrode through Mary's vagina and attached it to her baby's scalp. "So much for 'natural' childbirth," Mary wrote later. "I was attached to modern technology by an IV with a contraction-inducing drug and a glucose bag; by a 3-inch belt fastened hard around my belly measuring mountains of contractions and I had a wire coming out of my crotch measuring my baby's heartbeat." And now doctors threatened her with something else: "one more hour to go or they would cut me open." The contractions grew in strength. Mary tried to relax, but each contraction made her startle "in a sort of maniacal terror."[30]

At 6 p.m., "in came the doctor again. . . . It was clear that a caesarean was the only way out. . . . A weasel of an anesthesiologist came to 'discuss' the virtues of spinal vs. epidural anesthetics." The anesthesiologist told Mary he preferred spinals, so she chose a spinal. "I thought if he doesn't like epidurals perhaps he would fuck it up—better go with the spinal." Michael left the room to don scrubs in preparation for the surgery. "He was so much my mainstay that just having him away for a short period of time was unnerving and unpleasant."[31]

In the operating room, "15–20 people whirring about doing things" surrounded Mary. Someone strapped her arms down. The anesthesiologist administered the spinal. "I more or less shut out the fact that it was *me* that all these people were milling about for & it was me they were operating on." Suddenly she heard a baby cry. Someone held up her son for her to see. "I was shocked, where did they get this baby?" Then they whisked him away. They put an oxygen mask over Mary's face. She threw up. When nurses brought her son back, Michael held him "close & high on his chest: we both cried—he was beautiful." Later, in a letter to her newborn son, Mary summed up the birth this way: "I went into labor, went to the hospital, things did not progress normally so after several hours and various attempts to induce dilation by artificial means, a caesarean was done on me & [you were] born."[32]

Four years later, when Mary gave birth to her second child by emergency cesarean section, she approached birth with a markedly different attitude. After her son was born, she suffered two early miscarriages that influenced her desires for the course of her next birth far more than the disappointment she felt about having a cesarean. When a doctor confirmed her latest pregnancy, "I wanted to have the baby so bad I did not care how she was born." Michael noticed her transformed outlook immediately, observing that this time Mary was indeed "happy to answer" to the doctors and nurses. "Yep," Mary agreed, I "just let them do what they wanted. . . . Maybe if I had not had those miscarriages . . . I would have been more adamant again about giving birth vaginally."[33]

During labor, the fetal monitor indicated an abnormal fetal heart rate. The obstetrician on duty applied forceps. "And that was like, oh God, that was hell!" After forceps failed to deliver the baby, the doctor decided to perform a cesarean, deeming the situation so urgent that she told Michael he could not be present. Mary did not care. Two miscarriages put her second cesarean in a different light than the first. After her daughter was born, Mary was delighted when she "saw her straight away—they put her on my chest."[34]

Mothers Are Resigned

Just as Mary had resigned herself during her second pregnancy to whatever treatments doctors and nurses thought best, negative experiences impelled other mothers to accept medical procedures they might otherwise have questioned. Although Joan had never had a miscarriage before she became pregnant at age 38 in 1992 with her first child, a difficult pregnancy prompted her to put herself in doctors' hands. An early, routine ultrasound examination revealed placenta previa. Her obstetrician immediately referred her to a colleague specializing in high-risk pregnancies. That doctor told Joan that placenta previa required a cesarean, and during their numerous appointments he helped her to accept that. Joan liked him; they had a good rapport. Whenever she came in for her monthly prenatal exam, she announced herself by joking, "It's your elderly primipara." She always made him laugh. "We enjoyed each other. It was a good match."[35]

Despite her solid relationship with her obstetrician, Joan could not help but worry. At 10 weeks' gestation, she underwent chorionic villus sampling (CVS) to check the fetus for genetic disorders and chromosomal abnormalities. A week later, a story linking CVS to abnormal finger development in fetuses was national news. After the story broke, whenever Joan had an ultrasound she begged the technician to pay close attention to the baby's hands. Each time, the technician assured her that everything looked fine. Joan was not mollified. "Oh it was horrible! . . . I was just trudging forward to an uncertain outcome. . . . I might not survive. The baby might not survive. It may not have fingers."[36]

After a bleeding episode at the beginning of her third trimester, a common side effect of placenta previa, Joan's obstetrician hospitalized her for observation. Upon releasing her, he ordered her to stay in bed. Joan found bed rest especially difficult. "I was worried every single second." Although she had neither Google nor laptop to enhance her fears—"This was all before the Internet!"—she had spent time in the library early in her pregnancy to learn about placenta previa. Her diligence "over-prepared" her for everything that could go wrong.[37]

At 39 weeks, Joan checked into the hospital for a scheduled c-section. She was "speechless with fear, but I knew I was going to get some kind of relaxing drug or something like that." The epidural did not take full effect, however—her husband said later that he thought the anesthetic had been weakened by Joan's adrenalin-fueled terror—so when her obstetrician made his incision, she felt "terrible pain."

Despite the pain, she kept asking "what's the baby like, what's the baby like?" When she heard someone say, "Apgar 9," she knew everything was fine. After the delivery, the anesthesiologist administered general anesthesia so the obstetrician could stitch Joan up. She awoke later with a scratchy throat. Her husband was watching television. When one of the residents came in to check on her, he admired her abdominal scar: "Oooh, fancy." Joan remembered thinking that there was a "bright side to all this—I have a beautiful scar . . . sewn to perfection."[38]

Joan had no regrets about the experience. "I had a fleeting moment of 'jeez, many women get to have this great, alert birth experience,' but that was just so irrelevant because my son was there and he looked great." And, ultimately, she credited the surgery with her success breastfeeding. She had to stay in the hospital for five days, and her son did not start breastfeeding until the last day, with the help of a "brilliant lactation consultant" who worked on the maternity floor. Joan thinks that, if not for the cesarean and the lengthy hospital stay it demanded, the "whole nursing thing, which was the one thing that worked great . . . might not have happened."[39]

"Saving Me and My Baby"

As the cesarean rate increased, women became accustomed to anticipating that their birth might end in a c-section. Increasingly, they characterized their surgeries as life-saving, no matter the reason doctors performed them. "The pioneer woman would have died in my situation" was how Joan summed up her son's birth. Karen, who gave birth to her first child in 1996, felt similarly. Although she had expected to "go natural," she was not afraid of a cesarean. She herself had been born by cesarean section due to a placental abruption, so she knew that the surgery had likely saved her own, and possibly her mother's, life.[40]

During a routine prenatal exam, Karen's doctor told her that she had "very small pelvic bones" and probably would not be able to deliver any baby weighing more than eight pounds. She did not question his assessment. "I really trusted this doctor. He had the lowest c-section rate in the area"—21 percent. Karen contacted her older siblings who already had children, and learned that big babies ran in the family. At that point, she "knew darn well I wasn't going to have an eight-pound baby. I knew it was going to be more than that." From the start, a cesarean seemed to be a distinct possibility.[41]

A week past her baby's due date, Karen went to the hospital for a routine ultrasound. Her baby's heart rate appeared to be problematic. "And they said, 'you know, it's time. We're going to need to induce.'" Karen was disappointed. She had been hoping to avoid pain medication, and "I knew that the labor is more intense when it's induced versus not induced." Adding to her stress, months earlier one of her sisters asked to be at the birth. At the last minute, though, her sister decided not to come and told their mother to go in her place. "Without asking me! So my Mom shows up and . . . I really don't want to give birth with my mother in the room!" So, when doctors announced that they would perform a cesarean after Pitocin failed, and that her mother would not be allowed in the operating room, Karen was relieved. "I was like 'FINE, go for it!'" The baby, at 9 pounds 2 ounces, was well over the 8-pound limit set by Karen's doctor.[42]

Pregnant again three years later, Karen told her obstetrician that she wanted a VBAC. "He said 'as long as the baby is less than eight pounds you will be fine.'" Toward the end of the pregnancy, the doctor estimated Karen's baby weighed "around" 8 pounds. But he told her he would not permit a vaginal birth after the baby's due date. Consequently, Karen gave birth via a planned cesarean section to a baby weighing 9 pounds 12 ounces on the baby's due date. Today, she characterizes each cesarean as "saving me and my baby. . . . I really do feel strongly that I would have been one of those women who would have died in childbirth. I feel that . . . based on the fact that [my doctor] said that I have small pelvic bones." By the turn of the twenty-first century, the cesarean rate had been high for 20 years, and many women, like Karen, tended to accept their cesareans with equanimity—as either the way their babies had to be born or simply the way they had been born.[43]

Ashley typified those women. She gave birth to three children by cesarean, the first in 2003 when she was 30 and the last in 2012. At her first birth, nurses and doctors forbade her to eat during the 12 "long, boring" hours of labor. At the 12-hour mark, a doctor told her she was not progressing. Although he encouraged her to labor a little longer, he "also talked about the size of [the baby's] head" and advised her to talk to her husband about having a cesarean. Ashley deemed his suggestion absurd. "I would be the one that would be cut." She immediately consented to the surgery. "My feeling was that if we're just going to lay here the rest of the night and not progress, let's get this over with." In the operating room, attending physicians described each step of the surgery to Ashley. Even though she could not see what they were doing, she felt involved. The baby's Apgar scores were 9 and 10. Later, Ashley had no regrets about the birth; quite the contrary. "I was very happy with it."[44]

Four years later, at an early prenatal appointment, she asked her physician about having a vaginal delivery. Her assured her that he would monitor her closely and promised to discuss with her the viability of vaginal birth toward the end of the pregnancy. Eventually, she asked point blank what type of birth the doctor thought would be best. He responded, "cesarean section." If he had recommended a vaginal birth, she said later, "I would have done it." Her second son, just like her first, had Apgars of 9 and 10.[45]

When she was pregnant with her third baby, Ashley had high blood pressure and anemia; her platelets kept dropping. Although the baby was due in mid-August, the doctor decided to perform a cesarean at the end of the third week in July. Even if she had wanted a VBAC, doctors would have nixed it. The obstetric practice she used for all three of her births forbade vaginal birth after two cesareans. In any event, "it was not an issue" for her.[46]

Mitigating Risk, Providing Choice, or Pathologizing Birth?

By the end of the twentieth century, books and articles about cesarean section presented a perspective contrary to the angry pieces penned by birth reformers two and three decades earlier. Rather than denounce unnecessary medical interventions and the technologies that might have prompted them, the publications urged women to prepare themselves for "the strong possibility of unplanned cesarean birth." Although all childbirth educators, no matter their stance on cesareans, agreed on at least one message—"The right way to give birth is any way that minimizes the risk of harm to you and your baby"—by the 1990s, many of the authors of childbirth education material focusing on cesareans associated minimizing risk with cesarean surgery; at least one author argued that any risks associated with a first cesarean were so exaggerated as to be misleading.[47]

The prevailing messages about risk and cesarean surgery—one predominating in the 1970s, the other by the late 1990s—reflected two schools of thought that should not have been mutually exclusive. Childbirth educators in the earlier era tended to favor "natural" childbirth—that is, no medical intervention during labor without medical justification. Authors writing in the later era focused on respecting and validating the experience of women who had given birth by cesarean, whatever the reason. Although the two positions were not inherently contradictory, the two factions found themselves at odds. One group wanted a lower cesarean rate; the other called for acceptance of cesarean birth and, by implication, approval of the status quo. The latter position prevailed as cesarean surgery came to be characterized as a valid option, not to be questioned once chosen.[48]

Representing a cesarean section as a reproductive choice changed the nature of the conversation. In the context of human reproduction, American feminists have called for what they now term "women's right to choose" several times in US history. In the late nineteenth and early twentieth centuries, Progressive Era activists implied a right to reproductive choice when they dubbed women's demand for ready access to reliable contraceptive devices "voluntary motherhood." Decades later, in objecting to the rigid, involuntary nature of postwar obstetric treatments, women demanded options: home birth, hospital birth, birth at freestanding birthing centers, midwife-attended birth, obstetrician-attended birth, family-physician-attended birth, and, especially, the right to accept, or reject, any diagnostic tool and medical treatment offered during pregnancy and labor. Most famously today, feminists coined the descriptor "pro-choice" to counter the "pro-life" terminology used in the late-twentieth-century political arena by opponents of legal access to abortion. In invoking this terminology, feminists employed the concept of "choice" in the same way nineteenth-century feminists used the word "voluntary"—to indicate that women needed options, particularly in matters relating to reproduction, if they were to keep themselves and their children safe and well.[49]

Second-wave feminists employed the concept of "choice" so effectively that in the 1990s physicians and their professional organizations adopted the terminology to serve their own interests. When insurance companies began to deny women's claims for epidural anesthesia if there was no medical justification for its use, the American College of Obstetricians and Gynecologists (ACOG) and the American Society of Anesthesiologists (ASA) issued a joint *Committee Opinion* stating, "Maternal request is a sufficient justification for pain relief during labor." Two years later, after studies demonstrated that administering epidural anesthesia before the cervix had dilated five centimeters increased the likelihood of cesarean delivery, many doctors and hospitals responded by refusing to administer an epidural before the five-centimeter benchmark. The two organizations reiterated their position that doctors should accede to a maternal request for an epidural at any point during labor. In sanctioning the maternal-choice epidural, the two organizations paved the way for what became known in the medical literature as cesarean delivery by maternal request (CDMR).[50]

With cesarean section now characterized as a "choice," some in the medical community began to use the classification to quash public and medical debate about the cesarean rate. After the US Public Health Service (USPHS) listed a 15 percent cesarean rate as one of its goals in *Healthy People 2000*—a compendium of health objectives for the US populace to be achieved by the new millennium—the *New England Journal of Medicine* editorialized that the target represented "an authoritarian approach to health care delivery" that implied "women should have no say in their own care." By invoking feminist rhetoric, the physicians and organizations denouncing the 15 percent goal effectively cowed those who believed performing medically unnecessary surgery on women was no boon to women's rights. The dual charges of authoritarianism and chauvinism appealed not only to the faction of obstetricians who did not consider the cesarean rate to be a problem but also to a generation of women who had grown up in a world where the concept of reproductive choice was a given. *Vogue* magazine referred to elective c-sections as "the *other* debate over a woman's right to choose."[51]

Some leaders in the obstetric field were especially supportive of the concept of maternal-request cesareans. Benson Harer, the president of ACOG in 2000, used his bully pulpit to explicitly sanction it. In his ACOG presidential address, he celebrated an array of hard-won women's rights—suffrage, owning property, broadened economic and political opportunities, access to effective contraception, and safe, legal abortions. The "only remaining exception," he contended, was "a woman's right to choose, after being informed of risks and benefits, whether to deliver her baby by the vaginal or cesarean route." While the feminists who employed "choice" rhetoric in the late 1970s to champion birth reform would never have endorsed maternal-choice cesareans—they demanded fewer medical interventions, not more—times had changed.[52]

Some female physicians specializing in women's health joined Harer in endorsing CDMR. A New York plastic surgeon who gave birth to her second child by elective cesarean section decried "this whole crazy movement . . . toward natural childbirth—getting no anesthesia, getting no medicine, because somehow medicine is bad." She characterized vaginal birth as a "barbaric ritual, and I think it's insane." In what was becoming the prevailing tone in both lay and medical discussions about "choice" in relation to childbirth, the New York surgeon first championed choice and then immediately condemned any choice other than her own.[53]

While ACOG never officially endorsed Harer's stance, the organization issued a *Committee Opinion* in 2003 defending the right of well-informed patients to choose a cesarean section. Four years later, the organization issued a second opinion that described one benefit of CDMR (a decreased risk of maternal hemorrhage) and several risks (longer stays in the hospital, newborn respiratory problems, and complications in subsequent pregnancies, including life-threatening ones such as uterine rupture and placental anomalies) but did not outright condemn the practice.[54]

Not until 2013 did ACOG's guidelines on CDMR change in tone and emphasis. In contrast to the 2007 document, this time the organization listed risks before benefits and described any benefits as merely "short-term." Because no study had ever objectively or systematically assessed the risks and benefits of vaginal birth versus CDMR, but the medical community well knew that major surgery always carries risks, ACOG now urged obstetricians to recommend vaginal delivery to mothers seeking a cesarean in the absence of maternal or fetal indications.[55]

Despite the prolonged, public debate, CDMR appears to be an insignificant practice. Surveys of mothers indicate that primary cesareans prompted solely by maternal request, without any medical indication, represent only about 1 percent of all primary cesareans. What makes maternal-choice cesareans noteworthy is not their number, which is small, but the public conversations the concept has promoted. Indeed, CDMR has been used quite effectively as a red herring, whether intentionally or not, by the physicians who defend it. Characterizing any surgery that is associated with dangerous side effects as simply "a choice" downplays the seriousness of the procedure. And the very concept of maternal-choice cesareans implies that mothers share responsibility for the effects of the high cesarean rate.[56]

Privately, obstetricians remain divided on the issue. "If this was the only pregnancy in a 42-year-old who had been trying to get pregnant for the last seven years, no problem with that," said one obstetrician. A younger patient would be a different matter, however. "If this was a 22-year-old who is just concerned that she may have pain, then I'd try and say, 'We have things to deal with pain.'" Yet the physician admitted that she would agree to the surgery if any patient insisted, no matter their age or circumstance. "I would say now, versus 25 years ago, I wouldn't force someone to go into labor and refuse her a c-section." Another obstetrician, while regretting "encouraging that degree of medicalization" of childbirth, likewise affirmed the right of her patients to make an informed decision even if she disagreed with it.[57]

Other obstetricians, however, refused to equivocate about CDMR. A second-year obstetric resident said, "We were taught that that was bad . . . from day one of intern year. Hospitals should not do that, not good." Maternal-choice cesareans were "unacceptable," she explained, because the complications arising from any unnecessary surgery could never be justified. "We have seen horrific wound infections, I mean people whose skin stays open for months, packed with gauze and smelling terrible, who are in so much pain." Another obstetrician was equally adamant. "Elective primaries? No. I never did one and I never would." Just as in the nineteenth and early twentieth centuries, fundamental disagreements among obstetricians remain ongoing. The argument about the cesarean section rate is only the latest controversy.[58]

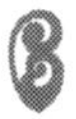

In the nineteenth century, physicians viewed cesarean section as the riskiest of surgeries. Only a few ever performed one, and even then, exceedingly rarely. As late as 1960, doctors were still performing the surgery infrequently enough that whenever a writer mentioned a cesarean in a newspaper or magazine article, he made sure that the strange word was accompanied by a definition. By 1970, however, the surgery was common knowledge. Ten years later, obstetricians were performing cesareans so often that federal government agencies issued several alarming reports about the phenomenon. Although the reports offered some suggestions to lower the rate, any efforts adopted by obstetricians and hospitals to stem c-sections were ultimately abandoned. By the early twenty-first century, cesarean section had become the most commonly performed surgery in the country.[59]

On its face, this trend is puzzling. In the eighteenth, nineteenth, and early twentieth centuries, when lifespans were shorter, diets poorer, environments less sanitary, and effective medical treatments scarce to nonexistent, only about 5 percent of births ran into trouble according to midwives', physicians', and hospitals' birth records. Today, in contrast, American doctors deem 32 percent of births to be so difficult they demand major abdominal surgery. Yet the extraordinary number of births ending in cesarean section since the mid-1980s has not resulted in improved maternal and infant outcomes; quite the contrary.

Many factors have contributed to the current numbers, few related to medical need. Instead, social and cultural phenomena in both the medical and lay communities have been the primary drivers of the cesarean rate. Medical and public embrace of diagnostic tools, such as the Friedman curve and the electronic fetal monitor, led to seemingly dire diagnoses despite the acknowledged high false positive rate for fetal hypoxia. An unsettling malpractice climate, prompted in no small part by the raft of dire diagnoses, created the concept of "defensive medicine." Reliance on machines weakened obstetricians' hands-on skills. The ubiquitous fetal monitor created what one physician characterized as a "default invasiveness" during even the most uneventful births, encouraging the view that childbirth is a naturally trouble-prone process requiring routine medical interventions. With the risks of vaginal birth and VBACs exaggerated, cesareans came to be viewed by doctors and patients alike as normal and necessary. As women's lives became busier and more complicated, the medical interventions that offered opportunities to schedule births and reduce pain and discomfort during labor seemed to be far more helpful than invasive. Some of the interventions, particularly labor induction, led to more cesareans. In this environment, a high cesarean section rate became a medical solution, not a medical problem.[60]

Cesarean sections have become so prevalent that the surgery, particularly the notion that it can be an elective surgery, is often satirized. In an episode of *Gilmore Girls*, first aired in the 2002–2003 television season, Sherry Tinsdale is pregnant with her first child. As a largely undeveloped minor character, she is the perfect target for mockery—the show's writers have not bothered to exhibit her strengths, only her easily ridiculed flaws. She is artificially perky and hyperfocused on her career, displaying a burning need to appear in control even when she is not. In the weeks before she is due to give birth, she sends invitations to friends heralding her upcoming elective cesarean section. As though the planned surgery were a wedding or a baby shower, she lists the place, date, and time her guests are to gather to witness and cheer her through the surgery. But Sherry's careful plans go awry when she goes into spontaneous labor the week before the scheduled celebration. One annoyed friend must take a break from her busy work day to call other invitees to explain the sudden glitch: "She screwed up. She's in labor. . . . She completely screwed up." In the meantime, Sherry, the would-be hostess of the cesarean party, lies in her hospital bed, sobbing between contractions: "I would love to go back to work, but I can't because I have to stay here. This wasn't supposed to happen until next week. I wrote it down. I can't just stop everything. . . . I had it planned." In this satire of the normalization of cesarean surgery, an unproblematic, spontaneous labor becomes the unforeseen, challenging emergency.[61]

As we became capable of controlling more—our food supply, indoor spaces, public health, and individual well-being—we began to magnify the threat of anything beyond our control. Macro-level fears of birth soon played out on a micro-level as first obstetricians, and eventually mothers, unintentionally created a synergy that ensured the normalization of cesarean section. One obstetrician explained the current high cesarean rate as being partly "patient-driven . . . because they see online . . . about the risk, that they don't want VBAC . . . they don't want to have vaginal twin delivery because of the risk." She acknowledged, however, that she and her colleagues play a far larger role than mothers. "We're all very comfortable doing c-sections." In the past, she observed, obstetricians did not hesitate to hold out for a vaginal birth. But, she admitted, "It's more common now, with the patient's input too, to say, 'Let's do a c-section.'"[62] As her words imply, the medical complacency toward cesareans eventually led to public complacency. Since 1970, obstetricians and pregnant women have gone from anticipating vaginal birth in virtually every instance to anticipating cesarean birth as a distinct possibility in every instance.

The consequences of this lax attitude toward cesareans are becoming clearer. The United States is currently an outlier among Western countries—maternal mortality is increasing rather than decreasing. From 7.2 maternal deaths per 100,000 births in 1987 to an estimated 23.8 in 2014, the upward trajectory has been described in newspaper headlines as "shocking" and a "national embarrassment." Admittedly, a portion of this increase is due to a change in data gathering. In 2003, the standard US death certificate added a series of checkbox questions to determine if the decedent had been pregnant at the time of death, within 42 days of death, or within a year of death. States slowly adopted the change; each year a few additional states added the questions, the last in 2017. While the questions have rectified at least some of the chronic underreporting of maternal deaths in the United States, the new checkboxes also created another problem. Researchers have found that the questions on pregnancy invariably produce false positive responses—deaths categorized as related to childbirth that were not. Doubt about the reliability of data has been so significant that at no time in the last decade has the US issued an official maternal mortality rate.[63]

US public health officials nevertheless admit that maternal mortality in the United States is significantly higher than in any other wealthy country. Texas's maternal death rate, at 35.8 per 100,000, is virtually identical to Malaysia's, Egypt's, and Mexico's. Indeed, the maternal mortality and morbidity rates in the United States are so uncharacteristically high for a wealthy nation that there have been calls to return "the 'M' to maternal-fetal medicine." Although in the nineteenth and first half of the twentieth centuries, obstetrics centered on ensuring mothers' well-being, public health professionals, physicians, and researchers alike now complain that while "the health care system focuses on babies [it] often ignores their mothers." The lack of official data has become a sign of the gravity of the problem. As Stacie Geller, an epidemiologist who is one of the most prominent scholars of women's health in the US, observes, "Preventable maternal deaths are not in the basement of our priorities, they are in the sub-basement." While it is impossible to know precisely how the 31.9 percent cesarean rate reported in 2015 contributes to the nation's maternal mortality—those statistics have never been compiled—one study found, after eliminating all deaths from prenatal morbidities, that the risk of postpartum death was 3.6 times higher after a cesarean birth than after a vaginal birth. Maternal morbidity rates also hold a clue to the effect of a high cesarean rate. Since 1999, postpartum complications have increased by 75 percent, and the most serious complications are related to cesarean surgery—pulmonary embolism, infection, hemorrhage, and placental anomalies.[64]

Obstetricians provide compelling anecdotal evidence of the seriousness of the problem. One obstetrician described a recent patient who exhibited "a really, really awful wound" after an elective cesarean. "She had to keep coming to the office over and over for packing and treatment and whatnot." The obstetrician worried most, though, about one of the deadliest downstream effects of cesarean surgery. "In my mind," she said, "I'm always thinking, 'my God, accretas.'" A retired obstetrician, who was still shaken by a maternal death at his hospital from an accreta caused by a previous cesarean, described the mother's death with horrifying succinctness: "72 units of blood, the entire hospital stopped." A cesarean today, he lamented, too often leads "to the complications [of] tomorrow." Another obstetrician likewise alluded to placenta accreta. "We're killing women with all these cesareans and it always comes back to the same thing." The only way to bring down the cesarean rate, she explained, is for birth attendants to have the skill to avoid a mother's first cesarean. "We've known this since the seventies. You prevent that first cesarean and that's how you prevent your cesarean delivery rate getting too high." She thought it was well past time for obstetricians' professional organizations "to come together and ban, or nearly ban, strategies and procedures that increase cesarean deliveries, like induction of labor." Another obstetrician, in describing how to avoid a cesarean, unwittingly repeated the advice that had appeared consistently in obstetric textbooks 150 years ago: be patient. Especially with first-time mothers, she said, "Allow them a little bit more time. As long as the baby looks ok, give them their chance to labor."[65]

By the end of the twentieth century, though, that advice was hard to follow. Increasingly, the threat to infants seemed to be in *not* doing the surgery. The medical perceptions of labor created by the Friedman curve and Apgar and Bishop scores demonstrated the power of a numerical standard. In judging the prevalence of risk according to a number—the amount of time spent in labor in the case of the Friedman curve, a newborn's condition in the case of the Apgar score, and the state of the cervix in the case of the Bishop score—the seemingly objective numbers dictated that an action had to be taken if any number veered from the standard, even if, especially in the case of the Friedman curve, physicians could not always be certain what the number signified.

Messages issued by the electronic fetal monitor were even more compelling. When the machine said the fetus was in distress, doctors responded by emotionally blackmailing mothers. To ensure consent for a cesarean they offered an impossible choice—do you want to risk damage to your baby's brain or its very life, or do you want a cesarean section? Though physicians did not intend the choice as blackmail, that nevertheless has been its effect. Time and again, obstetricians used their professional authority to steer women in one direction despite the dubious nature of the monitor's messages. As one obstetrician observed, "I think if you told a mother that you'd have to cut off her arm to get a healthy baby she'd say, 'Go ahead, just give me anesthesia.'"[66]

The fetal monitor not only heightened physicians' and patients' perception of the risk of childbirth, its use ensured that obstetricians would become less adept at executing the maneuvers that ensured a vaginal birth. When the monitor, rather than the obstetric resident, became the observer, obstetric residents had far fewer opportunities to learn about the rhythms of labor. As the electronic fetal monitor, and eventually ultrasound equipment, seemed to offer more, and more accurate, information than whatever an obstetrician could learn with her hands, external palpation became a lost, or at least a greatly diminished, art. As cesareans became safer, the use of forceps, a far more difficult skill to teach and learn than cesarean surgery, became passé. And "if you don't [use forceps]," noted one obstetrician, "you do a c-section."[67]

Thus far, physicians and hospitals have proven stubbornly resistant to changing the practices and tempering the views that maintain the cesarean rate and its ill effects. As Helen Marieskind noted in her 1979 study *An Evaluation of Caesarean Section in the United States*, the "interventionist approach" to obstetrics had become so pervasive and well-accepted by the 1970s that the cesarean rate, and the factors spurring its rise, were not conducive to objective study. While the first part of the history of cesarean sections in the United States—from the early nineteenth century through World War II—was one dominated by medical deliberation, with physicians determinedly keeping cesareans rare and taking pride in the skills allowing them to do so, the most recent portion of the history has been dominated by uncontrolled experimentation.[68]

Marieskind summed up this latter-day approach to the surgery in her report for the US Department of Health, Education, and Welfare: "Caesarean section appears to be a sometimes useful and much needed technology presently utilized in an undocumented, unclarified, and uncontrolled manner." Introducing electronic fetal monitoring without any proof of efficacy, and then ignoring studies demonstrating that the technology was largely ineffective and increased the cesarean rate to boot, exemplified that trend. The varied cesarean section rates around the country are another indication of the "uncontrolled manner" of cesarean surgeries—from 7.1 percent of all births in one hospital to 69.9 percent in another. The biggest risk for having a cesarean birth in the United States today is not a condition detected during pregnancy, or even during labor, but the hospital a mother enters to deliver her baby. Even among hospitals treating patients from similar socioeconomic backgrounds with similar forms of insurance coverage, the cesarean rates vary dramatically—from 53.5 percent in one hospital located in a largely white, affluent community in New York's Westchester County to 18.4 percent in another hospital also catering to a largely white, affluent community but this one on the New York–New Jersey border.[69]

In grappling with the multiple causes of the high rate of cesarean births in the late 1970s, a rate less than half what it is today, Marieskind wrote, "the question must be raised as to how much a climate accepting of C-sections, in and of itself promotes more Cesareans." Few in the medical community heeded her veiled warning. Rather than characterizing the unnecessary, or only marginally necessary, cesarean as risky for mothers and their infants, doctors instead came to view the surgery as both a safety net for the seemingly dangerous unpredictability of vaginal birth and an acceptable choice no matter the circumstance. Social factors that have influenced trends in medical and popular culture have shaped those perceptions, rather than the evidence-based medicine that physicians are taught to rely on.[70]

As part of a wider culture, medicine can never be truly value-free. But once a problem created by medicine has been recognized, it can and should be remedied. In the 1970s and early 1980s, some obstetricians and the public health community attempted to mitigate the cesarean rate, with only sporadic and temporary success. In questioning the need for their own cesareans, some mothers drew short-lived attention to the problem. Government agencies commissioned reports to little avail. Obstetricians' professional organizations have equivocated when confronted with the problem. Insurers have done nothing, perhaps due to the experience of the National Health Service in the United Kingdom—when the NHS attempted to eliminate medically unnecessary cesareans by withholding payment for them, the backlash was ferocious.

With physicians, professional organizations, patients, government agencies, and insurers unable to solve the problem individually or collectively thus far, perhaps widespread educational efforts that spark public discussion can. The United States has seen many largely successful public health campaigns that altered individual behaviors and views, both historically in the late nineteenth century (to bathe, to keep food on ice, not to spit in public) as well as more recently (to quit smoking, to use seat belts, not to drive drunk). One especially hopes that it will not require some high-profile deaths, or thus far undiscovered links to illnesses and conditions that can be precipitated by cesarean birth in susceptible children, to spark a robust conversation about the unnecessarily high cesarean section rate and its consequences.[71]

We are unlikely to be able to undo some of the steps that led us here. Obstetrics and gynecology, for example, are likely to remain conjoined despite the fact that the merger in the 1930s turned obstetrics into a surgical specialty. But we can enhance departments of obstetrics and gynecology by ensuring that all of them include experts in spontaneous vaginal birth. In other words, every department of obstetrics and gynecology at a medical school should have certified nurse-midwives on their faculty. Not only obstetrician/gynecologists but also midwives should participate in the training of obstetric residents. Obstetricians' professional societies can help mitigate the cesarean rate by issuing guidelines that clearly state that an elective cesarean, indeed any medically unnecessary surgery, comes with risks that cannot be justified. As such, elective cesareans are unethical. The criteria for medically necessary cesareans should be equally explicit. Obstetricians' professional organizations should ensure that their members neither embrace nor employ any medical technology or diagnostic tool until it has been tested according to the gold standard—the randomized, controlled trial. Medical interventions known to increase the cesarean rate, such as labor induction and the electronic fetal monitor, should be employed only for compelling medical reasons rather than routinely. And, recalling that when some hospitals in the 1980s required physicians to post their cesarean rates, the rates at those hospitals decreased significantly, each hospital in the United States should be instructed to make its cesarean rate, and the indications for all cesareans performed at the institution, public. Concrete data always contribute to the formulation of sound solutions. Emphasizing the realities of human birth can also help to alter attitudes and reshape the current American way of birth: Good outcomes are likely; bad outcomes are rare. Birth requires patience, for first-time mothers in particular. Physicians should not routinely employ medical interventions at all births in order to thwart the rare bad outcome; interventions carry their own (too often unnecessary) risks. All things being equal, a spontaneous labor ending in a vaginal birth benefits newborns as well as mothers and should be encouraged and nurtured by medical personnel. Instituting these basic guidelines would result in a tangible benefit for mothers, children, and the healthcare system: cesarean birth that is safe and rare.

Acknowledgments

This social history of cesarean sections in the United States is a complicated one. During the research phase of this book, the list of factors relevant to the increase in cesareans kept growing. Amassing that amount of data requires a good deal of help. On the most basic level, historians cannot find what they are looking for without the help of librarians and archivists. I am indebted to Debra Scarborough and Mary Hyde of the American College of Obstetricians and Gynecologists. On my many visits to their library, Debra gave me the run of ACOG's unparalleled collection of books and ephemera in women's health and medicine. Mary responded quickly over the years to my stream of requests for ACOG policies on everything from electronic fetal monitoring to maternity coverage to labor induction to vaginal birth after a previous cesarean. Elaine Challacombe, Lois Hendrickson, and Chris Herzberg helped make my visits to the Wangensteen Historical Library of Biology and Medicine at the University of Minnesota especially productive. Elaine had the foresight to purchase the marvelous Robert Harris papers and scanned items from the collection for me. At one point, while perusing the Harris papers, I made a stunning find: a letter written in the 1880s by a woman expressing gratitude for her unspecified 1843 surgery. Initially, I thought I had discovered a woman's description of her own cesarean section. Lois and Chris were on it immediately. Within minutes, Lois had verified that the woman's surgeon had graduated from the University of Pennsylvania medical school in 1820 and that the surgeon's son, the recipient of the woman's letter, was indeed the son of the original surgeon. Meanwhile, Chris went to track down the 1844 article about the woman's surgery written by the original surgeon. Alas, the surgery was not a cesarean section but an oophorectomy. Nevertheless, discovering a nineteenth-century patient's firsthand description of her reproductive surgery, without anesthesia, was thrilling. And watching a team of crackerjack archivists tracking down clues to substantiate the letter was equally exciting.

Stacey Peeples, lead archivist of the Pennsylvania Hospital historic collections, was unwavering in her attempts to open up as much of their collection to me as possible. She, too, was frustrated by HIPAA, a law which never considered the needs of the historian to study the medical records of people long dead, the obligation of institutions to share their archives with historians, and the care historians of medicine take to protect all patients' privacy. Sue Sacharski, the archivist at Northwestern Memorial Hospital in Chicago, is as delighted by the Joseph DeLee papers and the Chicago Maternity Center papers as the historians she guides through them. Russell Koonts, director of the Duke University Medical Center archives, pointed me to appropriate collections during my visits and, before I arrived, shepherded my application through the internal review board so that I could view those collections. His colleague, Rebecca Williams, quickly transcribed part of an oral history interview for me when I realized, long after I came home, that the original transcript was incomplete. Arlene Shaner, the historical collections librarian at the New York Academy of Medicine, directed me to some marvelous collections there. Brian McNerney at the Lyndon Baines Johnson Library and Museum patiently explained to me the art of "drilling down" to find what I was looking for in collections that did not appear immediately relevant to my work. Thanks, too, to Jim Gehrlich of New York–Presbyterian / Weil Cornell Medical Center Archives, who had dozens of cesarean section casebooks waiting for me upon my arrival. I am also indebted to Alex Welborn, head archivist at the University Kansas Medical Center, who made my brief time there so productive. Kristen Lynn Chinery at the Walter Reuther Library at Wayne State University was helpful, as were the reference staffs for the Sophia Smith Collection at Smith College and the Schlesinger Library at Harvard University.

Debi Orr, medical librarian extraordinaire at the Ohio University Heritage College of Osteopathic Medicine, has been my literature search hero. I only had to give her a topic, however vague, and she would find a trove of articles for me, often within hours. And then she would invariably follow up to see if I needed anything else.

Dozens of physicians in the Chicago area and in southern Ohio who performed cesareans between the 1940s and today, and dozens of mothers in the Chicago area and in southern Ohio who gave birth by cesarean between the early 1970s and today, generously shared their stories and perspectives with me. I would thank each by name, but the Ohio University Institutional Review Board insists that they remain anonymous.

I also received invaluable help from a stream of research assistants. Aalyia Sadruddin transcribed oral history interviews in her usual impeccable manner. Abby Huck spent a good part of the summer after her first year of medical school finding articles on childbirth and cesarean sections in popular magazines. Barbara Farley, a volunteer at Pennsylvania Hospital, took outstanding notes on the last four volumes of the maternity records I was allowed to view but did not have time to study during my visit. Oluwabukola Anuoluwapo Shaba took lists of daunting questions and found material that helped to answer those questions.

The patient, conscientious, and gifted Maryam Khaleghi Yazdi enhanced, and, in some instances, drew, the illustrations that dot this book. Working with her was a pleasure and very reassuring. From the moment we met, I knew the book's illustrations were in the best of hands.

My brother, Kevin Wolf, helped me not only with the Excel spreadsheets that logged cesarean and VBAC rates each year but with all things mathematical. Although not necessarily known for his patience, he was ever-patient with me, unfailingly responding to text messages that always asked some version of the following question: "If 33 percent of births are by cesarean, and 1 percent of cesareans are elective, what percentage of births are elective cesareans?" (I was sick during much of third grade and missed the arithmetic lessons on percentages, a deficiency that has dogged me ever since. Like a child raised by wild animals who missed the brief window to acquire language, no amount of explanation on how to figure percentages has ever sunk in, although Kevin has always gamely tried each time I ask for help.)

A three-year National Library of Medicine Scholarly Works in Biomedicine and Health Grant, an Ohio University College of Osteopathic Medicine Office of Research Direct Grant Award, and an Ohio University Research Challenge Grant all aided the research and writing of this book immeasurably.

Many colleagues and friends read all or part of this book, and the book has vastly improved thanks to their astute suggestions. Emily Abel, Wendy Kline, and Paul Milazzo each read several chapters. Paula Michaels, Steve Miner, Katherine Jellison, Jackie Wehmueller, Becky Kluchin, and Wanda Ronner read the entire book. To Steve and Katherine (and only recently Paul), who I have met with for years as the RRC (the Ruthless Readers' Club), I owe a special debt. Since we began our writers' group, we have produced among us four books and many articles and book chapters. I know my work would not be as good without their generosity, sharp eyes, talent, and honesty. Steve has been especially generous with his detailed suggestions, observations, and questions that sharpened the book's arguments, on call even on Sunday afternoons if I needed a quick assessment of any last-minute changes. Jackie Wehmueller, as my longtime (and now happily retired) editor at Johns Hopkins University Press, has always been generous, so generous that even in retirement she read my manuscript, tightened up language, and masterfully honed chapter titles and subheadings. Paula Michaels's comments were especially detailed, and the book has benefited from her smart page-by-page appraisal. It was my lucky day, after the two of us strangers had worked silently back to back for many hours doing research at the National Library of Medicine, when Steve Greenberg approached us to say that we really should talk to each other. Did we know that we were both working on the history of childbirth? And, finally and so importantly, historians of medicine depend on colleagues who are physicians to scan their books for medical accuracy. Wanda Ronner did that for this book, and her enthusiasm for the project was exactly what I needed to get me through the final months of rewriting.

Many medical historians will tell you that they did not attend graduate school with the intention of becoming a historian of medicine, nor did they specifically study the history of medicine in graduate school. Instead, many of us serendipitously tripped into the field. I owe that stumbling, rewarding entrance to my daughter, Cora. I was eight months pregnant when I sat for my master's exams in 1991 and still breastfeeding when I took my preliminary exams three years later. Caught in the midst of two activities—new motherhood and graduate school—that each suck time like a black hole sucks light, I melded the two by writing a dissertation on the history of breastfeeding practices in the United States in an unconscious effort to make life somewhat more coherent. And then there I was—a historian of women's health and medicine. Cora was my inspiration then; now that she has grown into a magnificent, wise, hard-working, compassionate, and generous young woman, she inspires me all the more.

Notes

INTRODUCTION: **From Risk to Remedy**

1. Cragin, "Conservatism in Obstetrics." Cragin has long been credited with this maxim, but there is evidence that it was medical custom long before 1916. Birch, "What You Should Know about Cesareans"; Gieske and Smith, "Boy Is Born to the Kennedys"; Perry, *Jacqueline Kennedy*, 63.

2. Placek and Taffel, "Recent Patterns in Cesarean Delivery"; Corea, "The Caesarean Epidemic"; Haseltine, "There Is No Mystery."

3. Leaming, *Mrs. Kennedy*, 13–14; Christopher Anderson, *Jack and Jackie*, 183; "How Many Caesareans?"; Marley, "Cesarean Baby Dangers."

4. Perry, *Jacqueline Kennedy*, 169–170; Smith, *Grace and Power*, 393–399; Leaming, *Mrs. Kennedy*, 296–304.

5. "The Whys of Caesareans." For a description of the effect of Patrick Kennedy's death on the development of a cure for hyaline membrane disease, see Haliday, "Surfactants," and Altman, "A Kennedy Baby's Life and Death." For a description of the public reaction to the birth and death of Patrick Kennedy, see Levingston, "For John and Jackie Kennedy."

6. The perspective of the few proponents of cesarean surgery in this era is best exemplified by Robert P. Harris's writings, discussed in chapter 1. The vast majority of physicians dismissed cesarean surgery as "sacrificial midwifery." Barnes, *Lectures on Obstetric Operations*, 312, 315.

7. David and David, "One in Five"; Placek and Taffel, "Recent Patterns"; Hamilton, Martin, and Ventura, "Births," 2; Grady, "Caesarean Births Are at a High"; for recent cesarean data consistently compiled from Centers for Disease Control statistics, see www.cdc.gov/nchs/fastats/delivery.htm.

8. Cord prolapse occurs in from 0.14 to 0.61 percent of births; most articles cite a 0.28 percent rate. See Uygur et al., "Risk Factors and Infant Outcomes." Placenta previa occurs in about 0.4 percent of births. See Faiz and Ananth, "Etiology and Risk Factors." Placental abruption occurs in 0.65 percent of births. See Ananth and Wilcox, "Placental Abruption and Perinatal Mortality." Transverse lie occurs in 0.12 percent of births. See Gardberg, Leonova, and Laakkonen, "Malpresentation"; Strong, *Expecting Trouble*, 3; Althabe and Belizán, "Caesarean Section." Some of the side effects of a high cesarean rate are discussed in World Health Organization, "WHO Statement on Caesarean Section Rates"; MacDorman et al., "Infant and Neonatal Mortality"; "Physiology of Fetal Lung Fluid Clearance"; Hansen et al., "Elective Caesarean Section"; Grolund et al., "Fecal Microflora in Healthy Infants"; Russell and Murch, "Could Peripartum Antibiotics Have

Delayed Health Consequences for the Infant?"; Penders et al., "Factors Influencing the Composition of the Intestinal Microbiota in Early Infancy"; Renz-Polster et al., "Caesarean Section Delivery"; Salam et al., "Mode of Delivery"; Deneux-Tharaux et al., "Postpartum Maternal Mortality and Cesarean Delivery."

9. Ulrich, *A Midwife's Tale*, 170–171; de Kruif, *The Fight for Life*, 100; Hooker and the New York Academy of Medicine Committee on Public Health Relations, *Maternal Mortality in New York City*, 116.

10. Cragin, "Conservatism in Obstetrics"; Williams, "Cesarean Section at the Johns Hopkins Hospital," 526.

11. Interview of obstetrician by author, Chicago physician interview 2, October 1, 2012, Chicago, IL, transcribed from digital recording.

12. Interview of mother by author, Chicago mother interview 2, March 13, 2012, Chicago, IL, transcribed from digital recording.

13. World Health Organization, "WHO Statement on Caesarean Section Rates"; MacDorman et al., "Infant and Neonatal Mortality"; Jain and Eaton, "Physiology of Fetal Lung Fluid Clearance"; Hansen et al., "Elective Caesarean Section"; Grolund et al., "Fecal Microflora in Healthy Infants"; Russell and Murch, "Could Peripartum Antibiotics Have Delayed Health Consequences for the Infant?"; Penders et al., "Factors Influencing the Composition of the Intestinal Microbiota in Early Infancy"; Renz-Polster et al., "Caesarean Section Delivery"; Salam et al., "Mode of Delivery." The importance of the human microbiome has now received so much attention that swabbing the newborn in a "vaginal microbial transfer" after a cesarean birth is under study. See Dominguez-Bello et al., "Partial Restoration of the Microbiota." On economic costs of cesareans, see Sakala and Corry, *Evidence-Based Maternity Care*.

14. Leth et al., "Risk of Selected Postpartum Infections"; MacDorman et al., "Infant and Neonatal Mortality"; Hansen et al., "Elective Cesarean Section"; Bréart, "Postpartum Maternal Mortality and Cesarean Delivery"; Nisenblat et al., "Maternal Complications Associated with Multiple Cesarean Deliveries"; Yang et al., "Association of Caesarean Delivery for First Birth." In 2002, the American College of Obstetricians and Gynecologists warned that the incidence of placenta accreta had increased and suggested that if a physician strongly suspected an accreta before delivery, the mother should be counseled about the likelihood of hysterectomy and blood transfusion ("Placenta Accreta"). Wu, Kocherginsky, and Hibbard, "Abnormal Placentation"; Gielchinsky et al., "Placenta Accreta"; Bretelle et al., "Management of Placenta Accrete"; interview of retired obstetrician by author, Chicago physician interview 8, October 5, 2012, Chicago, IL, transcribed from digital recording.

15. "Factbox: Ebola Cases in the United States"; Rothkopf, "Stephen Colbert." For a thorough analysis of how American physicians have come to focus more on alleviating risk than on illness, see Aronowitz, *Risky Medicine*.

16. Aronowitz, "The Converged Experience of Risk and Disease."

17. Williams, *Obstetrics* (1917), 712, 723, 729–733; McCloskey, Petitti, and Hobel, "Variations in the Use of Cesarean Delivery for Dystocia"; Gifford et al., "Lack of Progress in Labor as a Reason for Cesarean"; Nancy K. Lowe, "A Review of Factors"; Marieskind, *An Evaluation of Caesarean Section in the United States*, 9–10.

18. Strong, *Expecting Trouble*, 1–32; Lyerly et al., "Risk and the Pregnant Body," 35.

19. Kolata, "Panel Urges Mammograms at 50 Not 40"; USPSTF, "Breast Cancer Screening"; "Tamoxifen and Uterine Cancer." For a discussion of the extent of overtreatment in the United States, see Korenstein et al., "Overuse of Health Care Services in the United States."

20. Greene, *Prescribing by Numbers*; Lane, "The Medical Model of the Body."

21. Gabe, "Health, Medicine and Risk."

22. Douglas, "Risk as a Forensic Resource."

23. Starr, "Social Benefit versus Technological Risk"; Slovic et al., "Risk Perception of Prescription Drugs"; Slovic, "Perception of Risk."

24. Toto, "Choosing Caesarean"; Minkoff and Chervenak, "Elective Primary Cesarean Delivery"; Park, "Choosy Mothers Choose Caesareans"; Goff, "Birth by Appointment." Electronic fetal monitoring (EFM), with its high false positive rate for fetal hypoxia, has been instrumental in spurring the notion that vaginal birth is risky, another example of "mixed-up perception of risk." Although designed and implemented to reduce risk, in the more than 40 years of its use, EFM has not reduced the infant mortality, morbidity, or cerebral palsy rates. See Sartwelle, "Electronic Fetal Monitoring"; Lent, "The Medical and Legal Risks of the Electronic Fetal Monitor." On the other hand, cesarean section carries with it a host of well-known risks, particularly in a population at low risk for birth complications. See Hansen et al., "Elective Cesarean Section"; MacDorman et al., "Infant and Neonatal Mortality"; Deneux-Tharaux et al., "Postpartum Maternal Mortality and Cesarean Delivery."

25. Notzon, Placek, and Taffel, "Comparisons of National Cesarean-Section Rates." For an examination of the increase in cesareans in Canada, see Mennill, "Prepping the Cut." Brennan et al., "Comparative Analysis of International Cesarean Delivery Rates"; Notzon, "International Differences in the Use of Obstetric Interventions."

26. The infant mortality rate in the Netherlands in 2013 was 3 deaths for every 1,000 live births; in the United States the rate was 6/1,000. The 2013 maternal mortality rate in the Netherlands was 6/100,000 births; in the United States the rate was more than 4.5 times higher—28/100,000. World Health Organization, *World Health Statistics 2014*, 65, 67, 82, 86. Notzon, "International Differences"; Declercq et al., "Is a Rising Cesarean Delivery Rate Inevitable?"; World Health Organization, *World Health Statistics 2014*, 110.

27. Borquez and Wiegers, "A Comparison of Labour and Birth Experiences."

28. World Health Organization, *World Health Statistics 2014*, 106; Khazan, "Why Most Brazilian Women Get C-Sections"; "Brazil Unveils New Rules"; Hopkins, "Are Brazilian Women Really Choosing to Deliver by Cesarean?" The Brazilian healthcare system is a three-tiered system consisting of a public sector open to most Brazilians and financed with public funds, a private sector financed by a mix of public and private funds, and a private insurance sector. The public and private health sectors are distinct but also interconnected, in that any individual can use services in all three sectors but the private sector is effectively accessible only to those who are able to pay for it. Paim et al., "The Brazilian Health System."

29. Klimpel, "Performing Modernity through Birth," 82–85. To see how apt the American wedding/Brazilian cesarean video comparison is, see Jellison, *It's Our Day*.

30. Klimpel, "Performing Modernity through Birth." For more on birth in modern-day Brazil, see Declercq, "Is Medical Intervention in Childbirth Inevitable in Brazil?"; Chaves, "Birth as a Radical Experience of Change"; Domingues, "Process of Decision-Making Regarding the Mode of Birth in Brazil." These articles, and others, appear in both Portuguese and English in a special 2014 issue of *Cadernos de Saúde Pública, Rio de Janeiro,* devoted to birth in Brazil.

31. Feng et al., "Factors Influencing Rising Caesarean Section Rates in China." A study published in 2014 indicated that the cesarean rate in China is probably lower. While the WHO at one point reported a 46 percent rate, *JAMA* reported more recently that the national average in China is 35 percent, with Shanghai at the high end with a 68 percent rate and Tibet at the low end with a 4 percent rate. Li, Luo, and Trasande, "Geographic Variations and Temporal Trends."

32. Blumenthal and Hsiao, "Lessons from the East"; Sakala and Corry, *Evidence-Based Maternity Care.*

33. Feng et al., "Factors Influencing Rising Caesarean Section Rates in China." To use a state-by-state accounting in the United States as an example, rates in 2007 ranged from a low of 22.2 percent in Utah to a high of 38.3 percent in New Jersey. Menacker and Hamilton, "Recent Trends in Cesarean Delivery in the United States." In southwestern Pennsylvania rates vary from a low of 19.8 percent in Indiana County to a high of 36.7 percent in Armstrong Country; midway is Allegheny County at 28.5 percent. H. Miller, "Regional Insights."

34. Song, "Too Posh to Push?"; "Too Posh to Push?" *The Telegraph.* The phrase was popularized after Victoria Beckham (then better known as Posh Spice) revealed that she had chosen to give birth to her first child by cesarean section; her following three children were also born with "surgical assistance." BBC Trending, "C-Sections Are Not an Easy Way Out"; "All Women get Right to Caesarean Birth"; Emma Innes, "Soaring Number of Women."

35. See www.nice.org.uk/guidance/cg62; www.nice.org.uk/guidance/cg190/chapter/1-Recommendations#place-of-birth.

36. Xu et al., "Wide Variation Found in Hospital Facility Costs."

37. Between the early nineteenth century and 1871, only 85 cesareans are known to have been performed in the United States. Robert Harris, a physician and medical statistician, collected data on each one. These data are available in the Robert P. Harris papers, Wangensteen Historical Library of Biology and Medicine, University of Minnesota, Minneapolis. Nationwide rates of cesarean births in the 1940s and 1950s are estimates based on local rates. Cesareans at Duke University Hospital in Durham, North Carolina, for example, actually went down slightly between 1930 and 1950, from 2.5 to 2.3 percent of births. Obstetrics Logs, Book 1 January 1930–1 July 1932, Book 5 September 14, 1940–December 1941, and Book 15 August 29, 1949–17 June 1950, Duke University Medical Center Archives, Durham, North Carolina. Other estimates set the rate at between 1 and 6 percent nationwide, although most areas of the country hovered closer to the low end. Between 1941 and 1949 at Johns Hopkins Hospital, for example, doctors performed 1,000 cesareans in 21,739 deliveries, a rate of 4.6 percent; doctors at Hopkins admitted being on the high end of the spectrum. In Alabama, the overall rate was

1.32 percent from 1945 to 1947. Eastman, *Williams Obstetrics*, 1099–1101; Sakala and Corry, *Evidence-Based Maternity Care*, 41–48. An assessment of overused interventions in obstetrics today appears in Sakala and Corry, *Evidence-Based Maternity Care*. A prototypical medical decision-making strategy in obstetrics today is the "maximin" strategy, in which obstetricians routinely take aggressive preventive measures during all births to prevent bad outcomes in a slim minority of patients. As one attorney notes, the maximin strategy has become "almost synonymous with standard and accepted obstetrical practice." See Rhoden, "Informed Consent in Obstetrics," 72. Yet there is no evidence that the maximin strategy achieves better results. See Brody and Thompson, "The Maximin Strategy in Modern Obstetrics."

CHAPTER 1: **The Epitome of Risk: Cesarean Sections in the Nineteenth Century**

1. John L. Richmond, "History of a Successful Casarean Operation," 485. Richmond's was not the first cesarean performed in the United States. Rather, it was the first formally reported to the medical community. At least three other, unpublished cesareans occurred between "early" in the nineteenth century—the exact dates are unknown—and 1825. See Robert P. Harris, "The Caesarean Operations of the United States," bound, handwritten book, 1879, Robert Harris Collection, Wangensteen Historical Library of Biology and Medicine, University of Minnesota, Minneapolis, hereinafter referred to as the Harris Collection. There is also a published account of a self-inflicted cesarean occurring in 1822. See Francis and Beck, "Case of Self-Performed Caesarean Section," 1. According to the historian of medicine Fielding H. Garrison, the first cesarean section in the United States occurred in rural Virginia at an unspecified time but went unreported for many years. The case is not recorded in Harris's journal, so there is no means of corroborating the claim. The surgeon who claimed to have performed the surgery, Jesse Bennett, explained why he never reported it: "No doctor with any feelings of delicacy would report an operation that he had done on his own wife." Faced with either piecemeal extraction of the fetus or a cesarean section due to his wife's contracted pelvis, Bennett, with his wife's blessing, claimed to have performed the surgery and successfully extracted their daughter. Determined this would be their last child, he removed his wife's ovaries before stitching the wound. His daughter lived to be 73. An account of this surgery, along with accounts of other early cesareans in the United States and Europe, can be found in Guttmacher, *Into This Universe*.

2. Richmond, "History of a Successful Casarean Operation." The facts of this case are similar to the descriptions of subsequent nineteenth-century cesareans in Harris, bound handwritten journal, Harris Collection.

3. Richmond, "History of a Successful Casarean Operation." Physicians did not use ether as a surgical anesthesia until 1846, when William T. G. Morton first demonstrated its use at Massachusetts General Hospital. The first doctor to use ether as an anesthetic during childbirth was Nathan Cooley Keep, a Boston dentist. See Fenster, *Ether Day*. The chemical properties of sulphuric ether, however, were known well before Morton's discovery. See Dalton, "Memoir on Sulphuric Ether."

4. Richmond, "History of a Successful Casarean Operation."

5. Ibid.

6. Ibid.

7. Letter from Catharine E. Reitzel to William Aug Atlee, June 29, 1893, Harris Papers. Atlee's father described Reitzel's surgery in detail shortly after it occurred. See Atlee, "Case of Successful Peritoneal Section."

8. Richmond, "History of a Successful Casarean Operation."

9. Examples of obstetric texts that discussed difficult births while simultaneously suggesting that simple measures be employed to resolve serious problems include Davis, *The Principles and Practice of Obstetric Medicine,* and Ramsbotham, *The Principles and Practice of Obstetric Medicine.* Davis does not mention cesarean birth in his book, although he does describe at length how to use forceps safely. Ramsbotham warned colleagues away from cesarean surgery in most instances, stating that 90 percent of the cesareans performed in the British Isles had ended in a mother's death (225). Women used the phrase "living mother of a living child" to indicate both gratitude after a successful birth and their anxiety about birth. The phrase can be seen often in the letters and diaries of eighteenth- and nineteenth-century women. See, for example, Ulrich, " 'The Living Mother of a Living Child' "; Curtis, *The Cary Letters*, 335.

10. Harris, "History of a Pair of Obstetrical Forceps," 55; Prentiss, "A Report."

11. Ramsbotham, *The Principles and Practice of Obstetric Medicine*, 213–216; Meigs, *Obstetrics*, 320.

12. Ulrich, *A Midwife's Tale*, 170–171; Irvine Loudon, *Death in Childbirth*, 366, 375; King, "Maternal Mortality in the United States." Although today's maternal death rate in the United States is historically low, the rate has risen since the 1980s, a trend the public health community calls "troubling." For more on maternal mortality statistics in the US today and elsewhere in the world, see World Health Organization, *World Health Statistics 2014*, 65, 67, 82, 86.

13. Dunn, "Dr. Francis Ramsbotham"; Ramsbotham, *The Principles and Practice of Obstetric Medicine*, 231.

14. Kass, *Midwifery and Medicine in Boston*, 35. As late as 1900, midwives attended half of all births in the United States. For more on midwives' training and education, particularly as a "neighborly practice," see Borst, *Catching Babies*, 13–89.

15. Mayfair, *Midwifery Illustrated*, 144–147. The 1856 edition of Meigs's book did not contain a reference to cesarean section either. Meigs, *Obstetrics*; McLane, "The Sloane Maternity Hospital"; Speert, *Essays in Eponymy*, 567.

16. Uterine rupture was, and continues to be, a rare occurrence. In 1880, a Philadelphia physician estimated that "this most fearful accident" happened so infrequently that a physician who attended "several thousand" births in his lifetime would not encounter a rupture. See Harris, "If a Woman Has Ruptured"; Hacker and Moore, *Essentials of Obstetrics and Gynecology*, 187–195; DeLee, "Two Cases of Obstetrical Hemorrhage."

17. Prentiss, "A Report"; Philadelphia Lying-In Charity Patient Chart, volume 17 (1899), case 2532, Pennsylvania Hospital Archives, Philadelphia, PA.

18. Huff, "History and Prophylaxis of Puerperal Infection," 281; Loudon, *The Tragedy of Childbed Fever*, 5–6; Brickell, "A Successful Case of Caesarean Section," 454–466; Barnes, *Lectures on Obstetric Operations*, 330.

19. Philadelphia Lying-In Charity Patient Chart, volume 10 (1895–96), case 1412, Pennsylvania Hospital Archives, Philadelphia, PA.

20. Lusk, "The Prognosis of Cesarean Operations." For much of the nineteenth century, hospitals were largely charitable institutions intended for the sick poor, and most often they were a place for them to go to die. People of means, however meager those means were, were cared for at home. See Rosner, *A Once Charitable Enterprise*; Rosenberg, *The Care of Strangers*; Abel, *Hearts of Wisdom.*

21. Brickell, "A Successful Case of Caesarean Section," quotes on 454, 456, and 457; Lungren, "A Case of Cesarean Section."

22. Ramsbotham, *The Principles and Practice of Obstetric Medicine*, 191; Kass, *Midwifery and Medicine in Boston*, 81.

23. Harris, bound handwritten journal, Harris Collection.

24. Noble, "Memoir of Dr. Robert P. Harris"; Harris, bound handwritten journal, Harris Collection, 7. Harris noted in the journal each case that had been published, and where.

25. Harris, bound handwritten journal, Harris Collection, 9; Noble, "Memoir of Dr. Robert P. Harris"; Harris, bound handwritten journal, Harris Collection, 7.

26. Harris, bound handwritten journal, Harris Collection. The cases of women described by Harris as dwarfs are cases 11, 14, 16, 17, 19, 23, 38, 42, 44, 45, 46, 52, 53, 60, 71, and 81. Harris described only 9 of the 85 women as slaves, although this appears to be because he listed a woman as a slave only when he could name her owner. Historical population statistics appear in US Department of Commerce, *Historical Statistics*, 15, 17.

27. Harris, bound handwritten journal, Harris Collection, 10–11. Prevost was born in southern France in 1771; in 1800, he was listed as a public health official in Port-de-Paix, Haiti. In 1801 he migrated to Louisiana, settling on the west bank of the Mississippi River a hundred miles upstream from New Orleans, where he performed the first known cesarean surgery in Louisiana. Whether he learned the technique in Haiti is not known. Brasseaux and Conrad, *The Road to Louisiana*, 210–211.

28. Schwartz, *Birthing a Slave*, 164–167; McGregor, *From Midwives to Medicine*, 27, 31, 32, 42, 54, 55, 61, 63; Harris, bound handwritten journal, Harris Collection, 11–12.

29. Harris, bound handwritten journal, Harris Collection, cases 8, 22, and 27. Cases 22 and 27 are also described in Beck, "Caesarian Operation."

30. Robert P. Harris, "The Operation of Gastro-Hysterotomy."

31. Harris, bound handwritten journal, Harris Collection, 13; "A Case of Cæsarian Section."

32. Harris, bound handwritten journal, Harris Collection, cases 81 and 42.

33. Barnes, *Lectures on Obstetric Operations*, 312, 315; Harris, bound handwritten journal, Harris Collection; Ramsbotham, *The Principles and Practice of Obstetric Medicine*, 225.

34. Harris, "Cattle-Horn Lacerations," 675.

35. For example, see cases 9, 15, 34, 37, 43, 51, 63, 67, 68, 72, 74, 80, and 81 in Harris's casebook; Harris, "Cattle-Horn Lacerations."

36. Harris, "The Operation of Gastro-Hysterotomy"; Harris, bound handwritten journal, Harris Collection, cases 10, 38, and 82; Harris, "Lessons from a Study."

37. Harris, "The Operation of Gastro-Hysterotomy." This article, cited in obstetric texts, had influence beyond its appearance in the *American Journal of the Medical Sciences.* See, for example, Marsden, *Handbook of Practical Midwifery.*

38. Harris, bound handwritten journal, Harris Collection; Harris, "The Operation of Gastro-Hysterotomy," 332.

39. Harris, bound handwritten journal, Harris Collection, cases 6, 11, 12, 30, 35, 36, 42, and 49.

40. Weems, "Case of Caesarian Section," 257; Harris, "The Operation of Gastro-Hysterotomy." Harris, bound handwritten journal, Harris Collection, cases 6 and 69 (case 6 contains the "folly" quote).

41. Zabriskie, *Nurses Handbook of Obstetrics*; Williams and Sun, "A Statistical Study," 748.

42. Harris, "The Operation of Gastro-Hysterotomy," 335.

43. Hoag, "Progress in Obstetric Practice," 6; Quoted in Kass, *Midwifery and Medicine in Boston*, 83. A comprehensive history of the invention and use of forceps is Cie, *Obstetric Forceps*, originally published in 1929.

44. Obstetric texts devoted many dozens of heavily illustrated pages to the nuances and difficulties of the use of forceps. See, for example, Meigs, *Obstetrics*; DeLee, *The Principles and Practice of Obstetrics* (1918), 987–1016; Williams, *Obstetrics* (1924), 439–470; Davis, *The Principles and Practice of Obstetric Medicine*, 1159.

45. H. Williams, "A Comparison"; Philadelphia Lying-In Charity Patient Charts, volume 15 (1898), record 2266, October 1898, Pennsylvania Hospital Archives, Philadelphia, PA; Manhattan Maternity and Dispensary Cesarean Section Cases, July 30, 1905 to December 11, 1912, July 10, 1908, Application No. 1746 and case on July 10, 1908, Medical Center Archives of New York–Presbyterian / Weil Cornell, New York, NY.

46. Record of patient admitted at 4:15 p.m., November 12, 1892, Sloane Maternity Hospital Obstetric Records De Forest volume 1 (1892), New York Academy of Medicine Rare Book Room, New York Academy of Medicine, New York, NY.

47. Philadelphia Lying-In Charity Patient Charts, volumes 1–20, May 1891–April 1901, Pennsylvania Hospital Archives, Philadelphia, PA; Ulrich, *A Midwife's Tale*, 170–171.

48. Meigs, *Obstetrics: The Science and the Art*, 529–569; DeLee, *The Principles and Practice of Obstetrics* (1918); Eastman, *Williams Obstetrics*; Hibbard, *The Obstetrician's Armamentarium*. Hibbard's book contains hundreds of photographs and descriptions of historical obstetric instruments.

49. Barnes, *Lectures on Obstetric Operations*, ix; Harris, "History of a Pair of Obstetrical Forceps," 58.

50. DeLee, "Syllabus of Lectures on Operative Obstetrics."

51. Davis, *The Principles and Practice of Obstetric Medicine*, 1152–1159; Hibbard, *The Obstetrician's Armamentarium*, 219–259; Skene, "A Contribution to Obstetrical Surgery."

52. Davis, *The Principles and Practice of Obstetric Medicine*, 1152–1159; Reynolds, "Circumstances Which Render," 489; Donohue, "A Successful Case of Cesarean Section." For more on the relationship between infant mortality and feeding cows' milk to infants in the nineteenth century, see Wolf, *Don't Kill Your Baby*, 42–73. In a typical case, a Chicago physician described a woman who died of sepsis shortly after a cesarean birth. Her surviving infant died a few months later of diarrhea. "Discussion, Caesarean Section." Interestingly, according to Harris, while far more women died in Great Britain than in the United States after a cesarean, far more children died in the United States as a result of the surgery than

in Europe. See Harris, "The Operation of Gastro-Hysterotomy." Perhaps in Ireland, due to the influence of the Catholic Church, the primary motivation in performing a cesarean was to save the child, whereas in the United States it was a last-ditch effort to save the mother.

53. Quoted in Kass, *Midwifery and Medicine in Boston*, 83; Sloane Maternity Hospital Obstetric Records De Forest, volume 1 (1892), New York Academy of Medicine Rare Book Room.

54. Harris, bound handwritten journal, Harris Collection, cases 9, 10, 11, 28, 46, and 52; Cottman, "Caesarian Operation Successfully Performed," 337.

55. Philadelphia Lying-In Charity Patient Charts, volumes 1–20, May 1891–April 1901, Pennsylvania Hospital Archives, Philadelphia, PA; Barnes, *Lectures on Obstetric Operations*, 313; Harris, "The Operation of Gastro-Hysterotomy."

56. Letter from Sänger to Dr. Harris, 1887 (exact date indecipherable), and Letter from Sänger to Dr. Harris, December 15, 1887, Folder Correspondence 1880s-1890s, Max Sänger Correspondence, Harris Collection; Kachlik, Kästner, and Baca, "Christian Gerhard Leopold." Sänger was not the first physician to suture the uterus, only the first to perfect and demonstrate the safety of the technique. D. Warren Brickell of New Orleans sutured a uterus at least once. After a cesarean birth in 1867 that delivered a dead fetus, he found "the blood was running pretty freely, it would not do to close the abdomen with the uterus in this state, and it was at once determined to close the wound in the organ by means of silver sutures." The woman survived, and another physician attending the surgery reported later to Brickell that "the silver wires left in the uterine walls have given no trouble whatever." Brickell, "A Successful Case," 458, 466.

57. Letter from Sänger to Dr. Harris, 1887 (exact date indecipherable), Harris Collection; Kachlik, Kästner, and Baca, "Christian Gerhard Leopold."

58. Letter from Sänger to Dr. Harris, 1887 (exact date indecipherable), Harris Collection.

59. Ramsbotham, *The Principles and Practice of Obstetric Medicine*, 363; Barnes, *Lectures on Obstetric Operations*, 326.

60. Cragin, *Obstetrics*, 788; DeLee, *The Principles and Practice of Obstetrics* (1918), 1027; Speert and Guttmacher, *Obstetric Practice*, 331; Playfair, *A Treatise*.

61. Harris, "The Cesarean Operation"; Letter from Sänger to Dr. Harris, June 10, 1891, Folder Correspondence 1880s–1890s, Max Sänger Correspondence, Harris Collection.

62. Speert, *Essays in Eponymy*, 587–590, quotes on 589, 592; Guttmacher, *Into This Universe*, 259–262.

63. "Obituary Notice: Max Sänger," 292; Guttmacher, *Into This Universe*, 259–262.

64. Parvin, *The Science and Art of Obstetrics*, 680–687. Sänger's 200-page book, written in German in 1881, was titled *Der Kaiserschnitt* (The Cesarean) and is available at the American Congress of Obstetricians and Gynecologists historical collection in Washington, DC; Letter from Sänger to Dr. Harris, 1887 (exact date indecipherable), Harris Collection.

65. Cragin, *Obstetrics*, 788; "Discussion, Caesarean Section"; Guttmacher, *Into This Universe*, 259–262; "Obituary Notice: Max Sänger," 294.

66. J. Williams, "A Critical Analysis"; Miller, "A General Consideration."

67. Hoag, "Caesarean Section."
68. "Discussion, Caesarean Section."
69. Dudley, "The Cesarean Operation."

CHAPTER 2: **Still Too Risky? 1900–1930s**

1. For more on the history of the use of anesthesia see Pernick, *A Calculus of Suffering;* Fenster, *Ether Day*; Stratmann, *Chloroform.* For more on the history of obstetric anesthesia specifically see Caton, *What a Blessing She Had Chloroform;* Wolf, *Deliver Me from Pain.* Nancy Tomes discusses when and how the public came to understand the germ theory of disease in *The Gospel of Germs.*

2. Loudon, *The Tragedy of Childbed Fever,* 111–112; Nuland, *The Doctors' Plague,* 177.

3. Nuland, *The Doctors' Plague,* 179; Loudon, *The Tragedy of Childbed Fever,* 130–133, quote on 131.

4. Markoe and Davis, "Fifty Cases of Cesarean Section"; Cragin, *Obstetrics,* 795; Peterson, "The Present Status."

5. Hooker and the New York Academy of Medicine Committee on Public Health Relations, *Maternal Mortality in New York City,* 127–138; Williams, "A Critical Analysis"; Williams, "Cesarean Section at the Johns Hopkins Hospital"; Manhattan Maternity and Dispensary Annual Reports 1905–1932, Medical Center Archives of New York–Presbyterian / Weil Cornell Medical Center, New York, NY.

6. C. Miller, "A General Consideration."

7. Newell, *Cesarean Section,* 13; C. Miller, "A General Consideration," 745.

8. DeLee, *The Principles and Practice of Obstetrics* (1925), 1084, 1086; Williams, *Obstetrics* (1909), 377; Speert, *The Sloane Hospital Chronicle,* 109, 119–120. In 1922, Toronto obstetrician B. P. Watson outlined a precise protocol for induction that held sway for more than 20 years. His technique called for the administration of castor oil, quinine, and an enema in the evening, followed in the morning by periodic injections of pituitary extract. Only if labor had not started after several days did he then recommend reverting to the proverbial bags and bougies. Watson, "Further Experience with Pituitary Extract."

9. Zinke, "The Limitations of Cesarean Section"; Eli K. Price, "Preston Retreat Address on the Laying of the Cornerstone Made by Eli K. Price," July 1837, Preston Retreat Miscellaneous Papers 1835–1948, Pennsylvania Hospital Historic Collections, Philadelphia, PA; Norris, "The Ultimate Results," 290, 292.

10. Manhattan Maternity and Dispensary Cesarean Section Cases July 30, 1905, to December 11, 1912, Medical Center Archives of New York–Presbyterian / Weil Cornell, New York, NY. For a sampling of cesareans performed due to profuse hemorrhage, see the descriptions of the July 31 and September 20, 1905, births. For a sampling of cesareans performed due to pelvic anomalies, see the descriptions of the July 13, 1906, April 21 and May 21, 1907, and July 8 and August 22, 1910, births. The "united twins" birth occurred on November 21, 1905.

11. Allen, "A Plea"; Cragin, "Conservatism in Obstetrics"; Holmes, "Obstetrics, A Lost Art."

12. Williams, "The Abuse of Cæsarean Section"; C. Miller, "A General Consideration"; Lynch, "More Conservatism in Cesarean Section."

13. DeLee, *The Principles and Practice of Obstetrics* (1918), 1018.

14. DeLee, *The Principles and Practice of Obstetrics* (1929), 1061.

15. Greenhill, *Principles and Practice of Obstetrics*, 924–927.

16. Newell, *Cesarean Section*, unnumbered first page and 12; C. Miller, "A General Consideration."

17. Williams, "A Criticism of Certain Tendencies." This definition of elective cesarean persisted through the 1950s. See Safford, "Tell Me Doctor—Part 16."

18. Peterson, "The Present Status"; "Lectures on Obstetrics 1930 by Leroy A. Calkins," 85, Leroy A. Calkins, MD Papers, Kansas University Medical Center Archives, Kansas City, KS.

19. C. Miller, "The Limitations of Caesarean Section"; Allen, "A Plea"; Newell, *Cesarean Section*, unnumbered first page of preface.

20. For more on assorted Progressive Era movements, see Gould, *America in the Progressive Era*. For more on the efforts to lower maternal and infant morbidity and mortality, see Meigs, *Maternal Mortality;* Lindenmeyer, *"A Right to Childhood,"* 1–7. George Newman, a British physician and pioneer in the fields of public and child health who was influential on both sides of the Atlantic, made the explicit connection between the good health of mothers and the good health of their babies in his 1906 book *Infant Mortality: A Social Problem*, the first book-length publication to address infant mortality. Newman argued that infants' health was largely dependent on their mothers' ability to properly care for them. See Garrett et al., *Infant Mortality*. For more on efforts to lower infant mortality in the early twentieth century, see Meckel, *Save the Babies*, 40–91; Wolf, *Don't Kill Your Baby*, 42–73.

21. "History of Baby Week," March 15, 1924, Infant Welfare Society Papers, Chicago History Museum Archives, Chicago, IL; Meckel, *Save the Babies*, 200–203. For more on Sheppard-Towner see Lindenmeyer, *"A Right to Childhood,"* 92–107.

22. Williams, "Cesarean Section at the Johns Hopkins Hospital"; Williams, "The Abuse of Cæsarean Section." This practice long continued. After performing her third cesarean at a large Chicago hospital in 1977, an obstetrician told one of the mothers interviewed by the author that she had to have a hysterectomy. Interview of mother by author, Chicago mother interview 1, March 13, 2012, transcribed from digital recording.

23. Baker, "Maternal Mortality in the United States"; Bromley, "What Risk Motherhood?" 14; Polak, "What Is the Matter?"; Hooker, *Maternal Mortality in New York City*, 116, 125–126, 130, quote on 130. Between 1900 and 1920, infant deaths dropped from 130 to 76 per 1,000 live births, while maternal deaths rose from 13.3 to 16.9 per 100,000 population, peaking in 1918 and 1920 with rates of 22.3 and 19 deaths (deaths spiked in those years due to the influenza pandemic). For more detailed statistics on infant mortality in the early twentieth century, see Preston and Haines, *Fatal Years*, 77; Meckel, *Save the Babies*, 238; Wolf, *Don't Kill Your Baby*, 205–211. For maternal death statistics in this era, see Woodbury, *Infant Mortality and Its Causes*, 180–192. The geographical area of the United States in which deaths were recorded was slowly expanded from 40.5 percent of the population in 1900 to 82.2 percent in 1920. This expansion does not explain the increase in maternal deaths, however. In most of the added states, the maternal rate was higher in

1921 than in the year of admission to the death registration area. See Woodbury, *Infant Mortality and Its Causes*, 180–192.

24. Hooker, *Maternal Mortality in New York City*, 85; de Kruif, *The Fight for Life*, 122–123, quote on 123; de Kruif, "Saver of Mothers," 125; DeLee, "How Should the Maternity Be Isolated?" See also DeLee and Siedentopf, "The Maternity Ward of the General Hospital." The move from home to hospital occurred more rapidly in some parts of the country than others. The records of the Manhattan Maternity and Dispensary, an organization that ran a maternity hospital but also dispatched physicians to attend home births, demonstrate how rapidly hospital birth became the norm within that closed system. From 1908 through 1911, roughly twice as many women using the dispensary's services chose to give birth at home—597 home births versus 304 hospital births in 1908; 883 home versus 378 hospital births in 1909; 939 versus 478 in 1910; and 929 versus 457 in 1911. By 1922 the locales had begun to approach par—665 births at home and 763 births in the hospital. By 1928, however, hospital birth was the clear favorite—1,206 hospital births versus 302 births at home. *Manhattan Maternity and Dispensary Annual Reports 1908 through 1928*, Medical Center Archives of New York–Presbyterian / Weil Cornell Hospital, New York, NY. Nationwide, the preference for hospital birth took a bit longer to manifest. Home versus hospital births did not see a roughly 50–50 split until 1938. Leavitt, *Brought to Bed*, 269.

25. De Kruif, *The Fight for Life*, 39–62.

26. Robert P. Harris, bound handwritten journal, *The Caesarean Operations of the United States* (Philadelphia, 1879), Robert Harris Collection, Wangensteen Historical Library of Biology and Medicine, University of Minnesota, Minneapolis; DeLee, *The Principles and Practice of Obstetrics* (1918), 1024.

27. Allen, "A Plea"; Cragin, *Obstetrics*, 788; Zabriskie, *Nurses Handbook of Obstetrics*; McNeile, *Notes on Pathological and Operative Obstetrics*, 192–201; Green, "A Study of the First Series."

28. Lynch, "More Conservatism in Cesarean Section."

29. Green, "A Study of the First Series"; Cragin, "Cesarean Section"; Williams, "A Critical Analysis," 173.

30. Williams and Sun, "A Statistical Study"; Newell, *Cesarean Section*, 20.

31. Williams, *Obstetrics* (1924), 780–899; Zinke, "The Limitations of Cesarean Section."

32. Cragin, "Cesarean Section"; Friedman, "Types of Pelvic Deformity, Technique."

33. Interview of retired obstetrician by author, Chicago physician interview 8, October 5, 2012, Chicago, IL, transcribed from digital tape recording; 1985 card, Nancy Wainer Papers, box 1, folder MC656 1.11 Correspondence: Birth Announcements, 1984–86, Schlesinger Library, Radcliffe College, Cambridge, MA.

34. Colcher and Sussman, "Changing Concepts of X-Ray Pelvimetry"; Lilienfeld, Treptow, and Dixon, "A Study of Variations"; Isadore Dyer, "Clinical Evaluation of X-Ray Pelvimetry"; Interview of retired obstetrician by author, July 19, 2004, Chicago, IL, transcribed from tape recording; Varner, Cruikshank, and Laube, "X-Ray Pelvimetry in Clinical Obstetrics"; Campbell, "X-Ray Pelvimetry."

35. Williams, *Obstetrics* (1924), 1–25, 780–899; DeLee, *The Principles and Practice of Obstetrics* (1925), 247–261, 689–762, quote on 248.

36. Williams, "The Abuse of Cæsarean Section"; Williams, *Obstetrics* (1924), 782; Williams, "A Critical Analysis."

37. "Discussion of Rudolph W. Holmes"; Letter from Joseph DeLee to J. Whitridge Williams, February 23, 1923, Joseph B. DeLee, MD Papers, Northwestern Memorial Hospital Archives, Chicago, IL, hereinafter referred to as DeLee Papers. DeLee apparently wrote the letter in response to Williams's article, "A Criticism of Certain Tendencies in American Obstetrics"; Williams, "Cesarean Section at the Johns Hopkins Hospital," 519; Williams and Sun, "A Statistical Study," 735; Acosta-Sison, "Pelvimetry and Cephalometry among Filipinas," 493.

38. Lombardo, *Three Generations, No Imbeciles*, ix–x. For more on the eugenics movement in the United States and its widespread influence, see Pernick, *The Black Stork*; Stern, *Eugenic Nation*; Kline, *Building a Better Race*. Both Stern and Kline argue that eugenics remained influential long after World War II, shaping the social control of women's reproductive behavior, school segregation, the border patrol, and the environmental movement.

39. Quoted in Gordon, *Woman's Body, Woman's Right*, 133; Baker, "The High Cost of Babies"; Cragin, *Obstetrics*, 788; "Discussion, Caesarean Section"; Guttmacher, *Into This Universe*, 259–262; Williams, "A Critical Analysis."

40. Cragin, "Conservatism in Obstetrics." The pronouncement has long been attributed solely to Cragin, although there is evidence that it was a well-known mantra earlier. See Green, "Cesarean Section," 442. Green's article appeared three months before Cragin's iconic article.

41. Miller, "A General Consideration," 749.

42. Green, "A Study of the First Series," 805.

43. Williams, "Cesarean Section at the Johns Hopkins Hospital"; Williams, "The Abuse of Cæsarean Section"; Williams, "A Criticism of Certain Tendencies;" Cragin, *Obstetrics*, 790–791, 795–796.

44. DeLee, *The Principles and Practice of Obstetrics* (1929), 1060; Williams, *Obstetrics* (1924), 495; "Lectures on Obstetrics 1930 by Leroy A. Calkins," 85; Speert and Guttmacher, *Obstetric Practice*, 326–329, quote on 329; Pritchard and MacDonald, *Williams Obstetrics*, 1085; Barnes, "'Twilight Sleep.'" DeLee credits Osiander of Göttingen, Germany, for having performed the first low transverse cesarean in 1805. Osiander observed that uterine rupture rarely occurred and chances of infection were lessened when the incision was made lower on the uterus than was customary at the time, although the two women Osiander first used the technique on died. Two other physicians later experimented with a similar cut, and it was Fritz Frank of Cologne in 1906 who blended the experience of the three together in what DeLee later called the "improved Osiander-Joerg-Physik operation" and introduced it to a more receptive audience in the European medical community. See DeLee, "An Illustrated History." Examinations of obstetric texts prior to 1980 indicate that the classic cut was still very much in use in the United States.

45. Letter from Wisconsin physician M. A. Lee to *Journal of the American Medical Association*, May 20, 1914; Letter from Pennsylvania physician, Dr. Guy Hale McKinstry, July 27, 1914, AMA Health Fraud and Alternative Medicine Collection, box 867 folder 0867-05, American Medical Association Archives, Chicago, IL.

46. Leavitt, *Brought to Bed*, 110; "Discussion of Joseph DeLee"; Ziegler, "How Can We Best Solve the Midwifery Problem."

47. Mengert, "Our Maturing Specialty," 355–356; Joseph B. DeLee, "Motherhood: An Address before the Women's Society of Isaiah Temple January 4th 1898," DeLee Papers; Williams, "Why Is the Art of Obstetrics so Poorly Practised?" 171, 172; Flexner, *Medical Education in the United States and Canada*, 117–118.

48. "The Chicago Lying-In Hospital Dispensary Second Annual Report 1896–97," 5–6, Northwestern Memorial Hospital Archives, Chicago, IL; Tucker and Benaron, "Maternal Mortality of the Chicago Maternity Center"; "The Chicago Lying-In Hospital Dispensary First Annual Report."

49. "Discussion of Rudolph W. Holmes"; Williams, "The Abuse of Cæsarean Section"; Williams, "A Criticism of Certain Tendencies in American Obstetrics."

50. Letter from Joseph DeLee to Mr. Raymond Hurley, 208 S. La Salle St. Chicago, July 26, 1929, DeLee Papers; Holmes, "Obstetrics, A Lost Art"; Norris, "The Ultimate Results," 290, 292.

51. Hoag, "Progress in Obstetric Practice." In acknowledging the operator/nonoperator distinction, Hoag notes that "the two schools" likely began with the introduction of obstetric forceps, when, for the first time, physicians had a means of both hastening labor and assisting women in the throes of a difficult labor. Hoag observed that eventually the divisions became so meaningful that some obstetric teachers at medical schools sought to ensure that their particular philosophy would be handed down through multiple generations of students.

52. DeLee, "The Prophylactic Forceps Operation," 40–41. Williams and DeLee battled privately as well as publicly. In an exchange of letters, DeLee told Williams, "I feel that if medical students and the laity are allowed to believe that labor is a normal function when as a matter of fact it produces so many abnormalities, the dignity as a pathological entity will not be appreciated. The fundamental reason why obstetrics is on such a low place in the opinion of the profession and reflected from the profession in the minds of the public, is just because pregnancy and labor are considered normal, and therefore anybody a medical student, a midwife, or even a neighbor, knows enough to take care of such a function." Letter from Joseph B. DeLee to Dr. J. Whitridge Williams, February 23, 1923, DeLee Papers. Williams responded almost three weeks later: "Of course ordinary labor is not pathologic and only becomes so under abnormal conditions. Likewise to my mind all labors cannot be designated as pathogenic as only those which are capable of producing a pathological condition should receive such a designation." Letter from J. Whitridge Williams to Dr. Joseph B. DeLee, March 14, 1923, DeLee Papers.

53. "Discussion"; DeLee, "Progress toward Ideal Obstetrics," 407; Williams, "A Criticism of Certain Tendencies." Many, if not most, medical journal articles about birth authored by physicians in the nineteenth and early twentieth centuries pointedly denigrated midwives. For a representative glimpse of doctors' characterization of midwives, see Williams, "Medical Education and the Midwife Problem." For more on the transition from midwife-attended to physician-attended birth, see Borst, *Catching Babies*.

54. Leavitt, "Joseph B. DeLee"; "The Chicago Lying-In Hospital Dispensary Second Annual Report," 5–6, and "The Chicago Lying-In Hospital Dispensary First Annual Re-

port," Northwestern Memorial Hospital Archives, Chicago, IL; Tucker and Benaron, "Maternal Mortality"; de Kruif, *The Fight for Life*, 137–138.

55. De Kruif, *The Fight for Life*, 99–101.

56. "The Chicago Lying-In Hospital Dispensary Second Annual Report," 5–6, and "The Chicago Lying-In Hospital Dispensary First Annual Report."

57. Joseph DeLee to Ogden T. McClurg, August 8, 1922, DeLee Papers. For an interesting analysis of DeLee's contemporary reputation as an advocate for medical intervention during birth and his actual daily practice at his world-renowned birth dispensary, see Lewis, "The Gospel of Good Obstetrics."

58. Leavitt, "More about 'Twilight Sleep' in Labor," 314.

59. For more on the class-based dichotomy of DeLee's obstetric practices, see Leavitt, "Joseph B. DeLee."

60. Letter from DeLee to Williams, January 16, 1925; Letter from Williams to DeLee, January 23, 1925; "Case of Mrs. Nicholas Longworth July 1924," DeLee Papers; DeLee, "The Prophylactic Forceps Operation"; Letter from DeLee to Dr. Sofie A. Nordhuff-Jung, Washington, DC, February 21, 1925, DeLee Papers.

61. DeLee, "Progress toward Ideal Obstetrics," 407; Williams, "Why Is the Art of Obstetrics so Poorly Practised?" 171, 172. For a discussion of the rising maternal mortality rate in the early twentieth century, see Wolf, *Deliver Me from Pain*, 74–75.

62. Letter from Joseph B. DeLee to Dr. J. Whitridge Williams, February 23, 1923; Letter from J. Whitridge Williams to Dr. Joseph B. DeLee, March 14, 1923, DeLee Papers.

63. Williams, "A Criticism of Certain Tendencies"; Cragin, "Conservatism in Obstetrics," 123; Polak and Beck, "The Present Status of Operative Obstetrics."

64. Lynch, "More Conservatism in Cesarean Section."

65. Polak and Beck, "The Present Status of Operative Obstetrics."

66. For additional information on the implementation and effect of the Sheppard-Towner Act, see Lindenmeyer, "*A Right to Childhood*," 76–108, 237–247; Ladd-Taylor, "'Grannies' and 'Spinsters'"; Ladd-Taylor, "'My Work Came Out of My Agony and Grief'"; "Close of the EMIC Program."

67. Peterson, "The Present Status." The vital components of premature infant care were being perfected in the 1920s, particularly under the auspices of pediatrician Julius Hess and nurse Evelyn Lundeen at the Premature Infant Station at Michael Reese Hospital in Chicago. For more information on the history of premature infant care in general and the work of Hess and Lundeen specifically, see Baker, *The Machine in the Nursery*.

68. Williams, "A Critical Analysis."

CHAPTER 3: **Risk or Remedy? 1930s–1970**

1. Nationwide rates of cesarean births during this era are estimates based on local rates. Cesareans at Duke University Hospital in Durham, North Carolina, for example, went down slightly between 1930 and 1950, from 2.5 to 2.3 percent of births. Obstetrics Logs, Book 1 January 1930–July 1, 1932; Book 5 September 14, 1940–December 1941; and Book 15 August 29, 1949–June 17, 1950, Duke University Medical Center Archives, Durham, North Carolina. Another maternity center in North Carolina, the Charlotte Maternity Clinic, saw only 23 cesareans in 5,000 births—a 0.46 percent rate—and those were

for life-threatening indications that could only be alleviated by cesarean section, such as toxemia, central placenta previa, and polyhydramnios. Charlotte Maternity Clinic, Deliveries 1933–1937, Duke University Medical Center Archives, Durham, NC. Estimates from other sources set the rate at between 1 and 6 percent nationwide, although most areas of the country hovered closer to the low end. Between 1941 and 1949, for example, doctors at Johns Hopkins Hospital performed 1,000 cesareans in 21,739 deliveries, a rate of 4.6 percent; doctors at Hopkins admitted being on the high end of the spectrum. In Alabama, the overall rate was 1.32 percent from 1945 to 1947. Eastman, *Williams Obstetrics*, 1099–1101. Other outliers included a Tennessee hospital and a North Carolina hospital that reported 5 percent rates in the early 1950s. Letter from Samuel S. Lambeth, MD, Gynecology and Obstetrics, Maryville, Tennessee, to Dr. Bayard Carter, September 9, 1951; letter from O. Hunter Jones, MD, Charlotte, NC, March 24, 1954, to Dr. Bayard C. Carter, Francis Bayard Carter Papers, Duke University Medical Center Archives, Durham, NC, hereinafter referred to as Carter Papers. An obstetrician in New York worked at a hospital on the low end of the spectrum, reporting in 1956 that his institution had a cesarean rate "still under 1.5% even including '*repeats*.'" Letter from Bill Butler, 7520th USAF Hospital NY, NY, October 21, 1956, to Dr. Carter, Carter Papers.

2. "J. P. Greenhill 1895–1975"; Greenhill, *Obstetrics*, 996–1001. There are many examples of obstetricians referring to vaginal birth as "delivery from below." See Baron, "The Intravenous Use of Pituitrin," 325; Letter from J. R. Kernodle, MD, Kernodle Clinic, Inc., Burlington, NC, July 14, 1952, to Dr. Bayard Carter, Carter Papers. In the dozens of oral history interviews I conducted with obstetricians, particularly retired obstetricians trained originally in the 1940s, several used the phrase "from below" to describe vaginal birth. One described "teaching students how to deliver from below properly." Interview by author with retired obstetrician, June 30, 2006, Glenview, IL, transcribed from tape recording. Another, when asked how he avoided cesarean sections if a baby was in the breech position, responded, "Deliver the baby from below. Just let it come." Interview by author with retired family physician, October 11, 1999, River Forest, IL, transcribed from tape recording.

3. Letter from L. E. Swanson to Dr. Bayard Carter, Chairman Department of Obstetrics-Gynecology December 30, 1957, Carter Papers; Letter from Bayard Carter to Dr. Marion S. Brown July 12, 1950, Carter Papers. The admonition to consult with one or two other obstetricians before performing a cesarean, if it was ever widely enforced, was apparently short-lived. When the American Academy of Obstetrics and Gynecology attempted to require all its members to do just that, obstetricians orchestrated a protest. "It seems to me," wrote one obstetrician who led the opposition to the rule, "that if this rule is allowed to become law, obstetricians are allowing a noose to be placed around their necks." He pointed out that every cesarean section, tubal ligation, and therapeutic abortion in his hospital was subjected to "careful scrutiny" at semiweekly department meetings where "one gets honest, impersonal evaluation by this method—whereas the mandatory consultation rule may lead to exactly the opposite (i.e., 'rubber stamp concurrence', or 'I concur' type of consultation)." Letter from O. Hunter Jones, MD, Charlotte, NC, March 24, 1954, to Dr. Bayard C. Carter. The protest was an addendum to the letter titled "Letter to The Joint Commission on Accreditation," 660 Rush Street, Chicago, Illinois, Attention: Dr. Edwin L. Crosby, Director, March 18, 1954, Carter Papers.

4. Walker, *Shaping Our Mothers' World.*

5. “Baby, Born after Mother Perishes, in Good Health”; “Pen-Knife Surgery.” These types of stories appeared occasionally in assorted venues. See also “Baby Delivered after Runaway Car Kills Mother.”

6. “Camera in Hospital.”

7. Davis, “The Truth about Caesareans”; Safford, “Tell Me Doctor”; Pierson, “WHEN Caesarean Section?”; Speert and Guttmacher, *Obstetric Practice*, 322.

8. Safford, “Tell Me Doctor—Part 16,” 95.

9. McEvoy, “Our Streamlined Baby,” 16; Walker, *Shaping Our Mothers' World*, 114–116.

10. McEvoy, “Our Streamlined Baby,” 16.

11. De Kruif, “Forgotten Mothers,” 64; “Childbirth: Nature v. Drugs”; Bolotin, “‘Painless’ Childbirth.”

12. Tracy and Leupp, “Painless Childbirth”; Ver Beck, “The Painless Childbirth”; Wolf, *Deliver Me from Pain*, 44–72. Maternity hospitals readily acknowledged that only the most desperate women gave birth outside their homes. The New England Hospital, the only all-women's hospital and only maternity hospital in Boston in the 1860s, for example, described itself as for the woman who “is not so fortunate as to possess a good home and friends.” “Annual Report of the New-England Hospital for Women and Children for the Year Ending November 10, 1864,” New England Hospital Papers, Sophia Smith Collection, Neilson Library, Smith College, Northampton, MA. See also Drachman, *Hospital with a Heart*. For histories of the changing role of hospitals in the United States, see Rosenberg, *The Care of Strangers*, and Rosner, *A Once Charitable Enterprise*.

13. De Kruif, “Forgotten Mothers,” 13; Leavitt, *Brought to Bed*, 269. The experience of just one small-town clinic is indicative of women's reluctance to give birth in an institutional setting. Of the more than 5,000 babies (only 23 of them by cesarean) delivered from 1933 to 1937 by doctors at the Charlotte Maternity Clinic in North Carolina, almost all were still being born at home. Charlotte Maternity Clinic Logbooks, Deliveries 1933–1937, Duke University Medical Center Archives, Durham, NC.

14. Speert and Guttmacher, *Obstetric Practice*, 320; Loudon, *Death in Childbirth*, 365–397, figures on 365; Greenhill, *Obstetrics*, 996–1001. For the story of the first antibiotic, made available to civilians after World War II, see Lax, *The Mold in Dr. Florey's Coat*. For more on the history of the post–World War II global blood industry, see D. Starr, *Blood*, 121–143, 185–204.

15. Letter from Samuel S. Lambeth, MD, Maryville, Tennessee, January 30, 1949, to Nick, Carter Papers; Letter from Nick to S. S. Lambeth, February 21, 1949, Carter Papers. Carter was known as “Nick” to family, friends, and colleagues.

16. Interview of retired obstetrician by author, Chicago physician interview 12, October 1, 2012, Avon, IN, transcribed from digital recording; Interview of retired obstetrician by author, Chicago physician interview 8, October 5, 2012, Chicago, IL, transcribed from digital tape recording.

17. Letter from William M. Mallia, MD, Schenectady, NY, to Robert L. Faulkner, MD, Cleveland, OH, July 5, 1952, Carter Papers (Carter is copied on the letter); Letter from James Kowchak, Fresno County Hospital, Fresno, Calif., to Dr. Carter, undated including a response dated November 19, 1952, Carter Papers.

18. Letter from Keith M. Oliver, Puercellville, VA, to Dr. Carter, February 2, 1949, Carter Papers; Letter from James Kowchak, Fresno County Hospital, Fresno, Calif., to

Dr. Carter, undated circa November 1952, Carter Papers; Letter from Bayard Carter to Dr. James Kowchok, Carter Papers; Letter from J. R. Kernodle, MD, Kernodle Clinic, Inc., Burlington, NC, July 14, 1952, to Dr. Bayard Carter, Carter Papers.

19. Letter from J. R. Kernodle, MD, Kernodle Clinic, Inc., Burlington, NC, March 1, 1951, to Dr. Bayard Carter, Carter Papers.

20. James T. Cleland, "Francis Bayard Carter," tribute written for dinner honoring Carter and letter to Mr. Howard I. Wells, 116 South Michigan Avenue, Chicago 3, IL, from Bayard Carter, September 23, 1957, Carter Papers; Letter from Samuel S. Lambeth, MD, Maryville, Tennessee, December 29, 1948, to Dr. Carter, Carter Papers; Letter from Nick to Dr. S. S. Lambeth, January 10, 1949, Carter Papers; Letter from Nick to S. S. Lambeth, June 13, 1949, Carter Papers.

21. Letter from I. M. Wright to Dr. Carter, President, American Board of Obstetrics and Gynecology, May 16, 1958, Carter Papers.

22. Lynch, "More Conservatism in Cesarean Section." Lynch provides this list as an example of how undervalued obstetrics was.

23. Holmes, "Obstetrics, A Lost Art."

24. Holmes, "Obstetrics, A Lost Art"; Letter from Joseph DeLee to Ogden T. McClurg, August 8, 1922, Joseph B. DeLee Papers, Northwestern Memorial Hospital Archives, Chicago, IL, hereinafter referred to as DeLee Papers.

25. Johnson, "John Whitridge Williams, MD," 136.

26. Dally, *Women Under the Knife*, xvii; McGregor, *From Midwives to Medicine*, 1–7, 33–68; Holmes, "Obstetrics, A Lost Art."

27. Letter from Sänger to Dr. Harris, October 1890, Robert Harris Collection, Wangensteen Historical Library of Biology and Medicine, University of Minnesota, Minneapolis, MN, hereinafter referred to as Harris Collection; Letter from Sänger to Dr. Harris, October 1891, Harris Collection.

28. C. Miller, "A General Consideration of Cæsarean Section."

29. Mitchinson mentions this pairing of two medical specialties with contradictory underlying premises in *Giving Birth in Canada, 1900–1950*, 57–58.

30. Randall, *Developments in the Certification of Obstetricians and Gynecologists*; Starr, *The Social Transformation of American Medicine*, 356–357; Stevens, *American Medicine and the Public Interest*, 202.

31. Randall, *Developments in the Certification of Obstetricians and Gynecologists*; Paul Starr, *The Social Transformation of American Medicine*, 356–57; Stevens, *American Medicine and the Public Interest*, 202; Frank P. Albertson, interview by Patrick Ettinger, October 28, 1993, Indiana University Center for the History of Medicine Oral History Project, Indiana Historical Society, Indianapolis, IN.

32. Letter from William M. Mallia, MD, Schenectady, NY, to Robert L. Faulkner, MD, Cleveland, OH, July 5, 1952, Carter Papers (Carter is copied on the letter); Letter to William F. Mengert, MD, President, American Academy of Obstetrics and Gynecology, College of Medicine, University of Illinois, 1853 W. Polk, Chicago 12, IL, from Willis E. Brown, MD, undated circa 1950s, Carter Papers (Carter is copied on the letter).

33. "Hospitals Approved for Residencies in Specialties"; "Approved Residencies and Fellowships"; 1954 Report of the Assistant Secretary, American Board of Obstetrics and

Gynecology, Carter Papers; Letter from Paul Titus to Howard C. Taylor, Jr., MD, Department of Obstetrics and Gynecology, College of Physicians and Surgeons, NY, NY, December 28, 1949, Carter Papers.

34. Letter from Bayard Carter to Dr. J. D. Bateman, Augusta, GA, July 28, 1953, Carter Papers.

35. Letter from Kermit E. Krantz to Lolita F. Navarro, MD, January 29, 1970, Kermit E. Krantz, MD, November 1969–May 1970 Correspondence, Kermit E. Krantz Papers, Kansas University Medical Center Archives, Kansas City, KS.

36. J. B. DeLee, "Mother's Day Address," May 12, 1940, DeLee Papers. Feminist scholars who have studied childbirth and written critically of DeLee include Rothman, *In Labor*, 57–59, and Block, *Pushed*, 21–23, 216–217. Historians have begun to re-examine DeLee's practice and legacy. See, for example, Lewis, "The Gospel of Good Obstetrics."

37. Coontz, *The Way We Never Were*, 24; May, *Homeward Bound*, xii–xv. As May writes on pp. 120–121, "The postwar consensus was nowhere more evident than in the matter of having children."

38. Hingson, "The Control of Pain and Fear."

39. Davis-Floyd, *Birth as an American Rite of Passage*, 102. The claim that analgesia made women quiet and cooperative is sprinkled throughout the medical literature of the era. See, for example, Garcia, Waltman, and Lubin, "Continuous Intravenous Infusion of Demerol in Labor"; Black, "Psychorelaxation Management for Labor and Delivery," 110; Interview of retired obstetrician ("Gene Lawrence," a pseudonym) by author, Chicago, IL, July 12, 1996, transcribed from tape recording.

40. Guttmacher, "The Facts about Caesarean Section"; "The Doctor Talks about Caesareans"; Greenhill, *Obstetrics*, 1000.

41. Taves, "Cesarean Births."

42. "For Cesarean Births"; Dailey, "Mother Is Hypnotised for Birth"; Cooley, "One-Hour Childbirth"; Dailey, "Painless Childbirth Seen Boon to Future Mothers." The black press also reported regularly on the far higher maternal death rate in the black community compared to the white community. See "Childbirth Deaths Drop"; "Pregnancy Death Rate Twice That of Whites"; "Hail Decrease In Deaths during Childbirth"; and "Negro Health Reasons."

43. Hilliard, "A Woman Doctor Speaks Frankly about Childbirth"; "Childbirth Dangers Cut"; Mendels, "A Revolution in Childbirth?"

44. "The Doctor Talks about Cesareans"; Guttmacher, "The Facts about Caesarean Section"; "Health Talk. So You're Expecting A Baby?"; Burns, "It's a Caesarean Baby."

45. Schauffler, "Tell Me, Doctor."

46. All Americans expressed keen interest in President Kennedy, the first lady, and the births of their sons; the death of Patrick thus affected every community. For a description of the warm relationship between the black community and Jackie Kennedy, see Granton, "The Lady in Black." For more details on the births of John Jr. and Patrick Kennedy, see Leaming, *Mrs. Kennedy*, 13–14; Anderson, *Jack and Jackie*, 183.

47. Gieske and Smith, "Boy Is Born to the Kennedys."

48. Lawrence, "Kennedy Alters Schedule."

49. Ibid.

50. Haseltine, "There Is No Mystery About Caesarean Section"; Letter from Mrs. X, NY, to Dr. Bayard Carter, July 8, 1954, Carter Papers; Letter from Bayard Carter to Mrs. X, July 12, 1954, Carter Papers.

51. "How Many Caesareans?"

52. Blair, "Kennedys Mourning Baby Son."

53. Ibid.; Burd, "Requiem Mass Slated Today for Kennedy Boy"; Birch, "What You Should Know about Cesareans." For a detailed account of Patrick Kennedy's birth and death, see Clarke, "A Death in the First Family."

54. "The Whys of Caesareans." In the early twenty-first century in the United States, placental abruption occurs in only 0.65 percent of births. See Ananth and Wilcox, "Placental Abruption and Perinatal Mortality."

55. "Why Babies Die."

56. Tron et al., "Trends in Smoking Before, During, and After Pregnancy"; Perry, *Jacqueline Kennedy*, 13, 25–26.

57. Brandt, *The Cigarette Century*, 57–58, 65, 324–325, quote on 57.

58. Ibid., 65, 324–325.

59. Ibid., 57–58, 324–325.

60. Ibid., 57–58, 65, 324–325, quote on 57. In the late 1950s and early 1960s very few studies examined the effects of cigarettes on pregnancy and fetal development. The few that did were inconsistent in their design, including the definition of a smoker. The only uniform finding coming from those rare, flawed studies was that the incidence of premature birth was about double for mothers who smoked, and the likelihood of prematurity increased according to a mother's daily consumption of cigarettes. Goldstein et al., "Cigarette Smoking and Prematurity." One well-designed 1959 study found that the effect of smoking on birth weight "significantly" lowered the incidence of induction among smokers because "smoking during pregnancy substantially retards foetal growth." See Lowe, "Effect of Mothers' Smoking Habits," 676. Only one study conducted in 1935 seemed particularly ominous, concluding that the fetal heart rate increased markedly within eight minutes of a mother lighting up. The discovery alarmed the researchers who authored the study but apparently not the at-large obstetric community. Sontag and Wallace, "The Effect of Cigaret Smoking during Pregnancy."

61. *Smoking and Health*, 343. While a few doctors suspected a link between smoking during pregnancy and negative pregnancy outcomes, their suspicions were based on either anecdotal evidence or happenstance personal observation. When treating Alice Roosevelt Longworth during her first and only pregnancy in 1925, Joseph DeLee wrote to a colleague: "When Mrs. Longworth arrived in Chicago . . . I kept her in bed a great part of the time and prescribed a diet, also a reduction of the amount of cigarettes, as it occurred to me that perhaps the nicotine was causing the uterus to contract." Letter from DeLee to Dr. Sofie A. Nordhuff-Jung, Washington, DC, February 21, 1925, DeLee Papers. In 1927, Dr. Bertha Van Hoosen's disdain for cigarettes, coupled with years of medical practice, prompted her to warn colleagues that "motherhood and tobacco . . . [are] as antagonistic as water and fire." Van Hoosen, "Should Women Smoke."

62. Pinney et al., *The Health Consequences of Smoking for Women*, vii–viii; Cope, Lancaster, and Stevens, "Smoking in Pregnancy"; Meyer, Jonas, and Tonascia, "Perinatal

Events Associated with Maternal Smoking"; Luck and Nau, "Exposure of the Fetus"; Greenberg et al., "Measuring the Exposure of Infants to Tobacco Smoke."

63. Killilea, *Karen*; Killilea, *With Love from Karen*, 284–286.

64. Ibid.

65. Killilea, *Karen*, 10, 20, 33–34, 54; Killilea, *With Love from Karen*, 270.

66. Killilea, *With Love from Karen*, 270–276.

67. Russell, Taylor, and Law, "Smoking in Pregnancy," 124, 125; Barnes, "Reducing the Hazards of Birth."

68. Brandt, *The Cigarette Century*, 65, 324–325. The increase in cesareans is alluded to in "The Doctor Talks about Caesareans." Greenhill, *Obstetrics*, 1000.

69. "When a Cesarean Birth Is Necessary"; "The Whys of Caesareans."

70. Davidson, "The Case for and against Induced Labor."

71. Ibid.; Jewett, "When Is It Safe to Induce Labor?"; Davidson, "The Case for and against Induced Labor."

72. Philadelphia Lying-In Charity, Patient Charts, vol. 1 (1891), Pennsylvania Hospital Historic Collections, Philadelphia, PA; New England Hospital Maternity Records, vol. 1 Maternity 1872–1873 and vol. 30 Maternity 1896, Francis A. Countway Library of Medicine, Rare Books and Special Collections, Harvard University, Boston, MA.

73. Interview of retired obstetrician by author, July 12, 1996, Chicago area, IL, transcribed from tape recording. "Gene Lawrence" is a pseudonym.

CHAPTER 4: **Assessing Risk: 1950s–1970s**

1. DeLee, "The Prophylactic Forceps Operation." In the article, DeLee characterized childbirth as "a decidedly pathological process," a premise that served as the rationale for the medical interventions DeLee advised be routine at all births. For detailed descriptions of post–World War II births in the United States, see Wolf, *Deliver Me from Pain*, 105–135.

2. Interview of retired obstetrician by author, Chicago physician interview 1, October 1, 2012, Chicago area, transcribed from digital recording.

3. A Chicago obstetrician trained in the early 1950s characterized labor-sitting when he was a resident as "my job and part of my training." Interview of retired obstetrician by author, July 19, 2004, Chicago, IL, transcribed from tape recording; de Kruif, *The Fight for Life*; Interview of retired obstetrician by author, July 19, 2004, Chicago, IL, transcribed from tape recording.

4. A brief biographical description of Friedman and his experience at Sloane is available online as part of the finding aid for the Emanuel A. Friedman Papers, 1953–1989, Columbia University Libraries Archival Collection, New York, NY, http://library-archives.cumc.columbia.edu/finding-aid/emanuel-friedman-papers-1953–1989, accessed May 28, 2017. Friedman first described the curve in Friedman, "The Graphic Analysis of Labor."

5. Friedman, "The Graphic Analysis of Labor."

6. Ibid., 1570; Neal et al., "'Active Labor' Duration and Dilation Rates"; Interview by author of obstetrician, Ohio obstetrician interview 3, August 12, 2013, southern Ohio, transcribed from digital recording.

7. Friedman himself presented this view less than a decade after introducing his curve, and, given his name, his views held great sway. See Friedman and Sachtleben, "Dysfunctional

Labor: II," 566, 576; Ramsbotham, *The Principles and Practice of Obstetric Medicine*, 213–216.

8. Friedman described the curve for primiparas in Friedman, "The Graphic Analysis of Labor," and the curve for multiparas in Friedman, "Labor in Multiparas."

9. Evans, "Prolonged Labor"; Calkins, "Prolonged Labor," 333; Interview of retired obstetrician by author, Chicago physician interview 7, October 5, 2012, Chicago, IL, transcribed from digital recording.

10. Friedman, "The Graphic Analysis of Labor"; Greenhill, *Obstetrics*, 189.

11. Peyton, "Prolonged Labor"; Calkins, Irvine, and Horsley, "Variations in the Factors"; Calkins, "Prolonged Labor."

12. Klingensmith, "The Clinical Management of Dystocia," 1580; Interview of practicing obstetrician by author, Ohio obstetrician interview 1, August 24, 2012, southern Ohio area, transcribed from digital recording.

13. Alexander et al., "Epidural Analgesia"; Interview by author of obstetrician, June 28, 2006, Chicago, IL, transcribed from tape recording; Interview of retired obstetrician by author, Chicago physician interview 7, October 5, 2012, Chicago, IL, transcribed from digital recording.

14. In the index of the 1924 fifth edition of J. Whitridge Williams' *Obstetrics*, the word "dystocia" appears followed by 11 "due to" subentries that included "abnormalities of the cervix," "abnormalities of the expulsive forces," "abnormalities of the foetus," "abnormalities of the vagina," "contracted pelves," "tumors of birth canal," and "uterine displacements." Williams, *Obstetrics* (1924), 1053. The 1918 edition of Joseph B. DeLee's text contained a considerably longer list in its index that included dystocia due to "anomalies of bony pelvis," "anomalies of parturient canal," "anomalies of uterine action," "excessively large fetus," "stenosis of vulva," and "tumors of bladder," among many others. DeLee, *The Principles and Practice of Obstetrics* (1918), 1063; Richmond, "History of a Successful Casarean Operation."

15. Williams, *Obstetrics* (1917), 712, 713, 723, 729–733, 857; Williams, *Obstetrics* (1924), 767.

16. "Dystocia," *ACOG Committee Statement*; "Dystocia," *ACOG Technical Bulletin*; "Dystocia and Augmentation of Labor," *ACOG Practice Bulletin*; Friedman, *Labor*, 4–5.

17. Interview by author of obstetrician, Chicago physician interview 2, October 1, 2012, Chicago, IL, transcribed from digital recording; Interview of obstetrician by author, Chicago physician interview 4, October 3, 2012, Chicago, IL, transcribed from digital recording; Marieskind, *An Evaluation of Caesarean Section*, 9–10; Oláh and Neilson, "Failure to Progress;" Interview of retired obstetrician by author, July 12, 1996, Chicago area, transcribed from tape recording.

18. "Dystocia," *ACOG Committee Statement*; "Dystocia," *ACOG Technical Bulletin*. In 1995, ACOG also sanctioned low- or high-dose oxytocin regimens to correct "uterine forces." "Dystocia and the Augmentation of Labor," *ACOG Technical Bulletin*; Evans, "Prolonged Labor," 528.

19. Landesman, "New Promise of Easier Childbirth"; Student Birth Report from L. S., May 1964, Flora Hommel Papers, Archives of Labor and Urban Affairs, Wayne State University, Detroit, MI.

20. Landesman, "New Promise of Easier Childbirth," 116; "Birth by Appointment."

21. Doctors first observed this tendency in the late 1930s. Cron, Randall, and Kretzschmar, "A Report of the Committee." Physicians did not consider the connection between elective induction and cesarean birth a significant problem until the 1970s and 1980s, when elective inductions increased markedly and studies showed that the cesarean section rate among first-time mothers who were induced was twice as high as among first-time mothers who went into labor spontaneously. Smith et al., "Hazards and Benefits"; Interview of obstetrician by author, Chicago physician interview 5, October 4, 2012, Chicago, IL, transcribed from digital recording; Interview by author of obstetrician, Ohio obstetrician interview 3, August 12, 2013, southern Ohio, transcribed from digital recording.

22. Bishop, "Elective Induction of Labor"; Bishop, "Pelvic Scoring for Elective Induction"; Frank J. Zlatnik, "Elective Induction of Labor"; "Induction and Augmentation of Labor," *ACOG Technical Bulletin* (1987); "Induction and Augmentation of Labor," *ACOG Technical Bulletin* (1991).

23. Interview of obstetrician by author, Chicago physician interview 6, October 4, 2012, Chicago, IL, transcribed from digital recording.

24. For a complete description of the analgesic and anesthetic protocol used in hospitals during the baby boom, see Wolf, *Deliver Me from Pain*, 105–135; Stanley, "Eulogy for Virginia Apgar," September 15, 1974, Apgar Papers, National Library of Medicine, available online.

25. Montgomery, "Obstetric Amnesia, Analgesia, and Anesthesia," 1638. For a complete description of the history of pain relief during childbirth in the United States, see Wolf, *Deliver Me from Pain*. For a specific description of mid-twentieth-century drug protocol during birth, see pages 73–104; Interview of mother by author, November 1, 2005, Glencoe, IL, transcribed from tape recording. The reason this mother did not receive analgesics during her first birth was that she had read Grantly Dick-Read's book *Childbirth without Fear* during her pregnancy and practiced his breathing exercises during labor. She was so quiet in the labor room that nurses did not realize how far along she was in labor until she was ready to push. Then she was wheeled to delivery, only to face general anesthesia.

26. Virginia Apgar, unpublished paper titled "The Perinatal Problem," 1958, Virginia Apgar Papers, Mount Holyoke College, Archives and Special Collections, South Hadley, MA, hereinafter referred to as Apgar Papers; Apgar and Papper, "Transmission of Drugs across the Placenta."

27. For a history of medical specialization and its influence on medical education and practice, see Stevens, *American Medicine and the Public Interest*.

28. Apgar, "A Proposal for a New Method"; Apgar, "Method of Evaluation of Newborn"; Letter from Virginia Apgar to Dr. Murdina M. Desmond, Baylor University College of Medicine, October 7, 1960, Virginia Apgar Papers, Mount Holyoke College, Archives and Special Collections, South Hadley, MA.

29. Apgar, "A Proposal for a New Method." Journal articles and letters from colleagues indicate that after its introduction in the United States, physicians in European countries adopted the Apgar score within a decade. See, for example, letter from Virginia Apgar to

Dr. D. Keith McElroy, May 9, 1962, and letter from Virginia Apgar to Dr. Hans Karl Wendl, Frauenklinik Finkenau, Hamburg, West Germany, November 22, 1963, both in Apgar Papers; Memorandum from Louis G. Buttell, The National Foundation / The March of Dimes, to Dr. Virginia Apgar, undated circa 1963–65, and letter from Virginia Apgar to Dr. Hans Karl Wendl, Frauenklinik Finkenau, Hamburg, West Germany, November 22, 1963, both in Apgar Papers; "Second Apgar Rating."

30. Memorandum from Louis G. Buttell, The National Foundation / The March of Dimes, to Dr. Virginia Apgar, undated circa 1963–65, Apgar Papers; Drage and Berendes, "Apgar Scores and Outcome of the Newborn"; "Second Apgar Rating"; "Apgar Scores as a Predictor of Fetal Outcome"; "Use and Misuse of the Apgar Score"; "Use and Abuse of the Apgar Score"; "The Apgar Score."

31. Virginia Apgar, unpublished paper titled "The Perinatal Problem," 1958, Apgar Papers; Day, "Guardian of the Newborn." Letter from Virginia Apgar to Jaime Quintanilla, MD, Amarillo, TX, January 20, 1969, Apgar Papers. For a history of pediatrics, see Halpern, *American Pediatrics.*

32. Letter from Jean Husted to Virginia Apgar, Office of *Dorland's Illustrated Medical Dictionary*, W. B. Saunders Company, June 6, 1961; Letter from Jean Husted to Virginia Apgar, June 20, 1961, both in Apgar Papers.

33. Student Birth Reports, box 11, folder 11.21, student birth report from M. C., 1977, Flora Hommel Papers, Archives of Labor and Urban Affairs, Wayne State University, Detroit, MI, hereinafter referred to as Hommel Papers.

34. Apgar, "A Proposal for a New Method."

35. James, "Aspects of Fetal Monitoring."

36. Apgar, "A Proposal for a New Method."

37. Letter from Apgar to Dr. William L. Rumsey, March 15, 1966; Letter from Apgar to Dr. Mary E. McGarry, March 16, 1966; Letter from Virginia Apgar to Jaime Quintanilla, MD, Amarillo TX, January 20, 1969; Letter from Virginia Apgar to Dr. E. K. Ahvenainen and Dr. Ikonen, Central Hospital of Tampere, Tampere, Finland, May 7, 1969, all in Apgar Papers.

38. Drage and Berendes, "Apgar Scores and Outcome of the Newborn"; Letter from Apgar to Dr. Herbert E. Poch, February 25, 1966, Apgar Papers.

39. Altman, "Doctors Debate Value of Test."

40. Student Birth Reports, box 11, folder 11.21, student birth report from M. D., 1973; Box 12, folder 12.1, student birth report from C. S., April 29, 1974; box 12, folder 12.4, student birth report from O. M., May 6, 1977, Hommel Papers.

41. Letter from J. B. to Dr. Ralph H. Verploeg, December 16, 1960, Apgar Papers. See endnote 23 in chapter 2 for a discussion of infant mortality rates over time in the United States.

42. For a history of the March of Dimes and development of the polio vaccine, see Oshinsky, *Polio.* James, "Fond Memories of Virginia Apgar." During the 1960s, articles either by or about Apgar and her work on birth defects appeared in every major American magazine. A representative sampling includes Apgar, "They're Solving the Mysteries of Birth Defects"; Apgar, "New Ways to Save Your Unborn Child"; Day, "Guardian of the Newborn."

43. Watson, "How to Have a Perfect Baby."

44. Ibid. For a description of Apgar's life and work, see Calmes, "Virginia Apgar"; Gerl, "Out of the Back Rooms"; James, "Fond Memories."

45. Apgar, "New Ways to Save Your Unborn Child"; Commiff, "New Medical Specialty"; Letter from Mrs. I. T. to Public Affairs Pamphlet No. 272, March 13, 1969; Letter from Virginia Apgar to Mrs. I. T., March 21, 1969, Letter from Virginia Apgar to Mrs. I. T., July 1, 1969, all in Apgar Papers.

46. Watson, "How to Have a Perfect Baby"; Apgar, "New Ways to Save Your Unborn Child"; Apgar, "They're Solving the Mysteries of Birth Defects"; Day, "Guardian of the Newborn."

47. Eisenberg, "Genetics and the Survival of the Unfit"; Commiff, "New Medical Specialty"; Day, "Guardian of the Newborn." The Apgar Papers contain a folder devoted to Apgar's 1973 appearance on *Donahue*; mothers from all over the country wrote to her with their concerns after that show. Apgar responded to every letter.

48. Watson, "How to Have a Perfect Baby."

49. Apgar, "New Ways to Save Your Unborn Child"; Watson, "How to Have a Perfect Baby."

50. Office of NIH History, "A Thin Blue Line"; Apgar, "New Ways to Save Your Unborn Child." Although laws governing health insurance have always varied from state to state, before the early 1960s pregnancy was considered a voluntary condition not automatically covered by health insurance. Even the 1978 Pregnancy Discrimination Act had loopholes leaving many women without maternity coverage. Gold, Kenney, and Singh, "Paying for Maternity Care." Until passage of the Patient Protection and Affordable Care Act by Congress in 2010 and its full implementation in 2014, the law concerning maternity coverage did not apply to individually purchased policies.

51. Letter from Virginia Apgar to Mrs. W. S., NJ, June 23, 1967, Apgar Papers; Commiff, "New Medical Specialty."

52. Apgar and Beck, *Is My Baby All Right?*, 122–123.

53. For a description of American mothers' tranquilizer use, see Metzel, " 'Mother's Little Helper.' "

54. "The Untold Story of the Thalidomide Babies," 20; Ridgeway, "More about Thalidomide." The particular deformity, or set of deformities, seen in a child depended on which organ or limb had been in a crucial stage of development on the day, or days, a woman had ingested the drug. See Brynner and Stephens, *Dark Remedy*.

55. Brynner and Stephens, *Dark Remedy*, 53. American infants were not wholly spared from the effects of thalidomide because many American doctors agreed to test market the drug on patients for Richardson-Merrell, the pharmaceutical company seeking to market thalidomide in the United States. Those clinical tests involved at least 20,000 patients, more than 3,700 of whom were women of childbearing age; 207 were pregnant. Brynner and Stephens, *Dark Remedy*, 55–56. For more evidence of thalidomide consumption by pregnant women in the United States, see Nulsen, "Trial of Thalidomide." The letter that first alerted the medical community to thalidomide's potential dangers is Florence, "Is Thalidomide to Blame?" The American press widely reported the effects of thalidomide even though it was largely a European story. See, for example, "Sleeping Pill Nightmare"; "The Full Story"; "The Thalidomide Disaster"; "The Untold Story."

56. "Rubella Vaccines"; Brynner and Stephens, *Dark Remedy,* 56. For a history of German measles and the 1963–65 epidemic, see Reagan, *Dangerous Pregnancies.* For more on the history of therapeutic abortions, see Reagan, *When Abortion Was a Crime.*

57. See, for example, Spencer, "Attack on the Unborn"; "The Agony of Mothers"; "Rubella Vaccines."

58. "Narrative History of the National Institutes of Health," Administrative History, Department of Health, Education, and Welfare volume 1, parts XIII and XIV, box 7, papers of Lyndon Baines Johnson, 1963–1969, The Lyndon Baines Johnson Presidential Library, Austin, TX, hereinafter referred to as LBJ Library. "A Bill of Rights for Children," Task Force Reports, box 4, 1966, Report of the President's Task Force on Early Childhood Development, LBJ Library.

59. Memorandum July 17, 1973, to Dr. Apgar from D. H.; Letter from D. M., Bloomingdale, NJ, to Virginia Apgar, April 16, 1968; Letter from Apgar to Mrs. H. M., May 9, 1968; Letter from L. M., Birmingham, MI, March 21, 1973, to Virginia Apgar; Letter to Apgar from C. L., March 22, 1973, all in Apgar Papers.

60. Letter from D. M., Bloomingdale, NJ, to Virginia Apgar, April 16, 1968; Letter from Apgar to Mrs. H. M., May 9, 1968; Letter to Apgar from M. A., Columbus, OH, March 21, 1973; Letter from Apgar to Mrs. M. A., April 9, 1973; Letter from L. M., Birmingham, MI, March 21, 1973, to Virginia Apgar; Letter from Apgar to Mrs. L. M., April 6, 1973; Letter to Apgar from Mrs. L. D., April 11, 1973, all in Apgar Papers.

61. Barnes, "Reducing the Hazards of Birth."

62. Day, "Guardian of the Newborn."

63. Neuhoff, Burke, and Porreco, "Cesarean Birth."

64. The overall induction of labor in the United States more than doubled from 1990 to 2006 to 225 per 1,000 live births. "Induction of Labor"; Interview by author of obstetrician, Chicago physician interview 6, October 4, 2012, Chicago, IL, transcribed from digital recording.

65. "Presidential Address, Obstetrical Society of Philadelphia," February 12, 1981, J. Robert Willson, MD, presidential guest speaker, typed transcript, J. Robert Willson Papers, National Library of Medicine, History of Medicine Division, Bethesda, MD.

CHAPTER 5: **Inflating Risk: 1960s–1980s**

1. Irvine Loudon discusses the maternal death rate in the United States in *Death in Childbirth*, 365–397.

2. "Monitoring Childbirth."

3. Interviews by author of obstetrician, June 26 and June 28, 2006, Chicago, IL, both transcribed from tape recording.

4. Nicolson and Fleming, *Imaging and Imagining the Fetus*; Taylor, *Public Life of the Fetal Sonogram*, 30–35; Interview of Dr. Charles Hammond by Jessica Roseberry, June 2, 2004, Durham, NC, Duke University Medical Center Archives, Durham, NC.

5. Donald, MacVicar, and Brown, "Investigation of Abdominal Masses"; Nicolson and Fleming, *Imagining and Imaging the Fetus*, 240–245; Campbell, "A Short History of Sonography"; Interview of Dr. Charles Hammond.

6. Quoted in Becker, *The Elusive Embryo*, 165–166; Quoted in Rothman, *The Tentative Pregnancy*, 87–88; Rapp, *Testing Women, Testing the Fetus*, 119–121.

7. "Ultrasonography in Pregnancy," *ACOG Technical Bulletin*; "Ultrasonography in Pregnancy," *ACOG Practice Bulletin*.

8. Kolker and Burke, *Prenatal Testing*, 25–26; Interview by author of obstetrician, June 26, 2006, Chicago, IL, transcribed from tape recording. For more on the fetus as patient, see Casper, *The Making of the Unborn Patient*. Studies have consistently corroborated the observation that ultrasounds do not change pregnancy outcome. See Bricker and Nelson, "Routine Doppler Ultrasound in Pregnancy"; Alfirevic, Stanpalija, and Medley, "Fetal and Umbilical Doppler in Normal Pregnancy."

9. Twist, "Story of a Home VBAC"; copies of the newsletter are available as part of the Sophia Smith Collection, Smith College, Northampton, MA. Women active in the birth reform movement in the 1970s and 1980s complained of a host of suspected side effects of ultrasound, including reduced birth weight, neurological impairment, "cellular effects," "effects on red blood cells," dyslexia, and "abnormal grasp," among many others. None have been proven. See Oberhaus, "How Safe Is Ultrasound?" The Cesarean Prevention Movement published *The Clarion;* copies of the newsletter are available at the Schlesinger Library, Radcliffe Institute, Cambridge, MA.

10. Taylor, "The Public Fetus and the Family Car." The ad appeared in the February 1991 issue of *Harper's*.

11. Sartwelle, "Electronic Fetal Monitoring."

12. Hon, "The Electronic Evaluation"; Hon, "The Diagnosis of Fetal Distress"; Interview by author of obstetrician, Chicago physician interview 2, October 1, 2012, Chicago, IL, transcribed from digital recording.

13. Quilligan and Paul, "Fetal Monitoring: Is It Worth It?"

14. Paul and Hon, "A Clinical Fetal Monitor"; " 'Watching' the Unborn Inside the Womb"; Kelly and Kulkarni, "Experiences with Fetal Monitoring"; Block, *Pushed*, 32.

15. "Theresa" is a pseudonym. Interview of mother by author, Chicago mother interview 1, March 13, 2012, Chicago, IL, transcribed from digital recording.

16. Ibid.

17. Ibid.

18. Hon, "Fetal Monitoring for the Practicing Physician"; Corea, "The Caesarean Epidemic," 30; Lent, "The Medical and Legal Risks," 817.

19. " 'Watching' the Unborn Inside the Womb."

20. Paul and Hon, "A Clinical Fetal Monitor"; Hon and Petrie, "Clinical Value of Fetal Heart Monitoring." As early as 1973, however, Hon began to echo others around the country, speculating that universal monitoring might demonstrate the same benefit in uncomplicated as in complicated labors. See Hon, "Current Concepts of Fetal Monitoring."

21. Quilligan and Paul, "Fetal Monitoring: Is It Worth It?"; Haverkamp and Orleans, "An Assessment of Electronic Fetal Monitoring"; Boehm, Davidson, and Barrett, "The Effect of Electronic Fetal Monitoring." Routine testing for diseases and conditions in the entire population is not done because the less likely a disease will be present, the more likely a positive test result will be a false positive. The same rule applies to monitoring all laboring women with EFM. For any given test, as the prevalence of the disease or condition decreases, the positive predictive value of the test decreases even more dramatically. Frigoletto and Nadel, "Electronic Fetal Heart Rate Monitoring."

22. Steinfels, "New Childbirth Technology"; Check, "Electronic Fetal Monitoring"; Marieskind, *An Evaluation of Caesarean Section*, 3–18; Prentice and Lind, "Fetal Heart Rate Monitoring during Labour"; Haverkamp and Orleans, "An Assessment of Electronic Fetal Monitoring"; Gilfix, "Electronic Fetal Monitoring." Feminists active in birth reform wrote critically about the credit mistakenly given to the higher cesarean rate for the lowered infant death rate. See Daub and Daub, "Caesareans Credited for Lower Death Rate"; Hall and Alexander, "Fetal Monitoring in a Community Hospital."

23. Interview by author of obstetrician, Chicago physician interview 6, October 4, 2012, Chicago, IL, transcribed from digital recording; Lent, "The Medical and Legal Risks."

24. Hon and Quilligan, "Electronic Evaluation of Fetal Heart Rate"; Yeh, Betyar, and Hon, "Computer Diagnosis of Fetal Heart Rate Patterns"; Benson et al., "Fetal Heart Rate as a Predictor of Fetal Distress."

25. Koh et al., "Experience with Fetal Monitoring"; Lee and Baggish, "The Effect of Unselected Intrapartum Fetal Monitoring"; Boehm and Goss, "The Xerox 400 Telecopier"; Cohen, Klapholz, and Thompson, "Electronic Fetal Monitoring and Clinical Practice." Decades of additional experience failed to mitigate the problem. In a 2008 study, four obstetricians could agree on the meaning of 50 fetal heart rate tracings in only 22 percent of cases. See Parer, Ikeda, and King, "The 2008 National Institute"; Brody, "Updating a Standard."

26. Interview by author of obstetrician, Chicago physician interview 6, October 4, 2012, Chicago, IL, transcribed from digital recording; Interview by author of obstetrician, Ohio obstetrician interview 1, southern Ohio area, August 24, 2012, transcribed from digital recording; Quoted in Grisanti, "The Cesarean Epidemic."

27. See, for example, Pollack, "The Case for Natural Childbirth"; Juhl, "I Had This Baby Under Hypnosis"; Haggerty, "Childbirth Made Difficult"; Gardner, "Having Your Baby at Home."

28. Interview by author of mother, July 18, 2004, Chicago area, IL, transcribed from tape recording, Carol is a pseudonym; Haverkamp, Orleans, et al., "A Controlled Trial"; Haverkamp and Orleans, "An Assessment of Electronic Fetal Monitoring," 130.

29. Interview by author of mother, July 18, 2004, Chicago area, IL, transcribed from tape recording.

30. Hon, Zannini, and Quilligan, "The Neonatal Value of Fetal Monitoring," 125; Lee and Baggish, "The Effect of Unselected Intrapartum Fetal Monitoring." For a history of the introduction and use of medical technology, see Howell, *Technology in the Hospital*. For more on the postwar infatuation with science and medical technology, see Brynner and Stephens, *Dark Remedy*, 1–17.

31. Haverkamp, Thompson, et al., "The Evaluation."

32. Placek and Taffel, "One-Sixth of 1980 US Births"; Haverkamp and Orleans, "An Assessment of Electronic Fetal Monitoring"; MacDonald et al., "The Dublin Randomized Controlled Trial"; Thacker, "The Efficacy of Intrapartum Electronic Fetal Monitoring"; Leveno et al., "A Prospective Comparison"; Costaine and Saade, "The First Cesarean." Obstetricians observed this immediately. At a Salt Lake City hospital, for example, where 84.4 percent of patients were monitored in 1971 and 1972, cesarean section rates were

3.5 percent before EFM but rose to 6.0 percent during the first year of EFM and 9.5 percent during its second year. Gabert and Stenchever, "Electronic Fetal Monitoring." See also Check, "Electronic Fetal Monitoring"; Kelso et al., "An Assessment"; Haverkamp, Orleans, et al., "A Controlled Trial"; Leveno et al., "A Prospective Comparison"; Prentice and Lind, "Fetal Heart Rate Monitoring during Labour."

33. Cole, "Can Natural Childbirth Survive Technology?"; Interview by author of obstetrician, Chicago physician interview 4, October 3, 2012, Chicago, IL, transcribed from digital recording; Marieskind, *An Evaluation of Cesarean Section*, 195.

34. Interview by author of obstetrician, Chicago physician interview 6, October 4, 2012, Chicago, IL, transcribed from digital recording. Systematic studies demonstrated the same phenomenon. Most excess cesarean surgeries performed under EFM seemed to be unnecessary—between 71 and 95 percent of the babies delivered by cesarean for presumed fetal distress, as indicated by a reading of the EFM strip, demonstrated no clinical signs of distress at birth. Prentice and Lind, "Fetal Heart Rate Monitoring during Labour."

35. Interview by author of obstetrician, Chicago physician interview 6, October 4, 2012, Chicago, IL, transcribed from digital recording.

36. Myers and Gleicher, "A Successful Program"; Gina Kolata, "New York Is First State"; March of Dimes, "New York Cesarean Rates, 2013." The nationwide rate in 2010 was 32.8 percent.

37. "Labor-Saving Devices"; Banta and Thacker, "Assessing the Costs and Benefits." By 1988, 70 percent of births in the United States were under EFM surveillance. Frigoletto and Nadel, "Electronic Fetal Heart Rate Monitoring."

38. Callaghan, Creanga, and Kuklina, "Severe Maternal Morbidity." Not only are maternal and neonatal care an essential moneymaker for hospitals, women customarily make healthcare decisions for their families. When hospitalization for a medical condition becomes necessary, wherever their children were born tends to be women's hospital of choice for the current crisis. For a discussion of this phenomenon, see Erikson, "New Focus on Women." For a critique and explanation of the fee-for-service system in the United States, see Bodenheimer and Grumbach, *Understanding Health Policy*, 31–32. Gilfix, "Electronic Fetal Monitoring"; Interview by author of retired obstetrician, Chicago physician interview 8, October 5, 2012, Chicago, IL, transcribed from digital recording. Some studies likewise noted the lower cost of EFM compared to human monitoring. See, for example, Gabert and Stenchever, "The Results of a Five-Year Study." Others noted that women found the comfort provided by human contact more valuable than EFM. Orleans, "Lessons from the Dublin Study"; Interview by author of obstetrician, Chicago physician interview 6, October 4, 2012, Chicago, IL, transcribed from digital recording.

39. Interview by author of midwife, August 28, 2012, southern Ohio, transcribed from digital recording; Interview by author of obstetric resident, Chicago physician interview 10, October 27, 2013, Chicago, IL, transcribed from digital recording; Interview by author of obstetrician, Chicago physician interview 11, October 24, 2013, Chicago, IL, transcribed from digital recording. No records track how many American hospitals have adopted central monitoring stations. Research indicates only that "many" have. See, for example, Withiam-Leitch, Shelton, and Fleming, "Central Fetal Monitoring"; Heelan, "Fetal Monitoring."

40. "Fetal Heart Rate Monitoring"; "Intrapartum Fetal Monitoring"; "The Current Role."

41. "State-of-the-Art: Electronic Fetal Monitoring"; "Guidelines for the Use of Fetal Monitoring"; "Intrapartum Fetal Heart Rate Monitoring"; "Fetal Heart Rate Patterns"; "Vaginal Birth after Previous Cesarean Delivery"; "Intrapartum Fetal Heart Rate Monitoring: Nomenclature, Interpretation, and General Management Principles."

42. "Management of Intrapartum Fetal Heart Rate Tracings"; Brody, "Updating a Standard."

43. Barnes, "Supreme Court Sides with Employers"; "All Women Get Right to Caesarean Birth"; Interview by author of obstetrician, Chicago physician interview 6, October 4, 2012, Chicago, IL, transcribed from digital recording.

44. Boston Women's Health Book Collective, *Our Bodies, Ourselves*, 286; Smith, "Angry and Happy at the Same Time," 103–104.

45. Smith, "Angry and Happy at the Same Time," 103, 105; Regal, "Home Birth after Two Cesareans," 124. That mothers are not given the opportunity to consent to treatments during labor is implied by the conclusions of the "Listening to Mothers" surveys conducted by Childbirth Connection in partnership with Lamaze International. The national survey of US women who gave birth in 2005 found that most mothers believed in the value of avoiding unnecessary medical interference but were nevertheless given a broad array of interventions and were poorly informed about the complications that could accompany those interventions. See Declercq et al., "Listening to Mothers II."

46. Haverkamp, Orleans, et al., "A Controlled Trial"; Interview of retired obstetrician by author, Chicago physician interview 1, October 1, 2012, Avon, IN, transcribed from digital recording. Hon did specifically claim that EFM solved the problems created by Pitocin. Hon and Petrie, "Clinical Value of Fetal Heart Monitoring"; Cole, "Can Natural Childbirth Survive Technology?," 14. That EFM replaced the nurse and the doctor, women's traditional companionship during labor, is discussed in Whitbeck, "Fetal Imaging and Fetal Monitoring."

47. Interviews by author of retired obstetricians, July 19, 2004, and Chicago physician interview 8, October 5, 2012, Chicago, IL, transcribed from tape recording.

48. Interview by author of obstetrician, Chicago physician interview 6, October 4, 2012, Chicago, IL, transcribed from digital recording.

49. Interview by author of obstetrician, Chicago physician interview 11, October 24, 2013, Chicago, IL, transcribed from digital recording.

50. May, *Homeward Bound*, 120–121; Interview by author of retired obstetrician, July 12, 1996, Chicago area, transcribed from tape recording. "Gene Lawrence" is a pseudonym.

51. Interview by author of retired obstetrician, July 12, 1996, Chicago area, transcribed from tape recording. "Gene Lawrence" is a pseudonym.

52. Ibid.; "The Doctor Talks about Babies by Appointment." Twilight sleep, developed by German obstetricians in Freiburg, Germany, in the early twentieth century, was touted widely in American magazines beginning in 1914, thanks to a few wealthy American women who traveled to Freiburg to give birth. A movement ensued for the right of American women to give birth painlessly, as one of many Progressive Era crusades. After the

death (having nothing to do with twilight sleep) in childbirth in 1916 of one of the movement's most vocal American proponents, the orchestrated demand for the original form of twilight sleep faded, although the term, and the use of different drug combinations, remained for many decades. For a description of the original, ritualized use of twilight sleep—scopolamine/morphine accompanied by blindfolding and binding women—see Wolf, *Deliver Me from Pain*, 44–72. Scholars have documented the relatively recent medicalization of childbirth, often in a critical fashion. See, for example, Rothman, *In Labor*, 29–77. Women's health reform organizations in the 1970s spoke directly to the public as they criticized what had become routine obstetrical interventions and procedures. See, for example, *Our Bodies, Ourselves*, 267–296.

53. Interviews by author of retired obstetricians, Chicago physician interview 8, October 5, 2012, Chicago, IL, and Chicago physician interview 12, October 1, 2012, Avon, IN, both transcribed from digital recording.

54. Letter from L. M., October 25, 1973, student birth reports, Flora Hommel Papers, Archives of Labor and Urban Affairs, Wayne State University, Detroit, MI.

55. Shultz, "*Journal* Mothers Report on Cruelty."

56. Gaskin, *Spiritual Midwifery*; Arms, *Immaculate Deception*, 10–27, quotes on 11, 25; *Our Bodies, Ourselves*, 267–269; Barbara H. Kane papers, Schlesinger Library, Radcliffe College, Cambridge, MA; Boston Association for Childbirth Education papers, Schlesinger Library, Radcliffe College, Cambridge, MA; Midwives Alliance of North American papers, Sophia Smith Collection, Neilson Library, Smith College, Northampton, MA.

57. *Our Bodies, Ourselves*, 251–326, quotes on 287–288. For more on the history of the birth reform movement, see Wolf, *Deliver Me from Pain*, 136–167. Judith Walzer Leavitt describes the efforts to ensure fathers would be permitted in labor and delivery rooms in *Make Room for Daddy: The Journey from Waiting Room to Birthing Room.*

58. *The Unnecesarean* blog is located at www.theunnecesarean.com; E-mail correspondence from Jill Arnold to the author, September 17 and 21, 2017.

59. www.theunnecesarean.com/obos, accessed September 18, 2017.

60. Cane and Shearer, *Frankly Speaking*, unnumbered p. i. The C/SEC papers, consisting largely of published newsletters, are housed at the Schlesinger Library, Radcliffe Institute, Cambridge, MA. For more on C/SEC, see Cohen and Estner, *Silent Knife*. For a history of CPM, see www.ican-online.org/history and www.theunnecesarean.com, accessed June 8, 2017.

61. Letter from D. C., January 27, 1988, letter from Mrs. K., Sterling Hts, MI, undated, and letter from S., Akron, OH, undated, National Women's Health Network Records, Sophia Smith Archives, Nielson Library, Smith College, Northampton, MA.

62. "Cesarean 'Seed' Uprooted"; Rahima Baldwin, "Whatever Happened to Normal Birth?," typed manuscript, 1984, Informed Homebirth/Informed Birth and Parenting Papers, Sophia Smith Collection, Neilson Library, Smith College, Northampton, MA.

63. Interviews of retired obstetricians by author, Chicago physician interviews 7 and 8, October 5, 2015, Chicago, IL, transcribed from digital recordings; "MDs Admit They Put Babys [sic] At Risk."

64. Rosen and Thomas, *The Cesarean Myth*, ix–xiii, quote on 70–71; Yuncker, "Delivery Procedures That Endanger a Baby's Life."

65. Interview by author of retired obstetrician, Chicago physician interview 8, October 5, 2012, Chicago, IL, transcribed from digital recording; Cole, "Can Natural Childbirth Survive Technology?" Therapeutic privilege—the right of doctors, given their education and expertise, to make unilateral decisions on behalf of their patients, even competent, adult patients—was the norm in American medicine until the early 1970s, affecting everyone seeking medical care. The impact on women, however, was particularly pronounced. Indeed, physicians' paternalistic approach incentivized the women's health reform movement, of which childbirth reform was a part. Other than childbirth, breast cancer treatment was perhaps the starkest example of how women were sidelined during every step of their medical care, from diagnosis to decision-making to treatment. For more information on physician paternalism in women's health and breast cancer treatment specifically, see Leopold, *A Darker Ribbon*, 188–242; Lerner, *The Breast Cancer Wars*, 141–195.

66. Stone, "Presidential Address"; Ranney, "Responsibilities," 245.

67. Beecham, "Natural Childbirth—A Step Backward?," 37, 44; Schmitt, "Natural Childbirth Takes a Giant Step"; Caillowette, "To the Editor;" Frank C. Yartz, "To the Editor," both letters in *The Female Patient* 15 (March 1990): 16.

68. "Monitoring Childbirth."

69. Hon and Petrie, "Clinical Value"; Marieskind, "An Evaluation of Cesarean Section," 195.

70. By 1990, 73 percent of all births in the United States were electronically monitored. The widespread use of the electronic fetal monitor happened so quickly that the American College of Obstetricians and Gynecologists (ACOG) did not begin to collect nationwide data on the extent of monitoring until 1990, when they found 73 percent of all births in the United States were monitored. By 2003, the rate was 85 percent. The ACOG Resource Center in Washington, DC, collects these figures from *National Vital Statistics Reports* and *Monthly Vital Statistics Reports*—1990–92: *Vital Statistics of the United States*, table 151; 2003: *National Vital Statistics Reports* 54, no. 2, table 27. In 2008, 85 percent of the approximately 4,000,000 babies born were born under continuous fetal monitoring. Parer, Ikeda, and King, "The 2008 National Institute"; Brody, "Updating a Standard."

71. Interview by author of obstetrician, June 28, 2006, Chicago, IL, transcribed from tape recording.

CHAPTER 6: **Operating in a Culture of Risk: A Fraught Environment for Obstetricians**

1. Emanuel Friedman, the developer of the Friedman curve, described his colleagues during this era as a beleaguered lot. See Friedman, "The Obstetrician's Dilemma."

2. Sartwelle and Johnston, "Cerebral Palsy Litigation."

3. For a thorough analysis of institutions', mainly hospitals', response to the legal, economic, and political environment affecting obstetricians and laboring women, see Morris, *Cut It Out*.

4. "NIH Consensus Development Task Force Statement," 902; Marieskind, *An Evaluation of Caesarean Section*, 1–25.

5. Marieskind, *An Evaluation of Caesarean Section*, 3–18; Interview of Helen Marieskind by author, July 9, 2008, Chicago, IL, quote from personal notes taken by author; Corea, "The Caesarean Epidemic," 31.

6. Comptroller General, *Report to the Congress of the United States*, 13, 39, and 40.

7. US Department of Health and Human Services, *Cesarean Childbirth*. The *American Journal of Obstetrics and Gynecology* published a synopsis of the findings six months before the formal report was issued: "NIH Consensus Development Task Force Statement."

8. Sidrow, "The Cesarean Phoenix."

9. DeLee, *The Principles and Practice of Obstetrics* (1925), 1046; Eastman, *Williams Obstetrics*, 1102–1105.

10. Interview of retired obstetrician by author, Chicago doctor interview 1, October 1, 2012, Avon, IN, transcribed from digital recording; "Guidelines for Vaginal Delivery after a Previous Cesarean Birth" (1982).

11. Cohen and Estner, *Silent Knife*, xvi–xviii.

12. All cards and letters quoted were written in 1984 and 1985 to Nancy Wainer Cohen, box 1 1973–2008 (inclusive), Nancy Wainer Papers, Schlesinger Library, Radcliffe Institute, Cambridge, MA.

13. Cohen and Estner, *Silent Knife*, quote of "Deborah (Maryland)" on 46, quote of "Beth (Florida)" on 51, quote of "Terry (New Hampshire)" on 51; Undated mass letter from Nancy Wainer Cohen, Boston Association for Childbirth Education Records 1928–1993 (inclusive), 1953–1993 (bulk), Schlesinger Library, Radcliffe Institute, Cambridge, MA.

14. Pritchard and MacDonald, *Williams Obstetrics*, 1085; "Vaginal Birth after Previous Cesarean Delivery" (1998); "Vaginal Birth after Previous Cesarean Delivery" (1999).

15. "Guidelines for Vaginal Delivery after a Previous Cesarean Birth" (1982); "Guidelines for Vaginal Delivery after a Previous Cesarean Birth" (1988).

16. Interview of obstetrician by author, Chicago physician interview 2, October 1, 2012, Chicago, IL, transcribed from digital recording.

17. Ibid.; "Vaginal Delivery after a Previous Cesarean Birth" (1994); Interview of retired obstetrician by author, Chicago physician interview 8, October 5, 2012, Chicago, IL, transcribed from digital recording; "Vaginal Delivery after Previous Cesarean Birth" (1995); Wolf, *Deliver Me from Pain*, 179.

18. "Vaginal Birth after Previous Cesarean Delivery" (1998); "Vaginal Birth after Previous Cesarean Delivery" (1999), quote "small but" on 2. The risk of uterine rupture in women undergoing VBACs is increased by the induction of labor; inducing labor with prostaglandins confers the greatest risk. See Lydon-Rochelle et al., "Risk of Uterine Rupture." Articles examining uterine rupture during a VBAC include Leung et al., "Risk Factors Associated with Uterine Rupture." For an example of the articles describing lawsuits filed against obstetricians as the result of uterine rupture during a VBAC, see Phelan, "VBAC: Time to Consider?"

19. "Vaginal Birth after Previous Cesarean Delivery" (2004); Osterman and Martin, "Trends in Low-Risk Cesarean Delivery"; "Decline in Rate." In Maine, the VBAC rate tumbled more than 50 percent, from 30.1 percent to 13.1 percent, between 1998 and 2001. See Pinette et al., "Vaginal Birth after Cesarean Rates."

20. American Academy of Family Physicians, "Trial of Labor after Cesarean (TOLAC)," 37; "Vaginal Birth after Previous Cesarean Delivery" (2010). ACOG promulgated this position despite studies showing that outcomes were more favorable overall in birth by VBAC than in births by elective repeat cesarean sections. See, for example, Rossi and D'Addario, "Maternal Morbidity."

21. "New VBAC Guidelines"; Paul, "The Trouble with Repeat Cesareans."

22. Interview of obstetrician by author, June 28, 2006, Chicago, IL, transcribed from tape recording. While obstetricians have traditionally avoided VBAC in the United States due to fear of uterine rupture, studies now show that women who attempt a VBAC, even if unsuccessful, have decreased risk overall for major maternal morbidities than women who have a repeat cesarean, apparently due to the benefits of a trial of labor. See, for example, Cahill et al., "Is Vaginal Birth after Cesarean."

23. Stolberg, "A Risk Is Found"; Interview of obstetrician by author, Chicago physician interview 2, October 1, 2012, transcribed from digital recording. In a 2006 ACOG survey of 10,659 OB-GYNs, 26 percent said they had given up doing VBACs because insurance to cover these births was either unaffordable or unavailable; 33 percent said they had stopped doing VBACs out of their own fear of litigation. Paul, "The Trouble with Repeat Cesareans."

24. See "National Institutes of Health Consensus Development Conference Statement."

25. Gabe, "Health, Medicine and Risk"; Farthing, "The VBAC Current."

26. Marieskind, *An Evaluation of Caesarean Section*, 4; Corea, "The Caesarean Epidemic."

27. Thorpe, "The Medical Malpractice 'Crisis' "; Shearer, Raphael, and Cattani, "A Survey."

28. Sartwelle, Johnson, and Arda, "Perpetuating Myths, Fables, and Fairy Tales."

29. Interview of obstetrician by author, Chicago physician interview 6, October 4, 2012, Chicago, IL, transcribed from digital recording; Zuckman, "Medical Bill Debate." Malpractice claims surged with the introduction of EFM. See Lent, "The Medical and Legal Risks"; Sartwelle, "Electronic Fetal Monitoring," quotes on 335. Sartwelle contends in the article, "Fetuses are resistant to oxygen deprivation. The degree of hypoxia needed to produce brain damage is close to the degree of hypoxia that is lethal."

30. Davis, "Edwards's Career"; Hurt, "Edwards' Malpractice Suits"; Wagner, "The Advocate as Politician"; "Brooklyn Girl Awarded $35.6 Million"; "Brain-Damaged New York Teen," 47.

31. Haverkamp and Orleans, "An Assessment of Electronic Fetal Monitoring"; Sartwelle and Johnston, "Cerebral Palsy Litigation"; Beller, "A Guest Editorial"; Banta, "Medical Liability Crisis"; Freeman and Freeman, "No-Fault Cerebral Palsy Insurance"; McCarthy, "Cesareans Give Birth to a Bonanza"; Minkoff, "Fear of Litigation"; Sachs, "Is the Rising Rate," 38.

32. Beller, "A Guest Editorial"; Banta, "Medical Liability Crisis"; Freeman and Freeman, "No-Fault Cerebral Palsy Insurance"; McCarthy, "Cesareans Give Birth to a Bonanza"; MacLennan et al., "Who Will Deliver Our Grandchildren?"; Interview of Dr. Charles Hammond by Jessica Roseberry, June 2, 2004, Durham, NC, Duke University Medical Center Archives, Durham, NC.

33. Interviews of retired obstetricians by author, July 19, 2004, Chicago, IL, and October 1, 2012, Avon, IN, both transcribed from digital recording; Gilfix, "Electronic Fetal Monitoring," 79.

34. Interview of obstetrician by author, Chicago physician interview 4, October 3, 2012, Skokie, IL, transcribed from digital recording; Rosen and Thomas, *The Cesarean Myth*, x; Afriat, "Historical Perspective on Electronic Fetal Heart Monitoring."

35. Interviews of obstetricians by author, Chicago physician interview 4, October 3, 2012, Skokie, IL, and Chicago physician interview 2, October 1, 2012, Chicago, IL, both transcribed from digital recording.

36. Interviews of obstetricians by author, Chicago physician interview 6, October 4, 2012, Chicago, IL, and Chicago physician interview 5, October 4, 2012, Chicago, IL, both transcribed from digital recording.

37. Corea, "The Caesarean Epidemic," 33; Kolata, "New York Is First State"; Gruber and Owings, "Physician Financial Incentives." Gruber and Owings note that the relationship between low fertility and more cesareans is too complex to attribute to only one factor. As the fertility rate decreased, first births became a larger percentage of all births, and, given the directives implied by use of the Friedman curve, first-time mothers were the most likely candidates for cesareans simply because first births take longer than subsequent births. Then, given the discomfort with VBACs, secondary cesareans were destined to follow.

38. Hoffman, *Health Care for Some*, 98–99, 158; Brecher, "The Disgraceful Facts"; "Statement on Maternity Insurance Benefits for Women"; Kolata, "New York Is First State"; Gold, Kenney, and Singh, "Paying for Maternity Care." Even with the federal law, loopholes to avoid insuring for maternity care remained. The Pregnancy Discrimination Act exempted policies purchased by individuals and employers with 15 or fewer employees. And employers with more than 15 employees were required to cover only policyholders and their spouses, not employees' minor daughters.

39. Hoxha et al., "Caesarean Sections and For-Profit Status"; Dubay, Kaestner, and Waidman, "The Impact of Malpractice Fears"; Gruber, Kim, and Mayzlin, "Physician Fees and Procedure Intensity"; Gruber and Owings, "Physician Financial Incentives"; National Partnership for Women and Families, "Overdue."

40. Alexander, "Does Physician Pay Affect Procedure Choice"; Keeler and Brodie, "Economic Incentives"; Kolata, "New York Is First State"; de Regt et al., "Relation of Private or Clinic Care"; Gause, "Dear Doctor." To take one state, California, in 1986, cesarean rates were 29.1 percent among the privately insured, 22.9 percent among women insured by Medicaid, 19.7 percent among members of the Kaiser healthcare network, where physicians were salaried and had no financial incentive to manage births in any particular way, and 19.3 percent among uninsured women who are unlikely to pay in full, or at all, for health services. Keeler and Brodie, "Economic Incentives."

41. "Landmark Cesarean Study Published by US Government," *NAPSAC News* 5 (Fall 1980), 5, Sophia Smith Archives, Nielson Library, Smith College, Northampton, MA; McCarthy, "Cesareans Give Birth to a Bonanza"; Bodenheimer and Grumbach, *Understanding Health Policy*, 31–32.

42. Keeler and Brodie, "Economic Incentives"; Interviews of obstetricians by author, June 28, 2006, Chicago, IL, and Chicago physician interview 4, October 3, 2012, Skokie, IL, both transcribed from digital recording.

43. Interview of retired obstetrician by author, Chicago physician interview 1, October 1, 2012, Avon, IN, transcribed from digital recording. The 1979 HEW report expressed the same concern—that an increase in obstetric residencies had led to far fewer deliveries per each resident and thus far fewer opportunities for each resident to gain expertise. Marieskind, *An Evaluation of Caesarean Section*, 5–7.

44. Rubin, *What If I Have a C-Section?*, 126.

45. Interview of obstetric resident by author, Chicago physician interview 10, October 27, 2013, Chicago, IL, transcribed from digital recording.

46. Interview of obstetrician by author, Chicago physician interview 2, October 1, 2012, Chicago, IL, transcribed from digital recording; Interview of obstetrician by author, June 28, 2006, Chicago, IL, transcribed from tape recording; Interviews of retired obstetricians by author, Chicago physician interview 8, October 5, 2012, Chicago, IL, and Chicago physician interview 1, October 1, 2012, Avon, IN, transcribed from digital recordings. Retired obstetricians also pointed out that the propensity to administer either general or saddle-block anesthesia during second-stage labor required forceps because both forms of anesthesia rendered women unable to push. This provided doctors with plenty of forceps practice. Physicians adept at applying forceps also thought of low forceps as a prophylactic measure. "We thought . . . that the forceps actually provided a steel cradle for the baby's head, to protect the baby's head." Interview of retired obstetrician by author, Chicago physician interview 8, October 5, 2012, Chicago, IL, transcribed from digital tape recording.

47. Interviews of obstetricians by author, Chicago physician interview 6, October 4, 2012, Chicago, IL, and Ohio obstetrician interview 1, August 24, 2012, southern Ohio area, both transcribed from digital recording.

48. Interview of obstetrician by author, Chicago physician interview 6, October 4, 2012, Chicago, IL, transcribed from digital recording, and Chicago physician interview, June 26, 2006, Chicago, IL, transcribed from tape recording.

49. Interviews of obstetricians by author, Ohio obstetrician interview 1, August 24, 2012, southern Ohio area, Chicago physician interview 2, October 1, 2012, Chicago, IL, and Chicago physician interview 4, October 3, 2012, Skokie, IL, all transcribed from digital recordings. That obstetricians in their 40s and younger did not learn how to deliver breech babies vaginally was confirmed by all the obstetricians I interviewed. One physician who graduated from medical school in 1991 said that in her entire training she only delivered "maybe three" babies in the breech position. Helen Marieskind noted the lack of training in vaginal breech births in *An Evaluation of Caesarean Section*, 6.

50. Interview of retired obstetrician by author, Chicago physician interview 8, October 5, 2012, Chicago, IL, and interview of obstetrician by author, June 29, 2006, Evanston, IL, both transcribed from tape recordings; Ventura et al., "Births: Final Data for 1999," 1–100.

51. "Mode of Term Singleton Breech Delivery" (2006), 3. The studies that prompted ACOG's warning against vaginal breech births include Gifford et al., "A Meta-Analysis of Infant Outcomes"; Roman, Bakos, and Cnattingius, "Pregnancy Outcomes by Mode of Delivery"; Hannah et al., "Planned Caesarean Section." Interview of obstetrician by author, June 28, 2006, Chicago, IL, transcribed from tape recording; "Mode of Term Singleton Breech Delivery"(2001).

52. Marieskind, *An Evaluation of Caesarean Section*, 6; Haverkamp et al., "A Controlled Trial"; "Presidential Address, Obstetrical Society of Philadelphia," February 12, 1981, J. Robert Willson, MD, presidential guest speaker, typed transcript, J. Robert Willson Papers, National Library of Medicine, History of Medicine Division, Bethesda, MD.

53. Hardy, "Birthing Breech"; Letter from S. F., Idaho, undated, circa 1988, Women's Health Network Records, box 83, Sophia Smith Archives, Nielson Library, Smith College, Northampton, MA.

54. Interview of mother by author, Chicago mother interview 3, March 15, 2012, Chicago area, IL, transcribed from digital recording.

55. Ibid.

56. Ibid.

57. "April" is a pseudonym. Interview of mother by author, Ohio mother interview 1, June 5, 2013, southern Ohio area, transcribed from digital recording.

58. Ibid.

59. Ibid.

60. Ibid.

61. Ibid.

62. Ibid.

63. Ibid.

64. Kitzinger, *The Experience of Childbirth*, 22; Arms, *Immaculate Deception*, 10–27, quotes on 11, 25.

65. "ACOG Fellows, Junior Fellows, and Total Membership," Unpublished ACOG In-House Data, ACOG Resource Center, American College of Obstetricians and Gynecologists, Washington, DC.

66. Interviews of obstetricians by author, November 1, 2005, Chicago area, IL, Ohio obstetrician interview 1, August 24, 2012, southern Ohio area, and Chicago physician interview 5, October 4, 2012, Chicago, IL, all transcribed from digital recordings. Other obstetricians tell the same story—having spent years surgically reconstructing pelvic floor muscles and repairing leaky bladders that they attribute to difficult vaginal deliveries, they don't want to face the risks of labor when they give birth to their own children, and they discuss what they view as the downstream repercussions of vaginal birth with patients. See, for example, Song, "Too Posh to Push?"

67. Interview of obstetrician by author, Chicago physician interview 2, October 1, 2012, Chicago, IL, transcribed from digital recording, and interview of obstetrician by author, June 26, 2006, Chicago, IL, transcribed from tape recording. Physicians' recommendations influence the decisions made by their patients. See Simpson, Newman, and Chirino, "Patient Education to Reduce Elective Inductions."

68. Al-Mufti, McCarthy, and Fisk, "Survey of Obstetricians' Personal Preference," "interventionist attitudes" on 1, "liberal attitude" on 3, and "interventionist views" on 4. MacDonald, Pinion, and Macleod, "Scottish Female Obstetricians' Views." A similar study of physicians' attitude toward cesarean section for themselves is Gabbe and Holzman, "Obstetricians' Choice of Delivery." Another study showed urogynecologists were significantly more likely to support elective cesareans than obstetricians (80.4 percent vs. 55.4 percent). Wu, Hundley, and Visco, "Elective Primary Cesarean Delivery." In another study, researchers concluded that the attitudes of healthcare providers toward cesarean section were based more on their professional role than on their gender. Monari et al., "Obstetricians' and Midwives' Attitudes." A study indicating that the percentage of obstetricians who prefer vaginal delivery and external cephalic version are higher than

other studies reported without significant gender differences is Wright et al., "A Survey of Trainee Obstetricians' Preferences." The study indicating that physicians shape their patients' birth preferences is Goyert et al., "The Physician Factor." See also Luthy et al., "Physician Contribution."

69. Interviews of obstetricians by author, June 28, 2006, Chicago, IL, Chicago physician interview 6, October 4, 2012, and June 26, 2006, Chicago, IL, all transcribed from tape or digital recordings. The latter two interviews were with the same obstetrician recorded six years apart. Studies indicate that an obstetrician's "individual practice style" may explain why there is such a wide variation in the rate of cesarean delivery among obstetricians. See Goyert et al, "The Physician Factor." This study, of more than 1,500 women who gave birth at a single community hospital, saw an average 26.9 percent cesarean rate that ranged, depending on the physician, from 19.1 to 42.3 percent.

70. Willson, "Elective Induction of Labor"; Interview of obstetrician by author, Chicago physician interview 2, October 1, 2012, Chicago, IL, transcribed from digital recording.

71. Pritchard and MacDonald, *Williams Obstetrics*, 1085, 1081.

72. Interview of obstetrician by author, Ohio obstetrician interview 1, August 24, 2012, southern Ohio area, transcribed from digital recording.

73. Ibid.; Interview of obstetrician by author, Chicago physician interview 11, October 24, 2013, Chicago, IL, transcribed from digital recording.

74. Interview of retired obstetrician by author, July 19, 2004, Chicago, IL, and interview of obstetrician by author, Ohio obstetrician interview 3, August 12, 2013, southern Ohio area, both transcribed from digital recordings.

CHAPTER 7: **Giving Birth in a Culture of Risk: Consequences for Mothers**

1. The views of birth reformers can be seen in Haggerty, "Childbirth Made Difficult"; Williams, "Natural Childbirth Comes of Age"; and Arms, *Immaculate Deception*.

2. Interview of mother by author, October 29, 2005, Northfield, IL, transcribed from tape recording. See chapter 5, note 65, for a description of how physicians' paternalism shaped women's medical treatments specifically.

3. "Enraged about Hospital Birth."

4. For more on the argument that in their attempts to juggle full-time motherhood and full-time jobs, women became more oppressed than stay-at-home mothers, see Friedan, *The Second Stage*, and Warner, *Perfect Madness*. For more on the contrast between benefits for mothers in the United States and the rest of the industrialized world, see Demleitner, "Maternity Leave Policies"; Issacharoff and Rosenblum, "Women and the Workplace."

5. Kathryn Woodruff, letter in response to "Pay on Delivery"; Interview of mother by author, Chicago mother interview 5, March 15, 2012, Chicago area, IL, transcribed from digital recording.

6. Interview of mother by author, Chicago mother interview 1, March 13, 2012, Chicago, IL, transcribed from digital recording; International Cesarean Awareness Network, *Cesarean Voices*, 7.

7. Interview of mother by author, Chicago mother interview 5, March 15, 2012, Chicago area, IL, transcribed from digital recording.

8. Grisanti, "The Cesarean Epidemic"; Korelitz, "Special Delivery," 414.

9. Interview of mother by author, Chicago mother interview 1, March 13, 2012, Chicago, IL, transcribed from digital recording. "Theresa's" first birth is described in detail in chapter 5.

10. Ibid.

11. Ibid.

12. Ibid.

13. Ibid. On cesareans and allergies see, for example, Tollånes et al., "Cesarean Section and Risk of Severe Childhood Asthma"; Pistiner et al., "Birth by Cesarean Section." Scientists now posit that because babies born by cesarean are always born with wet lung (during vaginal birth, the amniotic fluid is squeezed out in the birth canal), their risk of asthma is increased, and because they are not exposed to the vaginal microbiome, their risk of allergy increases. Painful abdominal adhesions are a well-known, long-term side effect of cesarean surgery, particularly after multiple cesarean births. See, for example, Stark et al., "Post-Cesarean Adhesions."

14. Corea, "The Caesarean Epidemic," 34.

15. 1985 card, Nancy Wainer Papers, box 1, folder MC656 1.11 Correspondence: Birth Announcements, 1984–86, Schlesinger Library, Radcliffe College, Cambridge, MA, hereinafter referred to as Wainer Papers; Cohen and Estner, *Silent Knife*, xvi–xviii.

16. Cohen and Estner, *Silent Knife*, xvi–xviii; "Number of Caesareans on Rise at Hospitals."

17. Leaflet announcement 1985, box 1, folder MC656 1.11 Correspondence: Birth Announcements, 1984–86, Wainer Papers; 1986 leaflet with handwritten note, box 1, folder MC656 1.11 Correspondence: Birth Announcements, 1984–86, Wainer Papers.

18. Letter to Nancy from a VBAC mom in California, September 14, 1983, Wainer Papers.

19. Ibid.

20. International Cesarean Awareness Network, *Cesarean Voices*, 24, 62. Although studies have been few, both the chemical induction of labor and epidural anesthesia have been linked to a greater incidence of cesarean section. See, for example, Heffner, Elkin, and Fretts, "Impact of Labor Induction"; Thorp, Hu, et al., "The Effect of Intrapartum Epidural Analgesia"; Thorp, Eckert, et al., "Epidural Analgesia and Cesarean Section."

21. "Mary" and "Michael" are pseudonyms. The story of Mary's first birth is taken from two sources: a letter written by Mary to her newborn son, begun on August 6, 1990, and completed on September 10, 1990, and a letter written by Mary to a friend nine weeks after her son's birth. Copies of each letter were given to the author by Mary, who is also referred to in the endnotes as "Chicago mother interview 4."

22. Ibid.

23. Ibid. Researchers have verified in many studies that mobility hastens labor. See, for example, Lawrence et al., "Maternal Positions and Mobility."

24. "Mary's" letters.

25. Ibid.

26. Ibid.
27. Ibid.
28. Ibid.
29. Ibid.
30. Ibid.
31. Ibid.
32. Ibid.
33. Interview of "Mary" and "Michael" by author, Chicago mother interview 4, March 13, 2012, Oak Park, IL, transcribed from digital recording.
34. Ibid.
35. "Joan" is a pseudonym. Interview of mother by author, Chicago mother interview 6, March 14, 2012, Chicago, IL, transcribed from digital recording.
36. Ibid.
37. Ibid.
38. Ibid.
39. Ibid.
40. Ibid. "Karen" is a pseudonym. Interview of mother by author, Chicago mother interview 2, March 13, 2012, Chicago, IL, transcribed from digital recording.
41. Interview of mother by author, Chicago mother interview 2, March 13, 2012, Chicago, IL, transcribed from digital recording.
42. Ibid.
43. Ibid.
44. Interview of mother by author, Ohio mother interview 2, June 5, 2013, southern Ohio, transcribed from digital recording.
45. Ibid.
46. Ibid.
47. Rubin, *What If I Have a C-Section?*, xiii–xvii, quotes on ix and xvi. For an example of minimizing the seriousness of cesarean surgery, see Walters, *Just Take It Out!*, 29–39.
48. A typical book for consumers about cesareans written in the early twenty-first century is Rubin, *What If I Have a C-Section?*
49. For more on the history of abortion and women's "right to choose" in the context of reproduction, see Joffe, *Dispatches from the Abortion Wars*; Watkins, *On the Pill*; Reagan, *When Abortion was a Crime*; Joffe, *Doctors of Conscience*; Huston, *Motherhood by Choice*; Gordon, *Woman's Body, Woman's Right.*
50. "Pain Relief during Labor"; "Analgesia and Cesarean Delivery Rates." Some of the studies linking epidural anesthesia with dystocia and an increase in cesarean sections include Thorp, McNitt, and Leppert, "Effects of Epidural Analgesia"; Thorp, Hu, et al., "The Effect of Intrapartum Epidural Analgesia." In 2006, ACOG announced that recent studies indicated that epidural analgesia did not increase the risks of cesarean delivery. This announcement strengthened their defense of epidural anesthesia on demand. See "Analgesia and Cesarean Delivery Rates." The studies cited by ACOG include Wong et al., "The Risk of Cesarean Delivery"; Sharma et al., "Cesarean Delivery."

51. US Public Health Service, *Healthy People 2000*; Althabe and Belizán, "Caesarean Section"; Sachs et al., "The Risks of Lowering the Cesarean-Delivery Rate"; Korelitz, "Special Delivery," 414.

52. Harer, "Patient Choice Cesarean"; Shelton, "C-Sections Increasing"; Hale and Harer, "Editorial: Elective Prophylactic Cesarean Delivery"; Harer, "A Look Back," 1.

53. Snowbeck, "Is Elective C-Section Delivery a Good Idea?" An article that attempts to present a balanced view of CDMR is Brody, "With Childbirth."

54. ACOG Committee Opinion, "Surgery and Patient Choice"; "Cesarean Delivery on Maternal Request" (2007). For a discussion of limiting patient choice in birth, even as physicians and women invoke choice, see Leeman and Plante, "Patient-Choice Vaginal Delivery?"

55. "Cesarean Delivery on Maternal Request" (2013). Although ACOG did not cite the Cochrane review as the impetus for its 2013 *Committee Opinion*, in 2012 the *Cochrane Database* issued a report noting that they were unable to find any study that fit their inclusion criteria for a proposed review of randomized trials on elective cesareans. Cochrane authors concluded, "There is no evidence from randomized controlled trials upon which to base any practice recommendations regarding planned caesarean section for non-medical reasons at term." They declared "an urgent need" to "better assess the short- and long-term effects of caesarean section and vaginal birth." See Lavender et al., "Caesarean Section for Non-Medical Reasons." Earlier, the NIH convened a consensus conference on CDMR that reached the same conclusion—there was insufficient evidence to compare the benefits and risks of CDMR with vaginal delivery. "NIH State-of-the-Science Conference Statement."

56. Declercq et al., "Listening to Mothers II"; Declercq et al., "Listening to Mothers III"; Declercq, "Is Medical Intervention in Childbirth Inevitable in Brazil?" Other estimates of the incidence of CDMR in the US vary from 4 to 18 percent of primary cesareans, although the studies that produced these estimates were not as comprehensive as the "Listening to Mothers" surveys. See Meikle et al., "A National Estimate"; Wax et al., "Patient Choice Cesarean."

57. Interviews of obstetricians by author, Chicago physician interview 5, October 4, 2012, Chicago, IL, and Chicago physician interview 11, October 24, 2013, Chicago, IL, both transcribed from digital recordings.

58. Interview of obstetric resident by author, Chicago physician interview 10, October 27, 2013, Chicago, IL, and interview of obstetrician by author, Chicago physician interview 6, October 4, 2012, Chicago, IL, both transcribed from digital recordings.

59. At almost 1.3 million cesareans in 2015, the incidence of the surgery exceeds all other surgical procedures, including abortions. See Centers for Disease Control statistics, www.cdc.gov/nchs/fastats/delivery.htm, accessed July 11, 2017.

60. Interview of obstetrician by author, June 28, 2006, Chicago, IL, transcribed from tape recording. The number of human births that have run into trouble historically is discussed in the introduction of this book.

61. *Gilmore Girls*, season 3, episode 13, aired on The WB, 2002–2003 season.

62. Interview of obstetrician by author, June 28, 2006, Chicago, IL, transcribed from tape recording.

63. For more on the number of human births that have run into trouble historically, see the introduction of this book. For a complete list of the world's countries and their estimated maternal mortality rates from 1990 to 2015, see World Health Organization et al., *Trends in Maternal Mortality 1990 to 2015*. The numbers, at least for the United States, in this "executive summary" are not as accurate as CDC and other data cited in this chapter. The Centers for Disease Control attempts to track maternal mortality and other birth-related statistics in the United States. See www.cdc.gov/reproductivehealth/maternalinfanthealth/pmss.html. Editorial Board, "America's Shocking Maternal Deaths"; Tavernise, "Maternal Mortality Rate in US Rises"; Ingraham, "Our Maternal Mortality Rate"; Fields and Sexton, "How Many American Women Die." The 2014 rate is discussed in MacDorman et al., "Recent Increases."

64. MacDorman et al., "Recent Increases"; *Trends in Maternal Mortality 1990 to 2015*; Deneux-Tharaux et al., "Postpartum Maternal Mortality and Cesarean Delivery"; Simkin, "Is Anyone Listening?"; Villar et al., "Maternal and Neonatal Individual Risk and Benefits"; Callaghan et al., "Severe Maternal Morbidity," 1034; Martin and Montagne, "The Last Person"; Fields and Sexton, "How Many American Women Die." Researchers often cite the rise in chronic diseases and conditions among pregnant women as a primary cause of the rise in the maternal death rate; these include hypertension, diabetes, heart disease, and obesity, each of which amplify the likelihood of a birth ending in cesarean section. Creanga et al., "Pregnancy-Related Mortality"; Creanga et al., "Maternal Mortality and Morbidity." Most recently, drug and alcohol abuse, particularly in specific areas of the country, have been named as additional factors. Achenbach, "No longer 'Mayberry' "; Achenbach, "An Addiction Crisis." Prior to the relatively recent increase, lowering maternal mortality and morbidity was consistently cited as one of the greatest public health achievements of the twentieth century. "Ten Great Public Health Achievements." See also Wolf, "Saving Mothers and Babies."

65. Interview of obstetrician by author, Chicago physician interview 6, October 4, 2012, Chicago, IL, transcribed from digital recording. Nineteenth-century texts suggested that even difficult births were usually resolved using simple measures. See Davis, *The Principles and Practice of Obstetric Medicine*, vol. 2; Ramsbotham, *The Principles and Practice of Obstetric Medicine and Surgery*; Bretelle, "Management of Placenta Accrete"; Interview of retired obstetrician by author, Chicago physician interview 8, October 5, 2012, Chicago, IL, transcribed from digital recording; Interview of obstetrician by author, Chicago physician interview 4, October 3, 2012, Skokie, IL, transcribed from digital recording.

66. Sartwelle, "Electronic Fetal Monitoring"; Interview of obstetrician by author, Chicago physician interview 6, October 4, 2012, Chicago, IL, transcribed from digital recording.

67. Interview of obstetrician by author, Chicago physician interview 2, Chicago, IL, October 1, 2012, transcribed from digital recording; Interview of obstetrician by author, June 28, 2006, Chicago, IL, transcribed from tape recording; Interview of retired obstetrician by author, Chicago physician interview 8, October 5, 2012, Chicago, IL, transcribed from digital recording; Interview of retired obstetrician by author, Chicago physician interview 1, October 1, 2012, Avon, IN, transcribed from digital recording. On the

effects of administering general or saddle-block anesthesia in second-stage labor, see chapter 6, note 46.

68. Marieskind, *An Evaluation of Caesarean Section in the United States*, 21.

69. Ibid., 25; Xu et al., "Wide Variation Found"; Haelle, "Your Biggest C-Section Risk"; March of Dimes, "New York Cesarean Rates, 2013."

70. Marieskind, *An Evaluation of Caesarean Section in the United States*, 9. The normalization of cesarean surgery continues to manifest in unexpected ways long after Marieskind issued her warning. In December 2016, a group of scientists postulated that the many cesarean sections performed in the last 40 years might have affected human evolution. They found that the incidence of fetal-pelvic disproportion had increased 20 percent since 1960. Perhaps, the scientists (preposterously) theorized, because babies who otherwise would have died had been born by cesarean section, the genes for a large head or a small female pelvis were appearing in the human genome with even greater frequency, assuring ever more cesarean sections. Aside from the fact that, as this history of cesarean surgery has demonstrated, a physician's diagnosis of fetal-pelvic disproportion does not mean the diagnosis was correct, indeed, pelvimetry has now been dismissed as "medical nonsense," not even the most sophisticated modern-day scientist can measure, or accurately predict, evolutionary transformation based on changes in human behavior over 45 years. Human evolution manifests over many thousands of generations, not two. Nevertheless, these types of "findings" wield influence. They make cesarean surgery seem not just normal but increasingly necessary. The news of this alleged development in human evolution appeared in a number of venues. See, for example, Briggs, "Caesarean Births 'Affecting Human Evolution'"; Pearson, "The Rise in C-Sections."

71. This sort of public education has already made an erratic appearance. See, for example, Haelle, "Your Biggest C-Section Risk"; Redden, "'A Third of People.'"

Glossary of Medical Terminology

abdominal pregnancy a pregnancy in which the embryo or fetus grows, not in the uterus, but in the abdomen.

abnormal presentation *See* presentation.

accouchear from the French term meaning "to be delivered of a child" or "to take to the birthing bed," used to describe a birth attendant.

accrete to adhere or become attached to. *See also* placenta accreta.

acidosis accumulation of hydrogen in the blood and body tissues, resulting in a decrease in pH. *See also* pH.

ACOG *See* American College of Obstetricians and Gynecologists.

active labor the segment of first-stage labor when contractions intensify and the cervix dilates more rapidly. *See also* first-stage labor; latent phase of labor; transition.

adhesion *See* surgical adhesion.

air embolism the sudden blocking of a blood vessel by an air bubble, usually caused by a surgical procedure or trauma.

albuminuria presence in the urine of an excess of serum proteins, a possible sign of kidney disease or preeclampsia. *See also* preeclampsia.

American College of Obstetricians and Gynecologists the premiere professional organization for obstetricians and gynecologists in the United States. The organization recently changed its name to American Congress of Obstetricians and Gynecologists. Only physicians who limit their practice to women are permitted to be members.

amniocentesis a transabdominal puncture of the uterus to obtain amniotic fluid for prenatal diagnosis.

amnionitis inflammation of the membrane surrounding the fetus and the amniotic fluid. *See also* amniotic fluid; amniotic sac.

amniotic fluid the protective liquid contained in the amniotic sac. *See also* amniotic sac.

amniotic fluid embolism the sudden entrance of amniotic fluid or fetal debris into the maternal circulatory system, triggering cardiopulmonary collapse and bleeding. Also known as anaphylactoid syndrome of pregnancy.

amniotic sac the bag of fluid inside the uterus in which the fetus develops and grows, also known as the bag of waters or membranes. *See also* amniotic fluid.

amniotomy rupture of the amniotic sac by artificial means.

ankyloses immobility of a joint due to disease.

aorta the main artery of the body from which the body's entire arterial system proceeds, the aorta arises from the left ventricle of the heart.

Apgar score the scoring system devised by anesthesiologist Virginia Apgar to ascertain the well-being of a neonate at one minute and five minutes after birth.

artificial rupture of membranes *See* amniotomy and ruptured membranes.

asphyxia pathological changes in the body caused by lack of oxygen.

aspiration inhalation or removal by suction of excess body fluid.

atelectasis incomplete expansion of the lungs, a common condition in premature infants.

atresia *See* vaginal atresia.

augmentation *See* labor augmentation.

auscultation listening to the internal sounds made by the body, usually with a stethoscope, from the Latin verb "to listen." During childbirth, auscultation most often refers to listening to the fetal heartbeat with a fetal stethoscope.

bag of waters *See* amniotic sac.

bilious attack an array of symptoms that include nausea, abdominal discomfort, headache, and constipation, originally attributed to excessive secretion of bile.

bipolar version *See* version.

Bishop score the scoring system devised by obstetrician Edward Bishop in 1964 to ascertain a pregnant woman's readiness for childbirth. The Bishop score assigns points to five cervical characteristics: station, dilatation, effacement, position, and consistency. *See also* consistency; dilatation; effacement; position; station.

blue baby a baby with a blue tinge to the skin due to lack of oxygen in the blood because of a congenital defect, usually of the heart.

bougie in obstetrics, an object placed through the cervix to induce contractions.

bradycardia a slow heartbeat.

breech a fetus is in a breech position when the presenting part during birth is a foot or the buttocks rather than the head. *See also* cephalic; footling breech; frank breech; presentation; presenting part.

calcareous containing calcium.

caliper compass with curved legs, designed for measuring the thickness and diameter of a solid object.

caput the swelling of a baby's scalp after delivery due to a difficult birth.

carbolic acid common name for phenol, a volatile, white, crystalline solid.

carcinoma a type of cancer that originates in the skin or tissues that line or cover organs.

catecholamines a class of drugs; drugs in the catecholamine class include norepinephrine, epinephrine, and dopamine.

catgut a surgical suture naturally degraded by the body's enzymes.

catheter a hollow tube used to withdraw fluid from, or insert fluid into, a body cavity. *See also* catheterize.

catheterize to introduce a catheter into a body cavity, most often to drain urine from the bladder. *See also* catheter.

caudal analgesia injected through the caudal, i.e., the sacral, portion of the spinal canal to reduce or eliminate pain from the umbilicus down.

CDMR cesarean delivery on maternal request. *See also* elective cesarean.

cephalic relating to the head. In childbirth, when the fetus presents headfirst. *See also* breech; presentation; presenting part.

cephalopelvic disproportion in the nineteenth and first half of the twentieth centuries, a fetus too large to fit through the birth canal, often (but not necessarily) because of a pelvic deformity; increasingly, as the cesarean section rate began to rise in the late 1970s, a catch-all phrase indicating that the progression of labor has stalled.

cephalotribe a head crusher, used in difficult births; could also double as an extractor.

cephalotripsy *See* cephalotribe.

cerebral palsy an array of neurological disorders that appear in infancy or early childhood, permanently affect body movement or muscle coordination, and do not worsen over time.

cervical dilation the gradual opening of the cervical os, the entrance to the uterus, during childbirth. *See also* active labor; Bishop score; first-stage labor.

cervical dystocia slow, obstructed, or otherwise abnormal opening of the cervix during labor. *See also* cervical dilation.

cervical effacement the thinning of the cervix during childbirth. *See also* Bishop score.

cervical stenosis abnormal narrowing of the cervical os. *See also* os.

cervix the lower portion of the uterus connecting the uterus to the vagina.

cesarean section removal of the fetus from the uterus through surgical incisions in the uterine and abdominal walls.

childbed fever the nineteenth- and early-twentieth-century term for postpartum infection.

cholera infantum the nineteenth- and early-twentieth-century term for infant diarrhea, a sure and swift killer in an era before pasteurized milk, filtered and chemically treated water, and pure food laws.

chondrodystrophic abnormal development of cartilage.

chorea the occurrence of ceaseless, jerky, involuntary movements.

chorionic villi sampling a form of prenatal diagnosis that involves removing cells from placental tissue to determine genetic and chromosomal abnormalities, usually performed at 10 to 12 weeks' gestation.

classic cut the original, now seldom-used method to open the abdomen and uterus to perform a cesarean section. The classic cut entailed a long, vertical incision performed high on the uterus beginning at the umbilicus. The remaining scar is weak and prone to rupture during labor in subsequent pregnancies. *See also* low transverse cut, Sänger cesarean, uterine rupture.

consistency in the context of the Bishop score, the cervical characteristic measured on a scale from firm to soft. The softer the cervix, the better the chance of a vaginal delivery. *See also* Bishop score.

control the standard against which experimental observations are evaluated; a group of patients who differ from those under study in that they do not have the disease or condition, or are not receiving the treatment regimen, or are undergoing a different treatment regimen.

cord blood gases used to assess a newborn's metabolic condition at birth by clamping and cutting a section of the umbilical cord, then putting it on ice for later analysis of the gases and pH values in the infant's blood.

cord compression the obstruction of blood flow through the umbilical cord due to external pressure. *See also* cord prolapse.

cord prolapse when the umbilical cord enters the birth canal before or with the presenting part of the fetus, exposing the fetus to possible oxygen deprivation if the fetal head or other body part compresses the cord. Cord prolapse is an obstetric emergency. *See also* cord compression.

corpus luteum a structure in the ovarian follicle formed after ovulation that produces progesterone to sustain the pregnancy.

corrosive sublimate an old, discarded term for mercury chloride.

CPD cephalopelvic disproportion. *See also* cephalopelvic disproportion.

craniotomy a cut that opens the largest part of the fetus's body—the cranium—in order to extract a fetus stuck in the birth canal. Once commonly used in extremely difficult births to save a mother's life before cesarean section became a safe option. A physician punctured the fetal skull to remove brain matter and collapse the fetal head. *See also* embryotomy.

craniotomy forceps forceps used to crush the cranium in the birth canal in the process of performing a craniotomy. *See also* craniotomy.

cretinism a chronic condition caused by severe congenital hypothyroidism; manifestations include arrested physical development and mental retardation.

crowning the phase of second-stage labor when the majority of the fetal scalp is visible at the vaginal opening.

cyanotic bluish discoloration of the skin caused by inadequate oxygenation of the blood.

cystadenoma a common benign ovarian tumor.

decidua the endometrium of the pregnant uterus, shed at birth.

defensive medicine the practice of ordering a test or treatment, not because it is necessary, but because the physician fears liability unless the test or treatment is performed.

Demerol an opioid analgesic used to treat moderate to severe pain and delivered via tablet, syrup, or intramuscular or intravenous injection. Demerol is the brand name of the drug; meperidine is the generic name.

dilatation the act of dilating. *See also* cervical dilation.

dilation *See* cervical dilation.

distend to expand due to pressure from within.

downstream effect in medicine, the negative side effect of a treatment or diagnostic tool that appears long after the treatment has been administered.

Down syndrome a genetic disorder caused by the presence of a third copy of the 21st chromosome, named after John Down, the first physician to describe the syndrome. Also known as trisomy 21. Associated with characteristic facial features, mild to moderate intellectual disability, and shorter-than-average lifespan. *See also* mongolism.

dystocia traditionally, labor completely blocked by a tumor, a deformed pelvis, or an exceedingly large (12+ pound) infant. Today, dystocia is more broadly defined as abnormal, difficult, or prolonged labor and is the most common indication for a cesarean section.

eclampsia *See* preeclampsia.

effacement *See* cervical effacement.

EFM electronic fetal monitoring. *See also* electronic fetal monitor.

elective cesarean before the 1980s, an elective cesarean was a medically necessary surgery, so obviously necessary early in pregnancy that it was planned in advance. Today, an elective cesarean refers to a medically unnecessary operation, performed for the convenience of the mother, the physician, or both. *See also* CDMR.

elective induction the induction of labor for social rather than medical reasons. *See also* induction.

electrode in the case of electronic fetal monitoring, a small wire attached to the fetal scalp to continually monitor the fetal heart rate.

electronic fetal monitor a device that collects and records throughout labor the fetal heart rate and fetal heart rate changes in response to uterine contractions.

embryotomy the dismemberment of a fetus in utero so that it can be removed without harming the mother. *See also* craniotomy.

encephalopathy any degenerative disease or wasting condition affecting the brain.

engaged head *See* engagement.

engagement the entrance of the fetal presenting part, most often the head, into the upper portion of the birth canal. *See also* presentation; presenting part.

enostosis a bony growth developed within the bone cavity.

episiotomy an incision made in the perineum to widen the vagina before giving birth.

ergot a fungus that grows on rye, used in nineteenth- and early-twentieth-century obstetrics to stimulate labor, administered either orally or hypodermically. Depending on the dose, capable of producing violent contractions that could rupture the uterus. Also used after expulsion of the placenta as a prophylactic measure to prevent postpartum hemorrhage.

erythroblastosis hemolytic anemia in the fetus and neonate caused by Rh-factor incompatibility; can occur when an Rh-negative female has developed antibodies to fetal red blood cells in a previous pregnancy and is now pregnant with an Rh-positive fetus. *See also* Rh factor; Rh incompatibility; Rh sensitization.

eugenics an influential, early-twenty-first-century philosophy advocating forced sterilization, euthanasia, and segregation of classes, races, and ethnic groups in order to safeguard and improve the human gene pool. *See also* eugenics laws.

eugenics laws state laws that permitted court-ordered, involuntary sterilization of "defective," "socially inferior" citizens.

external cephalic version a manual procedure performed on the outside of the body, on the uterus, to turn a fetus from buttocks- or feet-first to head-first. Usually performed, as necessary, in the last two or three weeks of pregnancy.

fallopian tube named for the Italian anatomist Fallopius, in female mammals one of the two tubes from which the egg travels from the ovary to the uterus.

fee-for-service the predominant payment method in American health care, a payment model in which each service performed in the course of a medical episode is billed separately. Widely criticized as encouraging physicians to provide more treatments and order more tests because financial reimbursement is based on quantity of service rather than quality of service.

fetal pulse oximetry use of a photoelectric device to determine the oxygen saturation of arterial blood of a fetus.

fetal scalp blood sampling used in conjunction with fetal heart monitoring in the 1970s and 1980s to determine the need for a cesarean section. After sufficient dilation of the cervix, sampling required piercing of the fetal scalp to take a blood sample in order to test pH levels to determine oxygen saturation. An abnormal pH level indicated the need for a cesarean. The practice was largely abandoned due to poor predictive value for intrapartum hypoxia and its failure to reduce operative interventions.

fetal stethoscope a listening device resembling, and used similarly to, an ordinary stethoscope, designed specifically to listen to the fetus's heart in utero.

fetoscope original name for a fetal stethoscope. *See also* fetal stethoscope.

FHR fetal heart rate, today usually discerned during labor by electronic fetal monitoring. FHR patterns are classified as reassuring, nonreassuring, and ominous. Ominous patterns require immediate delivery. Nonreassuring patterns suggest fetal compromise or a growing inability of the fetus to cope with the stress of labor; critics of fetal monitoring argue that nonreassuring patterns are difficult to discern from reassuring ones. *See also* innocuous FHR pattern; electronic fetal monitor.

fibroid tumor benign tumors originating in the uterus. *See also* fibromyomata.

fibromyomata a benign tumor growing from smooth muscle, usually the uterus; commonly known as a fibroid tumor.

FIGO International Federation of Gynecologists and Obstetricians.

first-stage labor the initial portion of labor when the cervix effaces and dilates to allow passage of the fetus into the vagina. The first stage of labor ends with complete cervical dilation, i.e., 10 centimeters. *See also* second-stage labor; transition.

fistula an abnormal passage between two internal organs. In the case of obstetrics, a fistula most often refers to a tear between the vagina and rectum, causing feces to leak into the vagina, or a tear between the vagina and bladder, causing urine to leak into the vagina. In both instances, tears are due to unusually difficult, prolonged labor. *See also* vesico-vaginal fistula.

flooding nineteenth- and early-twentieth-century term for severe maternal hemorrhage.

flora the bacteria and fungi, usually normally occurring but can also refer to pathological occurrence, found in or on an organ.

footling breech a birth in which the foot or feet, rather than the head, is the presenting body part. *See also* breech.

forceps an instrument designed to aid a physician in manually extracting the fetus from the uterus or birth canal. Forceps are of four general types, outlet, low, median, and high, and were used historically depending on the stage of fetal descent—outlet to extract a fetus already visible at the vaginal opening, high to extract a fetus still in the womb after full dilation of the cervix. *See also* operative vaginal delivery.

frank breech a birth in which the buttocks, rather than the head, is the presenting body part, with the baby's legs sticking straight up in front of his or her body and the feet near the head. *See also* breech.

Friedman curve depiction of the progress of labor in the form of a sigmoid curve.

gastro-hysterectomy generic term used to describe a Porro cesarean. *See also* Porro cesarean.

gastro-hysterotomy the early, standard form of cesarean section in which the uterus remained in the abdominal cavity, unsutured, after the surgery. *See also* gastro-hysterectomy; Porro cesarean.

gastrotomy incision into the stomach.

German measles *See* rubella.

gestational the process of fetal development in the womb from fertilization to birth.

gestational diabetes diabetes developed during pregnancy, causing high maternal blood sugar that can affect fetal health. Gestational diabetes enhances the chance of cesarean section due to abnormal fetal weight gain, preeclampsia, and stillbirth if not controlled.

grand multipara a woman who has given birth to five or more infants.

high forceps *See* forceps.

HMO health maintenance organization, a health insurance organization that relies on annual fees from members to cover all costs; their employees, including physicians, are customarily on a fixed salary.

hyaline membrane disease known today as respiratory distress syndrome. The disease, commonly suffered by premature infants, is caused by lack of surfactant, a substance that allows the lungs to inflate properly. The fetus does not begin to produce surfactant until between 24 and 28 weeks' gestation, and surfactant remains insufficient until about 35 weeks' gestation. Research on the cause of hyaline membrane disease began in earnest after the death of Patrick Kennedy—the newborn son of President John F. Kennedy and his wife, Jackie—who lived only two days. As a result of that research, artificial surfactant became available in the 1980s and is now routinely used to treat premature infants suffering from respiratory distress syndrome. *See also* surfactant.

hydrogen peroxide a strong disinfectant and bleaching liquid.

hypoxia reduction of oxygen supply to tissue below normal physiological levels despite adequate perfusion.

hysterectomy the surgical removal of the uterus; the operation might also include, in addition to the uterus, removal of some combination of the cervix, ovaries, and fallopian tubes. *See also* supravaginal hysterectomy.

iatrogenic an undesirable condition caused by medical treatment.

indication a sign pointing to the cause or treatment of a disease or pathological condition.

induction starting labor by artificial means, either mechanically, by stripping the membranes or rupturing the amniotic sac for example, or chemically with the administration of Pitocin. *See also* bougie; labor augmentation; oxytocin; Pitocin; pituitary extract; pituitrin.

infant mortality the death of an infant before its first birthday; the number of infants under the age of 1 who died per 1,000 live births in a given year in a given locale. The infant mortality rate is often used to assess the well-being of a country's population and the state of its healthcare system. *See also* neonatal mortality; perinatal mortality.

infusion the administration of medicine through a needle or catheter.

innocuous FHR pattern a pattern produced by continual electronic fetal monitoring that indicates the fetal heart rate is normal.

integument a tough, outer, protective layer covering an organ or organism.

internal version *See* version.

intraductal carcinoma in situ the presence of abnormal cells inside the milk duct of a breast but the cells are noninvasive, that is, they have not spread outside the milk duct and there is little to no risk of metastasis.

intrapartum occurring during labor or delivery.

intrauterine bag a bag-shaped device placed within the uterus to induce labor. *See also* Voorhees bag.

intrauterine pressure catheter a device placed in the amniotic space during labor to measure the strength of uterine contractions.

involution the shrinkage of an organ when inactive, particularly the uterus after childbirth.

justo major an unusually large pelvis, with all its dimensions proportionally increased.

Kielland forceps obstetrical forceps with a marked cephalic curve and no pelvic curve and with gliding blades that adapt to the sides of the fetal head. Invented by Christian Kielland, an early-twentieth-century Norwegian obstetrician. *See also* forceps.

kyphoscoliotic an abnormal curvature of the spine in which the spinal column is convex both backward and sideways.

labor the process during childbirth in which the cervix thins and opens and the uterus pushes the fetus into and, eventually, out of the birth canal. *See also* first-stage labor; labor augmentation; labor induction; second-stage labor; transition.

labor augmentation either a mechanical means, such as breaking the bag of waters, or a chemical means, usually using Pitocin, of hastening labor after a woman has gone into labor spontaneously.

labor dystocia *See* dystocia.

laparotomy an incision to open the abdomen.

latent phase of labor the initial, least uncomfortable segment of first-stage labor when the cervix dilates from 0 to 3 or 4 centimeters. *See also* active labor; first-stage labor.

laudanum an opium-based painkiller.

LDRP room a single room in a hospital used for labor, delivery, recovery, and postpartum care.

LED light emitting diode.

Leopold maneuvers named after its inventor, German obstetrician Christian Gerhard Leopold, a systematic way to determine the position of a fetus by placing one's hands on the abdomen of the pregnant woman.

linea alba a fibrous structure running down the middle of the abdomen. *See also* median incision.

liquor amnii amniotic fluid.

local anesthesia anesthesia affecting a specific part of the body, making it insensible to pain or any other sensation.

lochia the vaginal discharge after giving birth.

lordosis abnormal increase in the curvature of the lumbar and cervical spine.

low-cervical cesarean *See* low transverse cut.

low forceps *See* forceps.

low transverse cut the surgical incision most commonly used today to perform a cesarean section. The horizontal cut is made at the bottom of the uterus and is less likely to rupture than the original "classic cut." *See also* classic cut.

macrosomia fetal macrosomia is a larger-than-average fetus, that is, a fetus weighing more than 8 pounds, 13 ounces.

magnesium sulfate an anticonvulsant and electrolyte replenisher.

malacosteon a disease of the bones that softens them and allows them to bend without breaking; inadequate mineralization of bone, the equivalent of rickets. *See also* rickets.

mastectomy the removal of the whole breast. *See also* radical mastectomy.

meconium the first feces expelled by a newborn. Meconium is the substance lining the fetal intestines in utero. Meconium staining during birth can be a signal of fetal distress.

median forceps *See* forceps.

median incision a vertical incision that follows the linea alba. *See also* linea alba.

membranes *See* amniotic sac; rupture of membranes.

microbiome all the microorganisms in a particular environment.

microcephaly congenitally abnormal small head, usually associated with mental disability.

modifiable risk factors contributing to the development of a disease or condition that can be changed.

mongolism nineteenth-century term for what is now called Down syndrome, derived from the phrase "mongoloid race" and based on the belief that the facial characteristics typical of the syndrome were a manifestation of "racial degeneration." The derogatory term is no longer in use.

multipara a woman who is pregnant and has had previous children; a woman who has given birth two or more times. *See also* grand multipara; nullipara; primipara.

Naline trademark name for nalorphine, a drug structurally related to morphine but acting as an antagonist to morphine and related narcotics.

near term close to the time of birth but falling short (usually by two or three weeks) of the full 40-week gestation period.

necrotizing fasciitis a rapidly spreading bacterial infection capable of destroying skin, fat, fascia (tissue surrounding muscle), and muscle tissue.

Nembutal trademark name for sodium pentobarbital.

neonatal mortality aggregate annual death rate of infants at or before four weeks of age in a specified geographical locale. *See also* infant mortality; perinatal mortality

neoplastic disease uncontrolled tissue growth.

nephritis inflammation of the kidney.

NICU neonatal intensive care unit.

Nisentil an opioid analgesic chemically related to meperidine but more potent, faster acting, and of shorter duration. Meperidine, also an opioid analgesic, is used to treat moderate to severe pain and is delivered via tablet, syrup, intramuscular injection, or intravenous injection.

nonoperator the informal philosophical camp of obstetricians in the nineteenth and early twentieth centuries espousing trust in the physiology of labor and birth and calling for medical intervention only if empirically necessary. *See also* operator.

nonreassuring FHR pattern a pattern resulting from electronic fetal monitoring suggesting possible fetal distress and indicating corrective treatment and ongoing vigilance are necessary. Customarily, in light of a nonreassuring FHR pattern, labor continues unless another clinical indication suggests the need for medical intervention.

nosocomial an illness or serious medical condition caused by medical treatment.

nullipara a woman who has never given birth. *See also* multipara; primipara.

occiput the back part of the head; a fetus presenting at birth with the back part of the head first.

occiput posterior description of the fetal position when the back of the fetal head is resting against the mother's back; in lay terms, "sunny side up."

occlusion the blockage or closing of a blood vessel or a hollow organ such as the uterus.

ominous FHR pattern a pattern produced by continual electronic fetal monitoring suggesting probable fetal distress. Prompt corrective treatment is indicated, and immediate delivery is often considered.

oophorectomy surgical removal of one or both ovaries.

operative vaginal delivery traditionally, refers to a birth in which the physician uses forceps to extract the infant from the birth canal. Today, the phrase also encompasses the use of vacuum extractors. *See also* forceps; vacuum extractor.

operator the informal philosophical camp of obstetricians in the nineteenth and early twentieth centuries that characterized childbirth as an inherently pathological process and called for routine medical intervention during labor and birth. *See also* nonoperator.

os the cervical opening connecting the uterus and vagina.

osteomalacia softening of the bones, often (but not always) caused by Vitamin D deficiency.

os uteri *See* os.

outlet forceps *See* forceps.

oximetry a procedure to measure the amount of oxygen in the blood.

oxytocic drug drug used to hasten evacuation of the uterus after birth by stimulating contractions.

oxytocin a hormone that aids cervical dilation, released naturally by the pituitary gland after distension of the cervix during labor. Synthetic oxytocin is sold under the trade name Pitocin, a drug used to trigger and augment labor. Also sometimes administered after delivery to aid in contraction of the uterus to prevent postpartum bleeding. *See also* pituitary extract; pituitrin.

parietal bones bones forming the sides and roof of the cranium.

parity the fact of having borne children.

parturient a woman in labor.

pelvimeter an instrument designed to measure the size and capacity of the female pelvis. *See also* pelvimetry; x-ray pelvimetry.

pelvimetry the "science" of measuring the size and capacity of a woman's pelvis. *See also* pelvimeter; x-ray pelvimetry.

percreta *See* placenta percreta.

perinatal mortality the annual number of stillbirths and deaths per 1,000 live births in a given locale beginning at 28 weeks' gestation through one to two weeks after birth. *See also* infant mortality; neonatal mortality.

perineal pertaining to the perineum, the region in the female between the vulva and anus. *See also* perineum.

perineum in the female, the region between the vulva and anus.

peritoneal cavity a hollow space in the body or one of its organs.

peritoneum the large membrane sheet lining the walls of the abdominal and pelvic cavity.

peritonitis infection of the peritoneum. *See also* peritoneum.

permanganate of potash a poisonous salt used as a disinfectant and antiseptic.

pH a measure of hydrogen ion concentration; a measure of the acidity or alkalinity of a solution. A value of 7 represents neutrality—above it alkalinity increases, and below it acidity increases.

phlebitis inflammation of leg or arm veins caused by prolonged inactivity.

phocomelia congenital defect characterized by the hands or feet attached directly to the trunk of the body with proximal portion of the limbs absent.

phthisis old, now discarded, name for pulmonary tuberculosis.

Pitocin *See* oxytocin.

pituitary extract hormone produced by the posterior pituitary gland that helps to trigger labor. In modern obstetrics, used most often by obstetricians to aid in placental expulsion rather than labor induction. *See also* oxytocin; pituitrin.

Pituitrin the trademark name for a hormone released by the posterior pituitary; oxytocin is a pituitrin. *See also* oxytocin; pituitary extract.

placebo effect a beneficial effect produced by a medical preparation having no pharmacological activity, therefore the effect is caused by the patient's belief in the treatment.

placenta abruptio *See* placental abruption.

placenta accreta one of the most serious conditions of pregnancy, when a portion of the placenta becomes deeply embedded in the uterine wall, sometimes causing life-threatening hemorrhage after a birth. An accreta is a known complication of a previous cesarean birth. In subsequent pregnancies, the placenta can grow into the uterine scar. The more cesarean births a woman has had, the greater her risk of an accreta in her next pregnancy.

placental abruption the separation of the placenta from the uterine wall before delivery.

placenta percreta a life-threatening abnormality of placental attachment in which the placenta penetrates the myometrium (the smooth muscle tissue of the uterus), ruptures the uterine wall, and attaches to other organs, such as the bladder or rectum. As with other placental anomalies, the risk of a percreta in a subsequent pregnancy increases with each cesarean.

placenta previa a placenta that develops in the lower part of the uterus and covers part or all of the cervical opening causing painless, and possibly dangerous, hemorrhage.

polyhydramnios an excess of amniotic fluid in the amniotic sac.

Porro cesarean the protocol for a cesarean developed by Edorado Porro, an Italian obstetrician, also known as a radical cesarean. The salient characteristic of the Porro procedure is the culmination of the surgery in amputation of the uterus, removal of the ovaries, and then stitching up the cervix to prevent hemorrhage and leakage of lochia into the abdomen. Porro's protocol lessened the incidence of post-operative hemorrhage and infection. *See also* gastro-hysterectomy.

port a medical device installed beneath the skin, useful for transmitting medicine directly into a vein for a prolonged period.

position in relation to the Bishop score, refers to the position of the cervix; if the cervix faces front (anterior) it is considered favorable for labor, if the cervix is posterior facing it is considered unfavorable for labor. *See also* Bishop score.

postmaturity a pregnancy that has gone beyond its due date, usually by a week or more.

postpartum after birth.

Pott's disease tuberculosis of the spine.

preeclampsia a serious complication of pregnancy. Symptoms include high blood pressure; marked swelling of the face, hands, and feet; severe headache; and significant amounts of protein in the urine. When these symptoms are accompanied by convulsions and coma, it is called eclampsia. Both preeclampsia and eclampsia most often require immediate delivery of the fetus, either via the chemical induction of labor or cesarean section.

prep in obstetrics, slang used to describe the initial steps taken in a hospital to prepare a woman for childbirth, specifically shaving the pubic hair and administering an enema.

presentation the portion of the fetus that can be felt by a finger through the cervix toward the end of second-stage labor. In a normal presentation, the head is the presenting body part. In an abnormal presentation, another body part—a foot, arm, or buttocks, for example—is the presenting part. *See also* breech; cephalic; presenting part.

presenting part the anatomical portion of the fetus that is leading during birth. Most commonly, and safely, the head (cephalic presentation), but other body parts can also be the presenting part. *See also* breech; cephalic; cord prolapse; transverse lie.

primary cesarean a woman's first birth to end in a cesarean section. In the early twentieth century some doctors used "primary cesarean section" to mean any cesarean executed before labor began. *See also* cesarean section; secondary cesarean.

primary uterine inertia absence of effective uterine contractions during first labor. *See also* secondary uterine inertia; uterine inertia.

primigravida woman pregnant for the first time.

primipara a woman who is pregnant and has not previously given birth; the mother of only one child. *See also* multipara; nullipara.

prolapsed cord *See* cord prolapse.

pronatalism the policy, usually the concerted government policy, of encouraging women to bear more children.

prophylactic a treatment intended to prevent a disease or undesirable physical condition.

prostaglandin a hormone-like substance that contracts and relaxes smooth muscles; sometimes used prior to labor in vaginal suppository form to soften the cervix before labor induction or to simply instigate labor.

pubiotomy surgical separation of the pubic bone lateral to the symphysis; in the nineteenth century performed to ensure a vaginal birth and avoid a cesarean section if a woman's pelvis was slightly deformed or small. Not performed if a physician deemed a pelvis severely deformed or impossibly small. *See also* symphysis.

pubis the portion of the body forming the front arch of the pelvis; the pubic bone.

puerperal referring to the period of time from the expulsion of the placenta until involution of the uterus is completed, usually three to six weeks after birth.

pulmonary edema a condition caused by excess fluid in the lungs.

quadroon a person having one black grandparent and three of another race.

quickening a nineteenth-century term for the first fetal movements that the mother feels, usually during the nineteenth to twentieth week of pregnancy.

rachitic pelves a contracted, deformed pelvis caused by rickets.

radical cesarean *See* Porro cesarean.

radical mastectomy a surgical treatment for breast cancer, now discarded, that entails removal of all breast tissue, underlying muscles in the chest wall, and lymph nodes in the armpit.

randomized, controlled trial a study in which people are assigned by chance alone to receive one of several medical interventions, one of which is either the standard treatment for the disease or condition or a placebo.

RCT *See* randomized, controlled trial.

rhachitic affected by rickets. *See also* rickets.

Rh factor an inherited trait referring to a protein on the surface of red blood cells. If the protein is present, an individual is Rh positive. If the protein is absent, the individual is Rh negative. First discovered in rhesus monkeys, hence the name. *See also* erythroblastosis; Rh incompatibility.

Rh incompatibility if an Rh-negative female is impregnated by an Rh-positive male and her fetus is Rh positive. *See also* erythroblastosis; Rh factor; Rh sensitization.

Rh sensitization Rh sensitization can occur during pregnancy if the mother is Rh negative and carrying a fetus whose blood is Rh positive. If the Rh-negative mother is exposed to her infant's Rh-positive blood during birth, her body will make antibodies that might attack fetuses with Rh-positive blood in subsequent pregnancies, causing anemia, jaundice, or worse. *See also* erythroblastosis.

rickets defective mineralization of bone in children and adolescents prompting softened and weakened bones and skeletal deformities. Usually caused by Vitamin D deficiency.

roentgenogram an x-ray.

roentgenologist in modern parlance, a radiologist, a person skilled at using x-rays diagnostically and therapeutically.

rooming-in the practice of keeping the newborn in the mother's room after birth during the hospital stay, rather than in the hospital nursery.

rubella customarily a mild childhood illness caused by a virus, now prevented by vaccination but serious if suffered by a pregnant woman. If contracted during the first trimester of pregnancy, the virus can cause an array of physical malformations in the fetus including deafness, malformation of the heart and eyes, and cognitive disabilities. Known colloquially as German measles.

ruptured membranes a hole or tear in the amniotic sac, either spontaneously at the start of or during labor, or done deliberately to start or hasten labor. *See also* amniotic sac and amniotomy.

ruptured uterus *See* uterine rupture.

saddle-block anesthesia a form of regional spinal anesthesia confined to the perineum, buttocks, and inner thighs.

salpingectomy surgical removal of one or both fallopian tubes.

Sänger cesarean also known as the classic cesarean, invented by gynecologist Max Sänger of Leipzig, Germany. Sänger rejected the uterine amputation invented by Edorado Porro after a cesarean and suggested instead sewing the uterine incision firmly before replacing the organ in the body to prevent hemorrhage.

scoliorhacitic affected with both scoliosis and rickets.

scopolamine a central nervous system depressant that causes amnesia and, often, delirium. Used during childbirth from the early to mid-twentieth century so that women would not be able to recall their labors.

secondary arrest of dilatation the cessation of cervical dilation for at least two hours despite a history of normal dilation previously. *See also* uterine inertia.

secondary cesarean birth by cesarean after a previous birth or births by cesarean. *See also* primary cesarean.

secondary infertility fertility problems that occur after a woman has conceived normally and given birth at least once.

secondary uterine inertia when uterine contractions are initially vigorous but then decrease in strength.

second-stage labor the portion of labor occurring after full cervical dilation, when the uterus acts like a piston to aid the mother in pushing the fetus out of the cervix and through the birth canal. *See also* first-stage labor.

sensitized Rh fetus *See* erythroblastosis; Rh sensitization.

septicemia also known as bacteremia or blood poisoning, occurs when a bacterial infection enters the bloodstream.

sequelae a pathological condition caused by a previous disease.

serous producing or containing serum, i.e., the clear portion of any bodily fluid.

shoulder dystocia an obstructed labor in which the shoulders get stuck in the birth canal after delivery of the fetal head. Shoulder dystocia is an obstetric emergency; if the baby is not quickly delivered, compression of the umbilical cord can cause fetal demise.

sickle-cell disease a severe, hereditary form of anemia in which red blood cells form a sickle shape, most common in people of African descent. Two recessive genes must be present to cause the disease.

sickle-cell trait a mild form of sickle-cell disease in which only one recessive gene is present and far fewer red blood cells form a sickle shape. Sickle-cell trait confers some resistance to malaria.

sigmoid curve an s-shaped curve.

Smellie's scissors a device used to pierce the fetal cranium in cases of obstructed labor, developed by William Smellie, a prominent eighteenth-century English obstetrician.

sonogram *See* ultrasound.

sonography *See* ultrasound.

spina bifida one of several neural tube defects. A congenital defect in which a portion of the spine is exposed through a gap in the backbone.

spondylolisthetic a type of deformed pelvis.

spontaneous labor vaginal delivery that occurs on its own.

station term used to describe how far the baby has descended into the pelvis for birth. *See also* Bishop score.

stenosis *See* cervical stenosis.

stripping membranes a method used to start labor in which a physician or midwife uses a gloved hand to separate the amniotic sac from the uterine wall.

subcutaneous applied under the skin.

sulphuric ether once used widely as an inhalation anesthetic, an explosive, strong-smelling liquid synthesized by mixing ethyl alcohol with sulfuric acid.

supracervical hysterectomy the removal of the uterus but not the cervix. *See also* hysterectomy.

surfactant a mix of phospholipids secreted into the respiratory air passages that contribute to the elasticity of pulmonary tissue. Surfactant does not reach normal levels until 37 weeks' gestation, making breathing difficult or impossible for an infant born extremely prematurely. *See also* hyaline membrane disease.

surgical adhesion scar tissue from a previous surgery or trauma that binds two parts of tissue or two organs together.

sutures stitches holding together a wound or a surgical incision.

symphysiotomy the division of the fibrocartilage of the pubis in order to facilitate delivery.

symphysis pubis a midline or secondary cartilaginous joint between the left and right pubic bones.

tamoxifen a selective estrogen receptor modulator drug used to treat or prevent breast cancer.

term traditionally, a pregnancy lasting 37 to 42 weeks. A term or full-term pregnancy is now defined as a pregnancy lasting 39 to 42 weeks.

tertiary care highly specialized medical care performed in a state-of-the-art facility.

tetanic contraction a sustained, powerful muscle contraction; in labor, refers to an abnormally powerful and prolonged uterine contraction usually prompted by chemical induction of labor.

thalidomide a drug manufactured in the late 1950s and early 1960s by a German pharmaceutical company and sold as a safe, nonaddictive sedative in almost 50 countries. The drug caused severe fetal deformities if ingested during the first trimester of pregnancy. Almost 10,000 babies were born between 1956 and 1962 with thalidomide-induced malformations, including stunted or missing limbs. Many more infants were stillborn or died shortly after birth due to malformations caused by the drug.

third-stage labor the phase of labor that begins after delivery of the infant and ends with delivery of the placenta.

toxemia also known in the nineteenth and early twentieth centuries as eclamptic toxemia or toxemia of pregnancy, today the condition is known as preeclampsia. *See also* preeclampsia.

transition the portion of active labor when the cervix dilates rapidly—usually in 10 to 20 minutes—from 8 to 10 centimeters (that is, becomes fully dilated). Women customarily describe transition as the most painful portion of labor. *See also* first-stage labor.

transverse lie sideways position of the fetus in the uterus.

trefine also spelled trephine, a surgical instrument with circular, sawlike edges. Used to cut out bone, usually portions of the skull, most commonly during craniotomy. *See also* craniotomy.

twilight sleep the phrase originally referred to a mixture of a narcotic and scopolamine given by hypodermic injection to laboring women; in the first decades of the twentieth century, elaborate medical ritual accompanied the treatment. The original form of twilight sleep reduced women's pain, erased their memory of birth, and often caused undesirable side effects, such as delirium, which women had no memory of later. In later years, twilight sleep described a combination of Demerol and a barbiturate to produce a state in which the woman may sleep between contractions and may become disoriented during contractions.

ultrasound sound or other vibrations used to create medical imaging, especially of a fetus during pregnancy and labor.

umbilicus a scar on the abdomen where the umbilical cord was once attached, commonly known as the belly button.

uterine growth restriction poor growth of the fetus during pregnancy, also known as intrauterine growth restriction.

uterine inertia absence of effective uterine contractions during labor. *See also* primary uterine inertia; secondary uterine inertia.

uterine prolapse when pelvic floor muscles and ligaments weaken, providing inadequate support of the uterus, and the uterus slips into the vagina.

uterine rupture a rare but serious complication of pregnancy and labor caused by the scar from a previous cesarean tearing either during the third trimester of pregnancy or, more commonly, during labor. A uterine rupture is comparatively rare today because the classic cut is no longer used to perform cesarean surgery. *See also* classic cut.

uterus the pear-shaped, hollow muscle organ in human females in which the fetus implants and grows.

vacuum extractor a cup-shaped appliance, largely replacing forceps, used to extract the fetus from the birth canal by applying suction to the fetal head. *See also* forceps; operative vaginal delivery.

vaginal atresia a congenital condition in which the vagina is abnormally closed.

vaginal flora microorganisms that colonize the vagina.

vasodilation dilation of a vessel.

VBAC acronym meaning "vaginal birth after cesarean"; a vaginal birth after a previous birth by cesarean section.

version the forcible, manual movement of the fetus, usually from breech to cephalic position. Version is usually performed externally but can be performed internally.

vertex presentation during childbirth, when the top of the baby's head appears first.

vesico vaginal fistula a tear between the vagina and bladder, causing urine to leak into the vagina, usually caused by an unusually difficult, prolonged labor. *See also* fistula.

Voorhees bag a rubberized, rigid bag once used to efface the cervix and induce labor. *See also* intrauterine bag.

vulva the female external genital organ.

wet lung a common condition in infants born by cesarean because their lungs are still full of the amniotic fluid normally squeezed out during labor, known medically as transient tachypnea of the newborn.

x-ray pelvimetry a radiographic examination of the pelvis of a pregnant woman, and often of the diameter of the fetal head as well, to determine the likelihood of the fetal head passing easily and safely through the birth canal during childbirth.

Works Cited

Archival Sources

AMA Health Fraud and Alternative Medicine Collection. American Medical Association Archives, Chicago, IL.

Apgar, Virginia. Papers. Mount Holyoke College, Archives and Special Collections, South Hadley, MA.

Apgar, Virginia. Papers. National Library of Medicine, Washington, DC.

Boston Association for Childbirth Education Records. Schlesinger Library, Radcliffe Institute, Cambridge, MA.

Calkins, Leroy A., MD. Papers. Kansas University Medical Center Archives, Kansas City, KS.

Carter, Francis Bayard. Papers. Duke University Medical Center Archives, Durham, NC.

Charlotte Maternity Clinic. Deliveries 1933–1937. Duke University Medical Center Archives, Durham, NC.

Chicago Maternity Center Papers. Northwestern Memorial Hospital Archives, Chicago, IL.

C/Sec, Inc. Papers. Schlesinger Library, Radcliffe Institute, Cambridge, MA.

DeLee, Joseph B., MD. Papers. Northwestern Memorial Hospital Archives, Chicago, IL.

DeLee, Joseph B. "Syllabus of Lectures on Operative Obstetrics." Senior Class of Northwestern University Medical School 1897–98, 16–33. American College of Obstetricians and Gynecologists Historical Collection, Washington, DC.

Duke University Hospital Obstetrics and Gynecology Records. 1930 to 1948. Duke University Medical Center Archives, Durham, NC.

Friedman, Emanuel A. Papers. 1953–1989. Columbia University Libraries Archival Collection, New York. http://library-archives.cumc.columbia.edu/finding-aid/emanuel-friedman-papers-1953-1989.

Harris, Robert. Collection. Wangensteen Historical Library of Biology and Medicine, University of Minnesota, Minneapolis, MN.

Hommel, Flora. Papers. Archives of Labor and Urban Affairs. Wayne State University, Detroit, MI.

Infant Welfare Society Papers. Chicago History Museum Archives, Chicago, IL.

Informed Homebirth/Informed Birth and Parenting Papers. Sophia Smith Collection of Women's History. Neilson Library, Smith College, Northampton, MA.

James, L. Stanley Papers. Mount Holyoke College, Archives and Special Collections, South Hadley, MA.

Johnson, Lyndon Baines. Papers. 1963–1969. The Lyndon Baines Johnson Presidential Library, Austin, TX.

Kane, Barbara H. Papers. Schlesinger Library, Radcliffe Institute, Cambridge, MA.
Krantz, Kermit E. Papers. Kansas University Medical Center Archives, Kansas City, KS.
Manhattan Maternity and Dispensary Cesarean Section Cases. New York–Presbyterian / Weil Cornell Medical Center Archives, New York.
Midwives Alliance of North America. Papers. Sophia Smith Collection of Women's History. Neilson Library, Smith College, Northampton, MA.
National Women's Health Network Records. Sophia Smith Collection of Women's History. Nielson Library, Smith College, Northampton, MA.
New England Hospital Maternity Records. Francis A. Countway Library of Medicine. Rare Books and Special Collections. Harvard University, Boston, MA.
New England Hospital Papers. Sophia Smith Collection of Women's History. Neilson Library, Smith College, Northampton, MA.
Philadelphia Lying-In Charity Patient Charts. Pennsylvania Hospital Archives, Philadelphia.
Preston Retreat Miscellaneous Papers. 1835–1948. Pennsylvania Hospital Historic Collections, Philadelphia.
Sloane Maternity Hospital Obstetric Records. New York Academy of Medicine Rare Book Room. New York Academy of Medicine, New York.
Wainer, Nancy. Papers. Schlesinger Library. Radcliffe College, Cambridge, MA.
Willson, J. Robert. Papers. National Library of Medicine, History of Medicine Division, Bethesda, MD.

Interviews

Albertson, Frank P. Interview by Patrick Ettinger. October 28, 1993. Indiana University Center for the History of Medicine Oral History Project. Indiana Historical Society, Indianapolis, IN.
Hammond, Charles. Interview by Jessica Roseberry. June 2, 2004. Duke University Medical Center Archives, Durham, NC.
Marieskind, Helen. Interview by author. July 9, 2008. Chicago, IL.
Interview by author of midwife in southern Ohio. 2012. Transcribed from digital recording.
Interviews by author of mothers in Chicago area. 2004–2012. Transcribed from tape and digital recordings.
Interviews by author of mothers in southern Ohio. 2013. Transcribed from tape and digital recordings.
Interviews by author of obstetric residents in Chicago area. 2013. Transcribed from digital recordings.
Interviews by author of obstetricians in Chicago area. 2004–2013. Transcribed from tape and digital recordings.
Interviews by author of obstetricians in southern Ohio. 2012–2013. Transcribed from digital recordings.
Interview by author of retired family physician in Chicago area. 1999. Transcribed from tape recording.
Interviews by author of retired obstetricians in Chicago area. 1996–2012. Transcribed from tape and digital recordings.

Primary Sources

Achenbach, Joel. "An Addiction Crisis along 'The Backbone of America.'" *Washington Post*, December 30, 2016.

———. "No Longer 'Mayberry': An Ohio City Fights an Epidemic of Self-Destruction." *Washington Post*, December 29, 2016.

ACOG Committee Opinion. "Surgery and Patient Choice: The Ethics of Decision Making." *Obstetrics and Gynecology* 102 (2003): 1101–1106.

"ACOG Fellows, Junior Fellows, and Total Membership." Unpublished ACOG In-House Data. ACOG Resource Center. American College of Obstetricians and Gynecologists, Washington, DC.

Acosta-Sison, Honoria. "Pelvimetry and Cephalometry among Filipinas." *The Philippine Journal of Science* 9, no. 6 (1914): 493–497.

Afriat, Cydney I. "Historical Perspective on Electronic Fetal Heart Monitoring: A Decade of Growth, a Decade of Conflict." *Journal of Perinatal and Neonatal Nursing* 1 (July 1987): 1–4.

"The Agony of Mothers about Their Unborn." *Life*, June 4, 1965, 24–31.

Alexander, James M., Shiv K. Sharma, Donald D. McIntire, and Kenneth J. Leveno. "Epidural Analgesia Lengthens the Friedman Active Phase of Labor." *Obstetrics & Gynecology* 100 (July 2002): 46–50.

Alfirevic, Zarko, Tamara Stanpalija, and Nancy Medley. "Fetal and Umbilical Doppler in Normal Pregnancy." *Cochrane Reviews*, April 15, 2015.

Allen, L. M. "A Plea for the More Frequent Performance of Cesarean Section." *The American Journal of Obstetrics and Diseases of Women and Children* (1909): 189–202.

"All Women Get Right to Caesarean Birth on the NHS . . . Even If They Don't Need It." *Daily Mail*, October 31, 2011.

Al-Mufti, Raghad, Andrew McCarthy, and Nicholas M. Fisk. "Survey of Obstetricians' Personal Preference and Discretionary Practice." *European Journal of Obstetrics & Gynecology and Reproductive Biology* 7 (1997): 1–4.

Althabe, Fernando, and José M. Belizán. "Caesarean Section: The Paradox." *Lancet* 368 (2006): 1472–1473.

Altman, Lawrence K. "Doctors Debate Value of Test that Gauges Health of a Newborn." *New York Times*, October 17, 1989.

American Academy of Family Physicians. "Trial of Labor After Cesarean (TOLAC), Formerly Trial of Labor Versus Elective Repeat Cesarean Section for the Woman with a Previous Cesarean Section." www.annfammed.org/content/suppl/2005/07/26/3.4.378.DC1/TOLAC_2005_Guideline.pdf.

"Analgesia and Cesarean Delivery Rates." *ACOG Committee Opinion* 269, February 2002.

"Analgesia and Cesarean Delivery Rates." *ACOG Committee Opinion* 339, June 2006.

Ananth, Cande V., and Allen J. Wilcox. "Placental Abruption and Perinatal Mortality." *American Journal of Epidemiology* 153 (2001): 332–337.

"The Apgar Score." *ACOG Committee Opinion* 333, May 2006.

"Apgar Scores as a Predictor of Fetal Outcome." *ACOG Committee Statement*, April 12, 1984.

Apgar, Virginia. "Method of Evaluation of Newborn." *Current Medical Digest* 20 (December 1953): 71–75.

———. "New Ways to Save Your Unborn Child." *Ladies' Home Journal*, August 1966, 46, 48–49.

———. "A Proposal for a New Method of Evaluation of the Newborn Infant." *Current Research in Anesthesiology* 32 (July–August 1953): 260–267.

———. "They're Solving the Mysteries of Birth Defects." *Family Circle*, January 1964, 48–49, 88–90.

Apgar, Virginia, and Joan Beck. *Is My Baby All Right?: A Guide to Birth Defects*. New York: Simon and Schuster, 1972.

Apgar, Virginia, and E. M. Papper. "Transmission of Drugs across the Placenta." *Current Research in Anesthesiology* (1952): 309–320.

"Approved Residencies and Fellowships for Veteran and Civilian Physicians." *Journal of the American Medical Association* 131 (August 17, 1946): 1322–1354.

Arms, Suzanne. *Immaculate Deception: A New Look at Women and Childbirth in America*. New York: Bantam Books, 1975.

Atlee, John L. "Case of Successful Peritoneal Section for the Removal of Two Diseased Ovaria Complicated with Ascites." *American Journal of Medical Sciences* 7 (January 1844): 44–64.

"Baby, Born after Mother Perishes, in Good Health." *Los Angeles Times*, October 26, 1932, 2.

"Baby Delivered after Runaway Car Kills Mother." *Washington Post*, January 19, 1951, 2.

Baker, S. Josephine. "The High Cost of Babies." *Ladies' Home Journal*, October 1923, 13.

———. "Maternal Mortality in the United States." *Journal of the American Medical Association* 89 (1927): 2016–2017.

Banta, H. David, and Stephen B. Thacker. "Assessing the Costs and Benefits of Electronic Fetal Monitoring." *Obstetrical and Gynecological Survey* 34 (1979): 627–642.

Banta, John V. "Medical Liability Crisis: An International Problem." *Developmental Medicine & Child Neurology* 45 (2003): 363.

Barnes, Allan C. "Reducing the Hazards of Birth." *Harper's Magazine*, January 1964, 31–37.

Barnes, Robert. *Lectures on Obstetric Operations, Including the Treatment of Haemorrhage, and Forming a Guide to the Management of Difficult Labor*. London: J. and A. Churchill, 1871.

Barnes, Robert. "Supreme Court Sides with Employers over Birth Control Mandate." *Washington Post*, June 30, 2014.

Baron, Henry A. "The Intravenous Use of Pituitrin in Obstetrics." *British Journal of Obstetrics and Gynaecology* 42 (April 1835): 322–326.

BBC Trending. "C-Sections Are Not an Easy Way Out." August 26, 2016.

Beck, J. E. "Caesarian Operation. Performed Twice on the Same Woman." *New Orleans Medical and Surgical Journal* 6 (1850–51): 355–356.

Beecham, Clayton T. "Natural Childbirth—A Step Backward?" *The Female Patient* 14 (December 1989): 37–38, 41, 44.

Beller, Fritz K. "A Guest Editorial, The Cerebral Palsy Story: A Catastrophic Misunderstanding in Obstetrics." *Obstetrics & Gynecology Survey* 50 (1995): 83.

Benson, Ralph C., Frank Shubeck, Jerome Deutschberger, William Weiss, and Heinz Berendes. "Fetal Heart Rate as a Predictor of Fetal Distress: A Report from the Collaborative Project." *Obstetrics and Gynecology* 32 (August 1968): 259–266.

Birch, William G. "What You Should Know about Cesareans." *Parents Magazine and Better Homemaking*, January 1965, 38, 88.
"Birth by Appointment." *Newsweek* 76 (July 20, 1970): 85.
Bishop, Edward H. "Elective Induction of Labor." *Obstetrics and Gynecology* 5 (1955): 519–527.
———. "Pelvic Scoring for Elective Induction." *Obstetrics and Gynecology* 24 (August 1964): 266–268.
Black, Marion E., "Psychorelaxation Management for Labor and Delivery." *Clinical Obstetrics and Gynecology* 4 (March 1961): 108–116.
Blair, William M. "Kennedys Mourning Baby Son; Funeral Today Will Be Private." *New York Times*, August 10, 1963, 1, 44.
Boehm, Frank H., Kathy K. Davidson, and Jeffrey M. Barrett. "The Effect of Electronic Fetal Monitoring on the Incidence of Cesarean Section." *American Journal of Obstetrics and Gynecology* 140 (June 1, 1981): 295–298.
Boehm, Frank H., and Donald A. Goss. "The Xerox 400 Telecopier and the Fetal Monitor." *Obstetrics and Gynecology* 42 (September 1973): 475–478.
Bolotin, Joseph T. "'Painless' Childbirth: A Doctor Comments." *American Mercury* 478 (June 1939): 220–224.
Borquez, Heather A., and Therese A. Wiegers. "A Comparison of Labour and Birth Experiences of Women Delivering in a Birth Centre and at Home in the Netherlands." *Midwifery* 22 (2006): 339–347.
Boston Women's Health Book Collective. *Our Bodies, Ourselves: A Book by and for Women*. New York: Simon and Schuster, 1976.
"Brain-Damaged New York Teen Is Awarded $29 Million Judgment in Hospital Lawsuit." *Jet*, December 7, 1998, 46–47.
"Brazil Unveils New Rules to Curb Country's Caesarean 'Epidemic.'" *Guardian*, January 7, 2015.
Bréart, Gérard. "Postpartum Maternal Mortality and Cesarean Delivery." *Obstetrics and Gynecology* 108 (September 2006): 541–548.
Brecher, Ruth, and Edward Brecher. "The Disgraceful Facts about Infant Deaths in the US." *McCall's*, February 1966, 82, 154–158.
Brennan, Donald J., Michael S. Robson, Martina Murphy, and Colm O'Herlihy. "Comparative Analysis of International Cesarean Delivery Rates Using 10-Group Classification Identifies Significant Variation in Spontaneous Labor." *American Journal of Obstetrics and Gynecology* 201 (September 2009): 308.e1–308.e8.
Bretelle, Florence, Blandine Courbière, Chafika Mazouni, Aubert Agostini, Ludovic Cravello, Léon Boubli, Marc Gamerre, and Claude D'Ercole. "Management of Placenta Accrete: Morbidity and Outcome." *European Journal of Obstetrics & Gynecology* 133 (2007): 34–39.
Brickell, D. Warren. "A Successful Case of Caesarean Section." *New Orleans Journal of Medicine* 21 (1868): 454–466.
Bricker, L., and J. P. Nelson. "Routine Doppler Ultrasound in Pregnancy." *Cochrane Reviews*, April 24, 2000.
Briggs, Helen. "Caesarean Births 'Affecting Human Evolution.'" *BBC News*, December 7, 2016.

Brody, Jane E. "Updating a Standard: Fetal Monitoring." *New York Times*, July 7, 2009.
———. "With Childbirth, Now It's What the Mother Orders." *New York Times*, December 9, 2003, F7.
Bromley, Dorothy Dunbar. "What Risk Motherhood?" *Harper's Magazine*, June 1929, 11–22.
"Brooklyn Girl Awarded $35.6 Million in Hospital Lawsuit." *Jet*, August 12, 1996, 9.
Burd, Laurence. "Requiem Mass Slated Today for Kennedy Boy." *Los Angeles Times*, August 10, 1963, 1, 7.
Burns, Ruth. "It's a Caesarean Baby." *Parents' Magazine*, April 1948, 19, 92–93.
Cahill, Alison G., et al. "Is Vaginal Birth After Cesarean (VBAC) or Elective Repeat Cesarean Safer in Women with a Prior Vaginal Delivery?" *Obstetrics & Gynecology* 195 (2006): 1143–1147.
Calkins, L. A. "Prolonged Labor." *Journal of the Kansas Medical Society* 42 (1941): 331–333.
Calkins, L. A., Jed H. Irvine, and Guy W. Horsley. "Variations in the Factors Affecting Length of Labor." *American Journal of Obstetrics and Gynecology* 19 (February 1930): 294–297.
Callaghan, William M., Andreea A. Creanga, and Elena V. Kuklina. "Severe Maternal Morbidity among Delivery and Postpartum Hospitalizations in the United States." *Obstetrics & Gynecology* 120 (November 2012): 1029–1036.
Calmes, Selma Harrison. "Virginia Apgar: A Woman Physician's Career in a Developing Specialty." *Journal of the American Medical Women's Association* 39, no. 6 (November/December 1984): 184–188.
"Camera in Hospital." *Time*, December 9, 1935, 43.
Campbell, I. A. "X-Ray Pelvimetry: Useful Procedure or Medical Nonsense." *Journal of the National Medical Association* 68 (November 1976): 514–520.
Campbell, S. "A Short History of Sonography in Obstetrics and Gynaecology." *Facts, Views & Vision in ObGyn* 5 (2013): 213–229.
Cane, Aleta Feinsod, and Beth Shearer. *Frankly Speaking: A Book for Cesarean Couples.* Framingham, MA: C/SEC, 1984.
"A Case of Cæsarian Section, Terminating Favourably to the Mother." *New York Journal of Medicine and Surgery* 1 (1839): 214–217.
"Cesarean Delivery on Maternal Request." *ACOG Committee Opinion* 386, November 2007.
"Cesarean Delivery on Maternal Request." *ACOG Committee Opinion* 559, April 2013.
"Cesarean 'Seed' Uprooted." *Clarion* 9 (Spring 1993): 8.
Chaves, Ricardo Lêdo. "Birth as a Radical Experience of Change." *Cadernos de Saúde Pública, Rio de Janeiro* 30 (2014): S1–S3.
Check, William A. "Electronic Fetal Monitoring: How Necessary?" *Journal of the American Medical Association* 241 (April 27, 1979): 1772–1774.
"Childbirth Dangers Cut." *Science News Letter* 80 (December 9, 1961): 379.
"Childbirth Deaths Drop." *Chicago Defender*, May 17, 1952, 1.
"Childbirth: Nature v. Drugs." *Time*, May 25, 1936, 40–44.
"Close of the EMIC Program." *American Journal of Public Health* 39 (December 1949): 1579–1581.

Cohen, Alan B., Henry Klapholz, and Mark S. Thompson. "Electronic Fetal Monitoring and Clinical Practice: A Survey of Obstetric Opinion." *Medical Decision Making* 2 (1982): 79–95.

Cohen, Nancy Wainer, and Lois J. Estner. *Silent Knife: Cesarean Prevention and Vaginal Birth After Cesarean (VBAC)*. South Hadley, MA: Bergin & Garvey, 1983.

Colcher, A. E., and Walter Sussman. "Changing Concepts of X-Ray Pelvimetry." *American Journal of Obstetrics and Gynecology* 57 (March 1949): 510–519.

Cole, K. C. "Can Natural Childbirth Survive Technology?" *Maternal Health and Childbirth Resource Guide* 4 (1980), 18–19.

Commiff, James C. G. "New Medical Specialty—Fetology: The World of the Unborn." *New York Times Magazine*, January 8, 1967, 41, 96–100.

Comptroller General. *Report to the Congress of the United States: Evaluating Benefits and Risks of Obstetric Practices—More Coordinated Federal and Private Efforts Needed.* September 24, 1979.

Cooley, Donald Gray. "One-Hour Childbirth." *Better Homes and Gardens*, June 1958, 116, 153.

Cope, I., P. Lancaster, and L. Stevens. "Smoking in Pregnancy." *Medical Journal of Australia* 2 (1975): 745–747.

Corea, Gena. "The Caesarean Epidemic: Who's Having This Baby, Anyway—You or the Doctor?" *Mother Jones*, July 1980, 28–35, 42.

Costaine, Maged M., and George R. Saade. "The First Cesarean: Role of 'Fetal Distress' Diagnosis." *Seminars in Perinatology* 36 (2012): 379–383.

Cottman, Thomas. "Caesarian Operation Successfully Performed." *New Orleans Medical and Surgical Journal* 6 (1850–51): 337–338.

Cragin, Edwin B. "Cesarean Section." In *Sloane Hospital for Women New York City Obstetrical and Gynecology Reports*. Vol. 1 (1913), edited by Wilbur Ward, 13–19.

———. "Conservatism in Obstetrics." *New York Medical Journal* 104 (July 1, 1916): 1–3.

———. *Obstetrics: A Practical Text-Book for Students and Practitioners*. Philadelphia: Lea & Febiger, 1916.

Creanga, Andreea A., Cynthia J. Berg, Jean Y. Ko, Sherry L. Farr, Van T. Tong, F. Carol Bruce, and William M. Callaghan. "Maternal Mortality and Morbidity in the United States: Where Are We Now?" *Journal of Women's Health* 23 (2014): 3–9.

Creanga, Andreea A., Cynthia J. Berg, Carla Syverson, Kristi Seed, F. Carol Bruce, and William A. Callaghan. "Pregnancy-Related Mortality in the United States, 2006–2010." *Obstetrics & Gynecology* 125 (January 2015): 5–12.

Cron, R. S., L. M. Randall, and N. R. Kretzschmar. "A Report of the Committee on the Induction of Labor." *American Journal of Obstetrics and Gynecology* 37 (1939): 873–877.

"The Current Role of Continuous Electronic Fetal Heart Rate Monitoring in Labor." *ACOG Committee Statement: State-of-the-Art Opinion in Obstetrics and Gynecology*, March 1979.

Curtis, Caroline G., ed. *The Cary Letters*. Cambridge, MA: Riverside Press, 1891.

Dailey, U. G. "Mother Is Hypnotised For Birth." *Chicago Defender*, April 4, 1959, 15.

———. "Painless Childbirth Seen Boon to Future Mothers." *Chicago Defender*, January 30, 1943, 9.

Dalton, John. "Memoir on Sulphuric Ether." *Memoirs and Proceedings Manchester Literary and Philosophical Society* (1820): 446–482.

Daub, Raysh, and Cathy Daub. "Caesareans Credited for Lower Death Rate." *Clarion* 1 (1983): 5.
David, Lester, and Irene David. "One in Five." *Health*, May 1984, 73–81.
Davidson, Bill. "The Case For and Against Induced Labor." *Good Housekeeping*, January 1964, 59, 114, 116.
Davis, David B. *The Principles and Practice of Obstetric Medicine.* Vol. 2. London: Taylor and Walton, 1836.
Davis, Edward P. *Operative Obstetrics Including the Surgery of the Newborn.* Philadelphia: W. B. Saunders, 1911.
Davis, Maxine. "The Truth about Caesareans." *Good Housekeeping*, November 1941, 38, 72–73.
Davis, Wendy. "Edwards's Career Tied to Jury Award Debate." *Boston Globe*, September 15, 2003.
Day, Beth. "Guardian of the Newborn." *Woman's Day*, September 1966, 46–47, 97–99.
Declerq, Eugene. "Is Medical Intervention in Childbirth Inevitable in Brazil?" *Cadernos de Saúde Pública* 30 (2014): 523–524.
Declercq, Eugene R., Carol Sakala, Maureen P. Corry, and Sandra Applebaum. "Listening to Mothers II: Report of the Second National US Survey of Women's Childbearing Experiences." *Journal of Perinatal Education* 16 (Fall 2007): 9–14.
Declercq, Eugene R., Carol Sakala, Maureen P. Corry, Sandra Applebaum, and Ariel Herrlich. "Listening to Mothers III: Pregnancy and Birth." *Childbirth Connection.* http://transform.childbirthconnection.org/wp-content/uploads/2013/06/LTM-III_Pregnancy-and-Birth.pdf.
Declercq, Eugene, Robin Young, Howard Cabral, and Jeffrey Ecker. "Is a Rising Cesarean Delivery Rate Inevitable? Trends in Industrialized Countries, 1987 to 2007." *Birth: Issues in Perinatal Care* 38 (June 2011): 99–104.
"Decline in Rate of Vaginal Birth after Cesarean Tied to Restrictive Policies." *UCLA Public Health Magazine*, June 2011. https://ph.ucla.edu/news/magazine/2011/june/article/decline-rate-vaginal-birth-after-cesarean-tied-restrictive-policies.
de Kruif, Paul. *The Fight for Life.* New York: Harcourt, Brace, 1938.
———. "Forgotten Mothers." *Ladies' Home Journal*, December 1936, 12–13, 64–68.
———. "Saver of Mothers." *Ladies' Home Journal*, March 1932, 6–7, 124–125.
DeLee, Joseph B. "How Should the Maternity Be Isolated?" *Modern Hospital* 29 (September 1927): 65–72.
———. "An Illustrated History of the Low or Cervical Cesarean Section." *American Journal of Obstetrics and Gynecology* 50 (1925): 90–109.
———. *The Principles and Practice of Obstetrics.* Philadelphia: W. B. Saunders, 1918.
———. *The Principles and Practice of Obstetrics.* Philadelphia: W. B. Saunders, 1925.
———. *The Principles and Practice of Obstetrics.* Philadelphia: W. B. Saunders, 1929.
———. "Progress Toward Ideal Obstetrics." *American Journal of Obstetrics and Diseases of Women and Children* 73 (March 1916): 407–415.
———. "The Prophylactic Forceps Operation." *American Journal of Obstetrics and Gynecology* 1 (October 1920): 34–44.
———. "Two Cases of Obstetrical Hemorrhage." *Chicago Medical Recorder* 11 (September 1896): 151–161.

DeLee, Joseph B., and Heinz Siedentopf. "The Maternity Ward of the General Hospital." *Journal of the American Medical Association* 100 (January 7, 1933): 6–14.

Deneux-Tharaux, Catherine, et al. "Postpartum Maternal Mortality and Cesarean Delivery." *Obstetrics and Gynecology* 108 (September 2006): 541–548.

de Regt, Roberta Haynes, Howard L. Minkoff, Joseph Feldman, and Richard H. Schwarz. "Relation of Private or Clinic Care to the Cesarean Birth Rate." *New England Journal of Medicine* 315 (September 4, 1986): 619–624.

"Discussion." *American Journal of Obstetrics and Gynecology* 1 (October 1920): 77–80.

"Discussion, Caesarean Section, with Report of a Successful Case." *Chicago Medical Recorder* 7 (August 1894): 115–119.

"Discussion of Joseph DeLee, 'The Early Recognition of Impending Obstetric Accidents.'" *Chicago Medical Recorder* 24 (June 1903): 440–442.

"Discussion of Rudolph W. Holmes, 'Obstetrics, A Lost Art: A Criticism of the Promiscuous Indications for Cæsarean Section.'" *Surgery, Gynecology, and Obstetrics* 21 (1915): 663–664.

"The Doctor Talks about Babies by Appointment." *McCall's*, January 1957, 4, 81.

"The Doctor Talks about Caesareans." *McCall's*, December 1958, 4, 71.

Domingues, Rosa Maria Soares Madeira, et al. "Process of Decision-Making Regarding the Mode of Birth in Brazil: From the Initial Preference of Women to the Final Mode of Birth." *Cadernos de Saúde Pública, Rio de Janeiro* 30 (2014): S1–S16.

Dominguez-Bello, Maria G., et al. "Partial Restoration of the Microbiota of Cesarean-Born Infants via Vaginal Microbial Transfer." *Nature Medicine* 22 (2016): 250–253.

Donald, I., J. MacVicar, and T. G. Brown. "Investigation of Abdominal Masses by Pulsed Ultrasound." *Lancet* 271 (1958): 1188–1195.

Donohue, Frank M. "A Successful Case of Cesarean Section." *American Journal of Obstetrics and Diseases of Women and Children* 23 (1890): 508–511.

Drage, J. S., and H. Berendes. "Apgar Scores and Outcome of the Newborn." *Pediatric Clinics of North America* 13 (1966): 635–643.

Dudley, A. Palmer. "The Cesarean Operation, with the Report of a Case." *American Journal of Obstetrics and Diseases of Women and Children* 23 (1890): 712–719.

Dyer, Isadore. "Clinical Evaluation of X-Ray Pelvimetry." *American Journal of Obstetrics and Gynecology* 60 (August 1950): 302–314.

"Dystocia." *ACOG Technical Bulletin* 137, December 1989.

"Dystocia and Augmentation of Labor." *ACOG Practice Bulletin* 49, December 2003.

"Dystocia: Etiology, Diagnosis, and Management Guidelines." *ACOG Committee Statement*, June 1982.

Eastman, Nicholson J. *Williams Obstetrics*. New York: Apple-Century-Crofts, 1950.

Editorial Board. "America's Shocking Maternal Deaths." *New York Times*, September 3, 2016.

Eisenberg, Lucy. "Genetics and the Survival of the Unfit." *Harper's Magazine*, February 1966, 53–58.

"Enraged about Hospital Birth." *NAPSAC News, The National Association of Parents & Professionals for Safe Alternatives in Childbirth* 2 (Fall 1977): 21.

Erikson, Jane. "New Focus on Women in Hospitals Here." *Arizona Daily Star*, January 3, 2006.

Evans, Tommy N. "Prolonged Labor." *Obstetrics and Gynecology* 6 (November 1955): 522–531.

"Factbox: Ebola Cases in the United States." *Reuters*, October 23, 2014. www.reuters.com/article/us-health-ebola-usa-factbox-idUSKCN0ID06S20141024.

Faiz, A. S., and C. V. Ananth. "Etiology and Risk Factors for Placenta Previa: An Overview and Meta-Analysis of Observational Studies." *Journal of Maternal-Fetal & Neonatal Medicine* 13 (2003): 175–190.

Farthing, Kathleen Gray. "The VBAC Current." *Clarion* 12 (September 1997): 2.

Feng, Xing Lin, Ling Xu, Yan Guo, and Carine Ronsmans. "Factors Influencing Rising Caesarean Section Rates in China between 1988 and 2008." *Bulletin of the World Health Organization* 90 (2012): 30–39.

"Fetal Heart Rate Monitoring: Guidelines for Monitoring, Terminology, and Instrumentation." *ACOG Technical Bulletin* 32, June 1975.

"Fetal Heart Rate Patterns: Monitoring, Interpretation, and Management." *ACOG Technical Bulletin* 207, July 1995.

Fields, Robin and Joe Sexton. "How Many American Women Die from Causes Related to Pregnancy or Childbirth? No One Knows." *ProPublica*, October 23, 2017.

Flexner, Abraham. *Medical Education in the United States and Canada: A Report to the Carnegie Foundation for the Advancement of Teaching.* Stanford, CA: Carnegie Foundation for the Advancement of Teaching, 1910.

Florence, A. Leslie. "Is Thalidomide to Blame?" *British Medical Journal* (December 31, 1960): 1954.

"For Cesarean Births." *Science News Letter* 45 (January 22, 1944): 52–53.

Francis and Beck, Drs. "Case of Self-Performed Caesarean Section." *New York Medical and Physical Journal* 2 (Jan.–Mar. 1823): 1.

Friedan, Betty. *The Second Stage.* New York: Summit Books, 1981.

Friedman, Emanuel A. "The Graphic Analysis of Labor." *American Journal of Obstetrics and Gynecology* 68 (December 1954): 1568–1575.

———. *Labor: Clinical Evaluation and Management.* New York: Appleton-Century-Crofts, 1978.

———. "Labor in Multiparas: A Graphicostatistical Analysis." *Obstetrics and Gynecology* 6 (1955): 567–589.

———. "The Obstetrician's Dilemma: How Much Fetal Monitoring and Cesarean Section Is Enough?" *New England Journal of Medicine* 315 (September 4, 1986): 641–643.

Friedman, Emanuel A., and Marlene R. Sachtleben. "Dysfunctional Labor: II. Protracted Active-Phase Dilatation in the Nullipara." *Obstetrics and Gynecology* 17 (May 1961): 566–578.

Friedman, Leo V. "Types of Pelvic Deformity, Technique." *Boston Medical and Surgical Journal* 161 (December 2, 1909): 809–812.

Frigoletto, Fredric D., and Allan S. Nadel. "Electronic Fetal Heart Rate Monitoring: Why the Dilemma?" *Clinical Obstetrics and Gynecology* 31 (March 1988): 179–183.

"The Full Story of the Drug Thalidomide." *Life*, August 10, 1962, 25–33.

Gabbe, G. S., and G. B. Holzman. "Obstetricians' Choice of Delivery." *Lancet* 357 (2001): 722.

Gabert, Harvey A., and Morton A. Stenchever. "Electronic Fetal Monitoring as a Routine Practice in an Obstetric Service: A Progress Report." *American Journal of Obstetrics and Gynecology* 118 (February 15, 1974): 534–537.

———. "The Results of a Five-Year Study of Continuous Fetal Monitoring on an Obstetric Service." *Obstetrics and Gynecology* 50 (September 1977): 275–279.

Garcia, Celso Ramon, Richard Waltman, and Samuel Lubin. "Continuous Intravenous Infusion of Demerol in Labor." *American Journal of Obstetrics and Gynecology* 66 (1953): 312–318.

Gardberg, Mikael, Yana Leonova, and Eero Laakkonen. "Malpresentation—Impact on Mode of Delivery." *ACTA Obstetrica et Gynecologica Scandinavica* 90 (2011): 540–542.

Gardner, Janet. "Having Your Baby at Home: A Clear-Headed Report to Help You Make Up Your Mind." *Glamour*, March 1979, 240–242, 244.

Gaskin, Ina May. *Spiritual Midwifery*. Summertown, TN: Book Publishing Co., 1980.

Gause, Ralph W. "Dear Doctor: Birth by Cesarean." *American Baby*, July 1987, 42, 45.

Gielchinsky, Y., N. Rojansky, S. J. Fasouliotis, and Y. Ezra, "Placenta Accreta—Summary of 10 Years: A Survey of 310 Cases." *Placenta* 23 (2002): 210–214.

Gieske, Tony, and Marie Smith. "Boy Is Born to the Kennedys." *Washington Post*, November 25, 1960, A1.

Gifford, D. S., S. C. Morton, M. Fiske, and K. Kahn. "A Meta-Analysis of Infant Outcomes after Breech Delivery." *Obstetrics and Gynecology* 85 (1995): 1047–1054.

Gifford, D. S., S. C. Morton, M. Fiske, J. Keesey, E. Keeler, and K. L. Kahn. "Lack of Progress in Labor as a Reason for Cesarean." *Obstetrics and Gynecology* 95 (2000): 589–595.

Gilfix, Myra Gerson. "Electronic Fetal Monitoring: Physician Liability and Informed Consent." *American Journal of Law and Medicine* 10 (Spring 1984): 31–90.

Goff, Karen Goldberg. "Birth by Appointment." *Washington Times*, April 15, 2009.

Gold, Rachel Benson, Asta M. Kenney, and Susheela Singh. "Paying for Maternity Care in the United States." *Family Planning Perspectives* 19 (September–October 1987): 190–193, 195–206.

Goldstein, Hyman, Irving D. Goldberg, Todd M. Frazier, and George E. Davis. "Cigarette Smoking and Prematurity." *Public Health Reports* 79 (July 1964): 553–560.

Goyert, Gregory L., Sidney F. Bottoms, Marjorie C. Treadwell, and Paul C. Nehra. "The Physician Factor in Cesarean Birth Rates." *New England Journal of Medicine* 320 (March 16, 1989): 706–709.

Grady, Denise. "Caesarean Births Are at a High in the US." *New York Times*, March 23, 2010.

Granton, E. Fannie. "The Lady In Black: US Negroes Look with Nostalgia on Former First Lady's White House Reign." *Ebony*, February 1964, 81–82, 84–86.

Green, Charles M. "Cesarean Section: A Consideration of Indications, Technique, and Time of Operating." *Boston Medical and Surgical Journal* 174 (March 30, 1916): 441–449.

———. "A Study of the First Series of One Hundred Caesarean Sections Performed in the Boston Lying-In Hospital." *Boston Medical and Surgical Journal* 161 (December 2, 1909): 803–809.

Greenberg, R., N. J. Haley, R. A. Etzel, and F.A. Loda. "Measuring the Exposure of Infants to Tobacco Smoke." *New England Journal of Medicine* 311 (1984): 672.

Greenhill, J. P. *Obstetrics: From the Original Text of Joseph P. DeLee*. Philadelphia: W. B. Saunders, 1960.

———. *Principles and Practice of Obstetrics*. Philadelphia: W. B. Saunders, 1951.

Grisanti, Mary Lee. "The Cesarean Epidemic." *New York Magazine*, February 20, 1989, 56–61.

Grolund, M. M., O. P. Lehtonen, E. Eerola, and P. Kero. "Fecal Microflora in Healthy Infants Born by Different Methods of Delivery: Permanent Changes in Intestinal Flora after Cesarean Delivery." *Journal of Pediatric Gastroenterology and Nutrition* 28 (1999): 19–25.

Gruber, Jon, John Kim, and Dina Mayzlin. "Physician Fees and Procedure Intensity: The Case of Cesarean Delivery." NBER Working Paper 6744. Cambridge, MA: National Bureau of Economic Research, October 1998.

Gruber, Jonathan, and Maria Owings. "Physician Financial Incentives and Cesarean Section Delivery." NBER Working Paper 4933. Cambridge, MA: National Bureau of Economic Research, November 1994.

"Guidelines for the Use of Fetal Monitoring." *International Journal of Gynaecology and Obstetrics* 25 (1987): 159–167.

"Guidelines for Vaginal Delivery after a Previous Cesarean Birth." *ACOG Committee Statement State-of-the-Art Opinion in Obstetrics and Gynecology*, January 1982.

"Guidelines for Vaginal Delivery after a Previous Cesarean Birth." *ACOG Committee Opinion* 64, October 1988.

Guttmacher, Alan Frank. "The Facts about Caesarean Section." *Parents Magazine and Better Homemaking*, January 1960, 52–53, 95.

———. *Into This Universe: The Story of Human Birth*. New York: Viking, 1937.

Hacker, Neville F., and J. George Moore. *Essentials of Obstetrics and Gynecology*. Philadelphia: W. B. Saunders, 1998.

Haelle, Tara. "Your Biggest C-Section Risk May Be Your Hospital." *Consumer Reports*, May 2017.

Haggerty, Joan. "Childbirth Made Difficult." *Ms.*, January 1973, 16–17.

"Hail Decrease in Deaths during Childbirth." *Chicago Defender*, December 13, 1958, 20.

Hale, Ralph W., and W. Benson Harer. "Editorial: Elective Prophylactic Cesarean Delivery." *ACOG Clinical Review* 10 (March–April 2005): 1, 15–16.

Hall, Michael L., and C. H. Alexander. "Fetal Monitoring in a Community Hospital: Analysis of Health Maintenance Organization, Fee-for-Service, and Clinic Populations." *American Journal of Obstetrics and Gynecology* 143 (June 1, 1982): 277–285.

Hamilton, Brady E., Joyce A. Martin, and Stephanie J. Ventura. "Births: Preliminary Data for 2010." *National Vital Statistics Report* 60 (November 17, 2011).

Hannah, Mary E., Walter J. Hannah, Sheila A. Hewson, Ellen D. Hodnett, Saroj Saigal, and Andrew R. Willan. "Planned Caesarean Section versus Planned Vaginal Birth for Breech Presentation at Term: A Randomised Multicentre Trial." *Lancet* 356 (October 21, 2000): 1375–1383.

Hansen, A. K., K. Wisborg, N. Uldbjerg, and T. B. Henriksen. "Elective Caesarean Section and Respiratory Morbidity in the Term and Near-Term Neonata." *Acta Obstetricia et Gynecologica Scandinavica* 86 (2007): 389–394.

Hardy, Gail. "Birthing Breech: A Lost Art?" *Clarion* 1, no. 3 (1983), 1.

Harer, W. Benson, Jr., "A Look Back at Women's Health and ACOG, a Look Forward to the Challenges of the Future." *Obstetrics & Gynecology* 97 (January 2001): 1–4.

———. "Patient Choice Cesarean." *ACOG Clinical Review* 5 (March/April 2000): 1, 13–16.

Harris, Robert P. "Cattle-Horn Lacerations of the Abdomen and Uterus in Pregnant Women." *American Journal of Obstetrics and Diseases of Women and Children* 20, no. 7 (1887): 673–685.

———. "The Cesarean Operation, According to Porro and Müller." *American Journal of Obstetrics and Diseases of Women and Children* 13 (1880): 148–154.

———. "History of a Pair of Obstetrical Forceps Sixty Years Old." *American Journal of Obstetrics and Diseases of Women and Children* 4 (1871): 55.

———. "If a Woman Has Ruptured her Uterus during Labor, What Should Be Done in Order to Save Her Life?" *American Journal of Obstetrics and Diseases of Women and Children* 8 (1880): 802–821.

———. "Lessons from a Study of the Cesarean Operation in the City and State of New York, and Their Bearing Upon the True Position of Gastro-Elytrotomy." *American Journal of Obstetrics and Diseases of Women and Children* 12 (1879): 82–91.

———. "The Operation of Gastro-Hysterotomy (True Caesarean Section), Viewed in the Light of American Experience and Success; with the History and Results of Sewing Up the Uterine Wound; and a Full Tabular Record of the Caesarean Operations Performed in the United States, Many of Them Not Hitherto Reported." *American Journal of the Medical Sciences* 75 (1878): 313–342.

Haseltine, Nate. "There Is No Mystery about Caesarean Section." *Washington Post*, November 26, 1960, A18.

Haverkamp, Albert D., and Miriam Orleans. "An Assessment of Electronic Fetal Monitoring." *Women and Health* 7 (Fall–Winter 1982): 115–134.

Haverkamp, Albert D., Miriam Orleans, Sharon Langendoerfer, John McFee, James Murphy, and Horace E. Thompson. "A Controlled Trial of the Differential Effects of Intrapartum Fetal Monitoring." *American Journal of Obstetrics and Gynecology* 134 (June 15, 1979): 399–412.

Haverkamp, Albert D., Horace E. Thompson, John G. McFee, and Curtis Cetrulo. "The Evaluation of Continuous Fetal Heart Rate Monitoring in High-Risk Pregnancy." *American Journal of Obstetrics and Gynecology* 125 (June 1, 1976): 310–320.

"Health Talk. So You're Expecting A Baby?" *Chicago Defender*, April 10, 1948.

Heelan, Lisa. "Fetal Monitoring: Creating a Culture of Safety with Informed Choice." *Journal of Perinatal Education* 22 (Summer 2013): 156–165.

Heffner, Linda, Elena Elkin, and Ruth Fretts. "Impact of Labor Induction, Gestational Age, and Maternal Age on Cesarean Delivery Rates." *Obstetrics & Gynecology* 102 (August 2003): 287–293.

Herman, G. Ernest. *Difficult Labour: A Guide to Its Management for Students and Practitioners*. London: Cassell, 1898.

Heyns, O. S. *Abdominal Decompression: A Monograph*. Johannesburg: Witwatersrand University Press, 1963.

Hilliard, Marion. "A Woman Doctor Speaks Frankly about Childbirth." *Chicago Defender*, September 19, 1959, 7.

Hingson, Robert A. "The Control of Pain and Fear in the Management of Labor and Delivery." *Surgical Clinics of North America* 25 (December 1945): 1352–1381.

Hoag, J. C. "Progress in Obstetric Practice." *Chicago Medical Recorder* 19 (July 1900): 1–9.

Hoag, Junius C. "Caesarean Section, with Report of a Case." *Chicago Medical Recorder* 7 (July 1894): 17–26.

Holmes, Rudolph Wieser. "Obstetrics, A Lost Art: A Criticism of the Promiscuous Indications for Cæsarean Section." *Surgery, Gynecology, and Obstetrics* 21 (1915): 636–643.

Hon, Edward H. "Current Concepts of Fetal Monitoring." *California Medicine* 119 (July 1973): 63–64.

———. "The Diagnosis of Fetal Distress." *Clinical Obstetrics and Gynecology* 3 (December 5, 1960): 860–873.

———. "The Electronic Evaluation of the Fetal Heart Rate." *American Journal of Obstetrics and Gynecology* 75 (1958): 1215–1230.

———. "Fetal Monitoring for the Practicing Physician." *California Medicine* 113 (December 1970): 46–47.

Hon, Edward H., and Roy H. Petrie. "Clinical Value of Fetal Heart Monitoring." *Clinical Obstetrics and Gynecology* 18 (December 1975): 1–23.

Hon, Edward H., and E. J. Quilligan. "Electronic Evaluation of Fetal Heart Rate." *Clinical Obstetrics and Gynecology* 11 (March 16, 1968): 145–167.

Hon, E. H., D. Zannini, and E. J. Quilligan. "The Neonatal Value of Fetal Monitoring." *Transactions of the Pacific Coast Obstetrical and Gynecological Society* 42 (1974): 115–126.

Hooker, Ransom S., and the New York Academy of Medicine Committee on Public Health Relations. *Maternal Mortality in New York City: A Study of All Puerperal Deaths 1930–32*. New York: The Commonwealth Fund, 1933.

Hopkins, Kristine. "Are Brazilian Women Really Choosing to Deliver by Cesarean?" *Social Science and Medicine* 51 (2000): 725–740.

"Hospitals Approved for Residencies in Specialties." *Journal of the American Medical Association* 107 (August 29, 1936): 703–715.

"How Many Caesareans?" *Time*, June 7, 1963, 52.

Hoxha, Ilir, et al. "Caesarean Sections and For-Profit Status of Hospitals: Systematic Review and Meta-Analysis." *BMJ Open* 7 (2017). http://bmjopen.bmj.com/content/7/2/e013670.

Huff, O. N. "History and Prophylaxis of Puerperal Infection." *Chicago Medical Recorder* 12 (June 1897): 381–394.

Hurt, Charles. "Edwards' Malpractice Suits Leave Bitter Taste." *Washington Times*, June 25, 2007.

"Induction and Augmentation of Labor." *ACOG Technical Bulletin* 110, November 1987.

"Induction and Augmentation of Labor." *ACOG Technical Bulletin* 157, July 1991.

"Induction of Labor." *ACOG Practice Bulletin* 107, August 2009.

Ingraham, Christopher. "Our Maternal Mortality Is a National Embarrassment." *Washington Post*, November 18, 2015.

Innes, Emma. "Soaring Number of Women Who Are 'Too Posh to Push' Is 'Costing Millions and Putting Pressure on the NHS.'" *Daily Mail*, June 3, 2013.

International Cesarean Awareness Network. *Cesarean Voices*. Redondo Beach, CA: International Cesarean Awareness Network, 2007.

"Intrapartum Fetal Heart Rate Monitoring." *ACOG Technical Bulletin* 132, September 1989.

"Intrapartum Fetal Heart Rate Monitoring: Nomenclature, Interpretation, and General Management Principles." *ACOG Practice Bulletin* 106, July 2009.

"Intrapartum Fetal Monitoring." *ACOG Technical Bulletin* 44, January 1977.

"J. P. Greenhill 1895–1975." *Anatomical Record* 18 (October 1976): 241–243.

Jain, L., and D. C. Eaton. "Physiology of Fetal Lung Fluid Clearance and the Effect of Labor." *Seminars in Perinatology* 30 (2006): 34–43.

James, L. Stanley. "Aspects of Fetal Monitoring." In *Obstetrical Anesthesia: The Mother and The Newborn* (1973), edited by Alexander J. Buttice and Andrew Mashberg, 23. Sizeable pamphlet sponsored by Pfizer Laboratories, L. Stanley James Papers, Mount Holyoke College, Archives and Special Collections, South Hadley, MA.

———. "Fond Memories of Virginia Apgar." *Pediatrics* 55 (January 1975): 1–4.

Jewett, John Figgis. "When Is It Safe to Induce Labor?" *Redbook* 122 (April 1964): 44, 46.

Juhl, Jacqueline. "I Had This Baby Under Hypnosis." *Better Homes and Gardens*, November 1959, 152–155.

Keeler, Emmett B., and Molyann Brodie. "Economic Incentives in the Choice between Vaginal Delivery and Cesarean Section." *Milbank Quarterly* 71 (1993): 365–404.

Kelly, Vernon C., and Durgadas Kulkarni. "Experiences with Fetal Monitoring in a Community Hospital." *Obstetrics and Gynecology* 41 (June 1973): 818–824.

Kelso, Ian M., R. John Parsons, Gordon F. Lawrence, Shyam S. Arora, D. Keith Edmonds, and Ian D. Cooke. "An Assessment of Continuous Fetal Heart Rate Monitoring in Labor." *American Journal of Obstetrics and Gynecology* 131 (July 1, 1978): 526–532.

Khazan, Olga. "Why Most Brazilian Women Get C-Sections." *Atlantic*, April 2014.

Kitzinger, Sheila. *The Experience of Childbirth*. New York: Penguin, 1987 [1972].

Killilea, Marie. *Karen*. New York: Dell, 1952.

———. *With Love from Karen*. Englewood Cliffs, NJ: Prentice-Hall, 1963.

Klingensmith, Paul W. "The Clinical Management of Dystocia." *Surgical Clinics of North America* 34 (1954): 1579–1589.

Koh, K. S., D. Greves, S. Yung, and L. J. Peddle. "Experience With Fetal Monitoring in a University Teaching Hospital." *Canadian Medical Journal* 112 (February 22, 1975): 455–460.

Kolata, Gina. "New York Is First State to Try to Curb Caesareans." *New York Times*, January 27, 1989, 1, 12.

———. "Panel Urges Mammograms at 50 Not 40." *New York Times*, November 16, 2009.

Korelitz, Jean Hanff. "Special Delivery." *Vogue*, November 2003, 414, 416, 422.

"Labor-Saving Devices." *Newsweek*, February 6, 1976, 84.

Landesman, Robert. "New Promise of Easier Childbirth." *Woman's Home Companion*, August 1955, 38–39, 116.

Lavender, Tina, G. Justus Hofmeyr, James P. Neilson, Carol Kingdon, and Gillian M. L. Gyte. "Caesarean Section for Non-Medical Reasons at Term (Review)." *Cochrane Library*, 2012.

Lawrence, Annemarie, Lucy Lewis, G. Justus Hofmeyr, Therese Dowswell, and Cathy Styles. "Maternal Positions and Mobility during First Stage Labour." *Cochrane Database of Systematic Reviews*, April 15, 2009.

Lawrence, W. H. "Kennedy Alters Schedule to Stay Close to New Son." *New York Times*, November 26, 1960, 1, 8.

Leavitt, Frederick. "More about 'Twilight Sleep' in Labor." *American Journal of Clinical Medicine* 22 (1915): 309–315.

Lee, Wing K., and Michael S. Baggish. "The Effect of Unselected Intrapartum Fetal Monitoring." *Obstetrics and Gynecology* 47 (May 1976): 516–520.

Leeman, Lawrence M., and Lauren A. Plante. "Patient-Choice Vaginal Delivery?" *Annals of Family Medicine* 4 (May–June 2006): 265–268.

Leth, Rita Andersen, Jens Kjølseth Møller, Reimar Wernich Thomsen, Niels Uldbjerg, and Mette Nørgaard. "Risk of Selected Postpartum Infections after Cesarean Section Compared with Vaginal Birth: A Five-Year Cohort Study of 32,468 Women." *Acta Obstetricia et Gynecologica* 88 (2009): 976–983.

Leung, A. S., R. M. Farmer, E. K. Leung, A. L. Medearis, and R. H. Paul. "Risk Factors Associated with Uterine Rupture during Trial of Labor after Cesarean Delivery." *American Journal of Obstetrics and Gynecology* 168 (1993): 1358–1363.

Leveno, Kenneth J., et al. "A Prospective Comparison of Selective and Universal Electronic Fetal Monitoring in 34,995 Pregnancies." *Obstetric and Gynecological Survey* 42 (March 1987): 155–157.

Li, Hong-Tian, Shusheng Luo, and Leonardo Trasande. "Geographic Variations and Temporal Trends in Cesarean Delivery Rates in China, 2008–2014." *JAMA* 317 (January 3, 2017): 69–75.

Lilienfeld, A. M., E. Treptow, and D. M. Dixon. "A Study of Variations in the Interpretation of X-Ray Pelvimetry." *Human Biology* 21 (September 1949): 143–162.

Lowe, C. R. "Effect of Mothers' Smoking Habits on Birth Weight of Their Children." *British Medical Journal* 2, no. 5153 (October 10, 1959): 673–676.

Lowe, Nancy K. "A Review of Factors Associated with Dystocia and Cesarean Section in Nulliparous Women." *Journal of Midwifery & Women's Health* 52 (May/June 2007): 216–228.

Luck, W., and H. Nau. "Exposure of the Fetus, Neonate and Nursed Infant to Nicotine and Cotinine from Maternal Smoking." *New England Journal of Medicine* 331 (1984): 672.

Lungren, S. S. "A Case of Cesarean Section Twice Successfully Performed on the Same Patient, with Remarks on the Time, Indications, and Details of the Operation." *American Journal of Obstetrics and Diseases of Women and Children* 14 (1881): 78–94.

Lusk, William T. "The Prognosis of Cesarean Operations." *American Journal of Obstetrics and Diseases of Women and Children* 13 (1880): 18–23.

Luthy, David A., Judith A. Malmgren, Rosalee W. Zingheim, and Christopher J. Leininger. "Physician Contribution to a Cesarean Delivery Risk Model." *American Journal of Obstetrics and Gynecology* 188 (June 2003): 1579–1587.

Lydon-Rochelle, Mona, Victoria L. Holt, Thomas R. Easterling, and Diane P. Martin. "Risk of Uterine Rupture during Labor among Women with a Prior Cesarean Delivery." *New England Journal of Medicine* 345 (July 5, 2001): 3–8.

Lynch, Frank W. "More Conservatism in Cesarean Section." *Surgery, Gynecology and Obstetrics* 64 (1937): 338–346.

MacDonald, Christine, Sheena B. Pinion, and Una M. Macleod. "Scottish Female Obstetricians' Views on Elective Caesarean Section and Personal Choice for Delivery." *Journal of Obstetrics and Gynaecology* 22 (2002): 586–589.

MacDonald, Dermot, Adrian Grant, Margaret Sheridan-Pereira, Peter Boyland, and Iain Chalmers. "The Dublin Randomized Controlled Trial of Intrapartum Fetal Heart Rate Monitoring." *American Journal of Obstetrics and Gynecology* 152 (July 1985): 524–539.

MacDorman, Marian F., Eugene Declercq, Howard Cabral, and Christine Morton. "Recent Increases in the US Maternal Mortality Rate." *Obstetrics & Gynecology* 128 (September 2016): 447–455.

MacDorman, Marian F., Eugene Declercq, Fay Menacker, and Michael H. Malloy. "Infant and Neonatal Mortality for Primary Cesarean and Vaginal Births to Women with 'No Indicated Risk,' United States, 1998–2001 Birth Cohorts." *Birth* 33 (September 2006): 175–182.

MacLennan, Alastair, Karin B. Nelson, Gary Hankins, and Michael Speer. "Who Will Deliver Our Grandchildren? Implications of Cerebral Palsy Litigation." *JAMA* 294 (October 5, 2005): 1688–1690.

"Management of Intrapartum Fetal Heart Rate Tracings." *ACOG Practice Bulletin* 116, November 2010, reaffirmed 2015.

March of Dimes. "New York Cesarean Rates, 2013." www.marchofdimes.org/pdf/newyork/newyork_cesarean_rates_report_2013.pdf.

Marieskind, Helen I. *An Evaluation of Caesarean Section in the United States: Executive Summary.* Department of Health, Education, and Welfare Office of the Assistant Secretary for Planning and Evaluation/Health, 1979.

Markoe, J. W., and Asa B. Davis. "Fifty Cases of Cesarean Section." *American Journal of Obstetrics and Diseases of Women and Children* 55 (1907): 252–255.

Marley, Fay. "Cesarean Baby Dangers." *Science News Letter* 84 (July 13, 1963): 22.

Marsden, J. H. *Handbook of Practical Midwifery, Including the Instruction for the Homœpathic Treatment of the Disorders of Pregnancy, and the Accidents and Diseases Incident to Labor and the Puerperal State.* New York: Boericke & Tafel, 1879.

Martin, Nina, and Renee Montagne. "The Last Person You'd Expect to Die in Childbirth." *ProPublica*, May 12, 2017.

Mayfair, J. P. *Midwifery Illustrated.* New York: J. K. Moore, 1833.

McCarthy, Colman. "Cesareans Give Birth to a Bonanza." *Detroit Free Press*, January 8, 1985.

McCloskey, Lois, Diana B. Petitti, and Calvin J. Hobel. "Variations in the Use of Cesarean Delivery for Dystocia: Lessons about the Source of Care." *Medical Care* 30 (February 1992): 126–135.

McEvoy, J. P. "Our Streamlined Baby." *Reader's Digest*, May 1938, 15–18.

McLane, James W. "The Sloane Maternity Hospital: Report of the First Series of One Thousand Successive Confinements from January 1st 1888 to October 1st 1890." New York: William Wood, 1891.

McNeile, Lyle G. *Notes on Pathological and Operative Obstetrics*. Los Angeles: Division of Obstetrics, College of Physicians and Surgeons, Medical Department of the University of Southern California, 1919.

"MDs Admit They Put Babys [sic] at Risk but Are Concerned about Safety." *NAPSAC News* 4 (Fall 1979): 24.

Meigs, Charles D. *Obstetrics: The Science and the Art*. Philadelphia: Blanchard and Lea, 1856.

Meigs, Grace L. *Maternal Mortality from All Conditions Connected with Childbirth in the United States and Certain Other Countries*. Washington, DC: Government Printing Office, 1917.

Meikle, S. F., C. A. Steiner, J. Zhang, et al. "A National Estimate of the Elective Primary Cesarean Delivery Rate." *Obstetrics and Gynecology* 105 (2005): 751–756.

Menacker, Fay, and Brady E. Hamilton. "Recent Trends in Cesarean Delivery in the United States." NCHS Data Brief, March 2010. US Department of Health and Human Services Centers for Disease Control and Prevention National Center for Health Statistics.

Mendels, Ora. "A Revolution in Childbirth?" *Ladies' Home Journal*, January 1963, 40.

Mengert, William F. "Our Maturing Specialty." *Obstetrics and Gynecology* 7 (March 1956): 353–359.

Meyer, M. B., B. S. Jonas, and J. A. Tonascia, "Perinatal Events Associated with Maternal Smoking during Pregnancy." *American Journal of Epidemiology* 103 (1976): 464–476.

Miller, C. Jeff. "A General Consideration of Cæsarean Section." *Surgery, Gynecology and Obstetrics* 48 (1929): 745–750.

———. "The Limitations of Caesarean Section." *Surgery, Gynecology, and Obstetrics* 36 (June 1923): 840–841.

Miller, Harold D. "Regional Insights: Better Maternity Care Can Reduce Health Care Costs." *Pittsburgh Post-Gazette*, March 6, 2011.

Minkoff, Howard. "Fear of Litigation and Cesarean Section Rates." *Seminars in Perinatology* 36 (2012): 390–394.

Minkoff, Howard, and Frank A. Chervenak. "Elective Primary Cesarean Delivery." *New England Journal of Medicine* 348 (March 6, 2003): 946–950.

"Mode of Term Singleton Breech Delivery." *ACOG Committee Opinion* 265, December 2001.

"Mode of Term Singleton Breech Delivery." *ACOG Committee Opinion* 340, July 2006.

Monari, Francesca, Simona Di Mario, Fabio Facchinetti, and Vittorio Basevi. "Obstetricians' and Midwives' Attitudes toward Cesarean Section." *Birth* 35 (June 2008): 129–135.

"Monitoring Childbirth." *Newsweek*, February 6, 1967, 84.

Montgomery, Thaddeus L. "Obstetric Amnesia, Analgesia, and Anesthesia: Their Relationship to Sudden Death in Labor." *Journal of the American Medical Association* 108 (May 15, 1937): 1679–1683.

Myers, Stephen A., and Norbert Gleicher. "A Successful Program to Lower Cesarean-Section Rates." *New England Journal of Medicine* 319 (December 8, 1988): 1511–1516.

"National Institutes of Health Consensus Development Conference Statement: Vaginal Birth after Cesarean: New Insights." March 8–10, 2010. https://consensus.nih.gov/2010/images/vbac/vbac_statement.pdf.

National Partnership for Women and Families. "Overdue: Medicaid and Private Insurance Coverage of Doula Care to Strengthen Maternal and Infant Health." January 2016. www.nationalpartnership.org/research-library/maternal-health/overdue-medicaid-and-private-insurance-coverage-of-doula-care-to-strengthen-maternal-and-infant-health-issue-brief.pdf.

Neal, J. L., N. K. Lowe, K. L. Ahijevych, T. E. Patrick, L. A. Cabbage, and E. J. Corwin. "'Active Labor' Duration and Dilation Rates among Low-Risk, Nulliparous Women with Spontaneous Labor Onset: A Systematic Review." *Journal of Midwifery and Women's Health* 55 (July–August 2010): 308–318.

"Negro Health Reasons." *Daily Defender,* April 7, 1967, 11.

Neuhoff, Douglas, Shannon M. Burke, and Richard P. Porreco. "Cesarean Birth for Failed Progress in Labor." *Obstetrics and Gynecology* 73 (June 1989): 915–920.

"New VBAC Guidelines: What They Mean to You and Your Patients." *ACOG Today,* August 2010, 6–7.

Newell, Franklin S. *Cesarean Section.* New York: D. Appleton, 1924.

NICE. "Antenatal Care for Uncomplicated Pregnancies." March 2008, updated January 2017. www.nice.org.uk/guidance/cg62.

———. "Intrapartum Care for Healthy Women and Babies." December 2014, updated February 2017. www.nice.org.uk/guidance/cg190/chapter/1-Recommendations#place-of-birth.

"NIH Consensus Development Task Force Statement on Cesarean Childbirth." *American Journal of Obstetrics and Gynecology* 139 (April 15, 1981): 902–909.

"NIH State-of-the-Science Conference Statement on Cesarean Delivery on Maternal Request." *NIH Consensus State Science Statements* 23 (2006): 1–29.

Nisenblat, Victoria, et al. "Maternal Complications Associated with Multiple Cesarean Deliveries." *Obstetrics & Gynecology* 108 (July 2006): 21–26.

Norris, Richard C. "The Ultimate Results of Induced Labor for Minor Degrees of Pelvic Contraction." *American Journal of Obstetrics and Diseases of Women and Children* 50 (September 1904): 289–301.

Notzon, Francis C. "International Differences in the Use of Obstetric Interventions." *JAMA* 263 (June 27, 1990): 3286–3291.

Notzon, Francis C., Paul J. Placek, and Selma M. Taffel. "Comparisons of National Cesarean-Section Rates." *New England Journal of Medicine* 316 (1987): 386–389.

Nulsen, R. O. "Trial of Thalidomide in Insomnia Associated with the Third Trimester." *American Journal of Obstetrics and Gynecology* 81 (June 1961): 1245–1248.

"Number of Caesareans on Rise at Hospitals." *Jet,* January 28, 1984, 25.

Oberhaus, Sherry. "How Safe Is Ultrasound?" *Clarion* 6 (Summer 1989): 1.

"Obituary Notice: Max Sänger." *Journal of Obstetrics and Gynaecology of the British Empire* 3 (1903): 292–294.

O'Driscoll, Kieran, Reginald J. A. Jackson, and John T. Gallagher. "Prevention of Prolonged Labor." *British Medical Journal* (May 24, 1969): 477–480.

Oláh, Karl S. J., and James P. Neilson. "Failure to Progress in the Management of Labour." *British Journal of Obstetrics and Gynaecology* 101 (January 1994): 1–3.

"Optional Cesareans without Medical Reason More Risky, Study Reports." *Jet*, April 16, 2007, 49–50.

Orleans, Miriam. "Lessons from the Dublin Study of Electronic Fetal Monitoring." *Birth* 12 (1985): 86.

Osterman, Michelle J. K., and Joyce A. Martin. "Trends in Low-Risk Cesarean Delivery in the United States, 1990–2013." *National Vital Statistics Reports* 63 (November 5, 2014).

"Pain Relief during Labor." *ACOG Committee Opinion* 118, January 1993.

Parer, Julian T., Tomoaki Ikeda, and Tekoa L. King. "The 2008 National Institute of Child Health and Human Development Report on Fetal Heart Rate Monitoring." *Obstetrics and Gynecology* 114 (July 2009): 136–138.

Park, Alice. "Choosy Mothers Choose Caesareans." *Time*, April 17, 2008.

Parvin, Theophilus. *The Science and Art of Obstetrics*. Philadelphia: Lea Brothers, 1890.

Paul, Pamela. "The Trouble with Repeat Cesareans." *Time*, February 19, 2009.

Paul, Richard H., and Edward H. Hon. "A Clinical Fetal Monitor." *Obstetrics and Gynecology* 35 (February 1970): 161–169.

Pearson, Catherine. "The Rise in C-Sections Could Be Changing Human Evolution." *Huffington Post*, December 9, 2016.

Penders, J., C. Thijs, C. Vink, F. F. Stelma, B. Snijders, I. Kummeling, P. A. Fan den Brandt, and E. E. Stobberingh. "Factors Influencing the Composition of the Intestinal Microbiota in Early Infancy." *Pediatrics* 118 (2006): 511–521.

"Pen-Knife Surgery: Baby Delivered after Bullet Kills Mother." *Los Angeles Times*, January 11, 1950, 6.

Peterson, Reuben. "The Present Status of Abdominal Cæsarean Section: When and How Should the Operation Be Performed." *Surgery, Gynecology and Obstetrics* 15 (1912): 32–39.

Peyton, Frank W. "Prolonged Labor." *Obstetrics and Gynecology* 3 (January 1954): 121–123.

Phelan, J. P. "VBAC: Time to Consider?" *OBG Management* (1996): 62–68.

Pierson, Richard N. "When Caesarean Section?" *Parents' Magazine*, May 1944, 109–111.

Pinette, M. G., J. Kahn, K. L. Gross, J. R. Wax, J. Blackstone, and A. Cartin. "Vaginal Birth after Cesarean Rates are Declining Rapidly in the State of Maine." *Journal of Maternal, Fetal, and Neonatal Medicine* 16 (July 2004): 37–43.

Pinney, John M., et al. *The Health Consequences of Smoking for Women: A Report of the Surgeon General*. US Department of Health and Human Services, 1979.

Pistiner, Michael, Diane R. Gold, Hassem Abdulkerin, Elaine Hoffman, and Juan C. Celedón. "Birth by Cesarean Section, Allergic Rhinitis, and Allergic Sensitization among Children with a Parental History of Atopy." *Journal of Allergy and Clinical Immunology* 112 (August 2008): 274–279.

Placek, P. J., and S. M. Taffel. "One-Sixth of 1980 US Births by Caesarean Section." *Public Health Reports* 97 (March–April 1982): 183.

———. "Recent Patterns in Cesarean Delivery in the United States." *Obstetrics and Gynecology Clinics of North America* 15 (December 1988): 607–627.

"Placenta Accreta." *ACOG Committee Opinion* 266, January 2002.

Playfair, W. S. *A Treatise on the Science and Practice of Midwifery with Notes and Additions by Robert P. Harris*. Philadelphia: Lea Brothers, 1889.

Polak, John Osborn. "What Is the Matter with American Obstetrics?" *American Journal of Obstetrics and Gynecology* 19 (1930): 598–599.

Polak, John Osborn, and A. C. Beck. "The Present Status of Operative Obstetrics Referring to the Abuse of Cæsarean Section." *Surgery, Gynecology, and Obstetrics* 34 (1922): 566–573.

Pollack, Jack Harrison. "The Case for Natural Childbirth." *Cosmopolitan*, July 1953, 38–43.

"Pregnancy Death Rate Twice That of Whites." *Chicago Defender*, January 17, 1953, 12.

Prentice, A., and T. Lind. "Fetal Heart Rate Monitoring during Labour—Too Frequent Intervention, Too Little Benefit?" *Lancet* 2 (December 12, 1987): 1375–1377.

Prentiss, D. W. "A Report of Five Hundred Consecutive Cases of Labor in Private Practice, in the District of Columbia, between the Years 1864 and 1888." *American Journal of Obstetrics and Diseases of Women and Children* 21 (1888): 956–970.

Pritchard, Jack A., and Paul C. MacDonald. *Williams Obstetrics*. New York: Appleton-Century-Crofts, 1980.

Quilligan, E. J., and R. H. Paul. "Fetal Monitoring: Is It Worth It?" *Obstetrics & Gynecology* 45 (1975): 96–100.

Rabin, Roni Caryn. "Getting Screened for Breast Cancer." *New York Times*, November 16, 2009.

———. "New Guidelines on Breast Cancer Draw Opposition." *New York Times*, November 16, 2009.

Ramsbotham, Francis H. *The Principles and Practice of Obstetric Medicine and Surgery, in Reference to the Process of Parturition*. London: John Churchill, 1841.

Ranney, Brooks. "Responsibilities, Ten Problems, and a Few Solutions." *Obstetrics and Gynecology* 61 (February 1983): 241–247.

Redden, Molly. "'A Third of People Get Major Surgery to Be Born': Why Are C-Sections Routine in the US?" *Guardian*, October 4, 2017.

Regal, Deborah. "Home Birth after Two Cesareans." In *Birth Stories: The Experience Remembered*, edited by Janet Isaacs Ashford, 124–129. Trumansburg, NY: The Crossing Press, 1984.

Renz-Polster, H., M. R. David, A. S. Buist, W. M. Vollmer, E. A. O'Connor, E. A. Frazier, and M. A. Wall. "Caesarean Section Delivery and the Risk of Allergic Disorders in Childhood." *Clinical and Experimental Allergy* 35 (2005): 1466–1472.

Reynolds, Edward. "Circumstances which Render the Elective Section Justifiable in the Interest of the Child Alone." *American Medicine* (September 28, 1901): 489–492.

Richmond, John L. "History of a Successful Casarean Operation." *Western Journal of the Medical and Physical Sciences* (January–March 1830): 485–489.

Ridgeway, James. "More about Thalidomide." *New Republic*, January 8, 1966, 12–15.

Roman, Josefin, Oddvar Bakos, and Sven Cnattingius. "Pregnancy Outcomes by Mode of Delivery among Term Breech Births: Swedish Experience 1987–1993." *Obstetrics & Gynecology* 92 (December 1998): 945–950.

Rosen, Mortimer, and Lillian Thomas. *The Cesarean Myth.* New York: Penguin, 1989.
Rossi, A. Cristina, and Vincenzo D'Addario. "Maternal Morbidity Following a Trial of Labor after Cesarean Section vs Elective Repeat Cesarean Delivery: A Systematic Review with Meta-Analysis." *American Journal of Obstetrics & Gynecology* (September 2008), 224–231.
Rothkopf, Joanna. "Stephen Colbert: 'Fox & Friends' has Ebola!" *Salon*, October 3, 2014. www.salon.com/2014/10/03/stephen_colbert_fox_friends_has_ebola.
"Rubella Vaccines." *Time*, November 1968, 84.
Rubin, Rita. *What If I Have a C-Section? How to Prepare, How to Decide, How to Recover Quickly.* Emmaus, PA: Rodale, 2004.
Russell, A. R. Bedford, and S. H. Murch. "Could Peripartum Antibiotics Have Delayed Health Consequences for the Infant?" *British Journal of Obstetrics and Gynaecology* 113 (2006): 758–765.
Russell, C. Scott, R. Taylor, and C. E. Law. "Smoking in Pregnancy, Maternal Blood Pressure, Pregnancy Outcome, Baby Weight and Growth, and Other Related Factors: A Prospective Study." *British Journal of Preventive and Social Medicine* 22 (1968): 119–126.
Sachs, Benjamin, Cindy Kobelin, Mary Ames Castro, and Fredric Frigoletto. "The Risks of Lowering the Cesarean-Delivery Rate." *New England Journal of Medicine* 340 (January 7, 1999): 54–57.
Safford, Henry B. "Tell Me Doctor." *Ladies' Home Journal*, April 1956, 54, 56, 59.
———. "Tell Me Doctor—Part 16: 'I've Always Been Frightened about Caesarean Operations.'" *Ladies' Home Journal*, May 1951, 31, 93, 95.
Sakala, Carol, and Maureen P. Corry. *Evidence-Based Maternity Care: What It Is and What It Can Achieve.* New York: Milbank Memorial Fund, 2008.
Salam, M. T., H. G. Margolis, R. McConnell, J. A. McGregor, E. L. Avol, and F. D. Gilliland. "Mode of Delivery Is Associated with Asthma and Allergy Occurrences in Children." *Annals of Epidemiology* 16 (2006): 341–346.
Schauffler, Goodrich C. "Tell Me, Doctor." *Ladies' Home Journal*, February 1960, 40, 42, 44.
Schmitt, Susan Ann. "Natural Childbirth Takes a Giant Step." *Female Patient* 15 (March 1990): 13.
"Second Apgar Rating Increases Test's Predictive Value." *Medical World News*, September 25, 1964.
Sharma, S. K., J. M. Alexander, G. Messick, S. L. Bloom, D. D. McIntire, J. Wiley, et al. "Cesarean Delivery: A Randomized Trial of Epidural Analgesia versus Intravenous Meperidine Analgesia during Labor in Nulliparous Women." *Anesthesiology* 96 (2002): 546–551.
Shearer, Madeleine H., Maile Raphael, and Maryellen Cattani. "A Survey of California OB-GYN Malpractice Verdicts in 1975 with Recommendations for Expediting Informed Consent." *Birth and the Family Journal* 3 (1976): 59–65.
Shelton, Deborah L. "C-Sections Increasing as Doctors, Patients Re-Evaluate the Risks." *American Medical News*, October 9, 2000.
Shultz, Gladys Denny. "*Journal* Mothers Report on Cruelty in Maternity Wards." *Ladies' Home Journal*, May 1958, 44–45, 152–155.
Sidrow, Theresa Rahe. "The Cesarean Phoenix." *Clarion* 4 (Summer 1986).

Simkin, Penny. "Is Anyone Listening? The Lack of Clinical Impact of Randomized Controlled Trials of Electronic Fetal Monitoring." *Birth* 13 (December 1986): 219–220.

Simpson, Kathleen Rich, Gloria Newman, and Octavio R. Chirino. "Patient Education to Reduce Elective Inductions." *Maternal Child Nursing* 35 (July/August 2010): 188–194.

Skene, Alex J. C. "A Contribution to Obstetrical Surgery." *American Journal of Obstetrics and Diseases of Women and Children* 8 (1875): 150–151.

"Sleeping Pill Nightmare." *Time*, February 23, 1962, 86.

Slovic, P., N. Kraus, H. Lappe, H. Letzel, and T. Malmfors. "Risk Perception of Prescription Drugs: Report on a Survey in Sweden." *Pharmaceutical Medicine* 4 (1989): 43–65.

Smith, Gayle. "Angry and Happy at the Same Time." In *Birth Stories: The Experience Remembered*, edited by Janet Isaacs Ashford, 101–106. Trumansburg, NY: The Crossing Press, 1984.

Smith, L. P., B. A. Nagourney, F. H. McLean, and R. H. Usher. "Hazards and Benefits of Elective Induction of Labor." *American Journal of Obstetrics and Gynecology* 148 (March 1, 1984): 579–585.

Smoking and Health: Report of the Advisory Committee to the Surgeon General of the Public Health Service. US Department of Health, Education, and Welfare, 1964.

Song, Sora. "Too Posh to Push?" *Time*, April 11, 2004.

Sontag, L. W., and Robert F. Wallace. "The Effect of Cigaret Smoking during Pregnancy upon the Fetal Heart Rate." *American Journal of Obstetrics and Gynecology* 29 (1935): 77–83.

Snowbeck, Christopher. "Is Elective C-Section Delivery a Good Idea?" *Pittsburgh Post-Gazette*, March 18, 2003.

Speert, Harold. *The Sloane Hospital Chronicle*. Philadelphia: F. A. Davis, 1963.

Speert, Harold, and Alan F. Guttmacher. *Obstetric Practice*. New York: Landsberger Medical Books, 1956.

Spencer, Steven M. "Attack on the Unborn." *Saturday Evening Post*, March 13, 1965, 82–85.

Stark, Michael, Udo B. Hoyne, Bernd Stubert, Dirk Kieback, and Gian Carol di Renza. "Post-Cesarean Adhesions—Are They a Unique Entity?" *Journal of Maternal-Fetal and Neonatal Medicine* 21 (2008): 513–516.

"State-of-the-Art: Electronic Fetal Monitoring." *ACOG Committee Statement: State-of-the-Art Opinion in Obstetrics and Gynecology*, April 12, 1984.

"Statement on Maternity Insurance Benefits for Women." *ACOG Statement of Policy*, August 1976.

Steinfels, Margaret O'Brien. "New Childbirth Technology: A Clash of Values." *Hastings Center Report* 8 (February 1978): 9–12.

Stolberg, Sheryl Gay. "A Risk Is Found in Natural Birth after Caesarean." *New York Times*, July 5, 2001.

Stone, Martin L. "Presidential Address." *ACOG Newsletter*, May 1979, 4–6.

Sweet, Gail Grenier. "Mothering Interviews: Nancy Wainer Cohen Vaginal Birth after Cesarean." *Mothering*, December 1982, 66–72.

"Tamoxifen and Uterine Cancer." *ACOG Committee Opinion* 60, June 2014.

Tavernise, Sabrina. "Maternal Mortality Rate in US Rises, Defying Global Trend, Study Finds." *New York Times*, September 21, 2016.

Taves, Isabella. "Cesarean Births: How Many Are Safe?" *Look*, August 27, 1963, 70–72.

Thacker, Stephen B. "The Efficacy of Intrapartum Electronic Fetal Monitoring." *American Journal of Obstetrics and Gynecology* 156 (January 1987): 24–30.

"The Thalidomide Disaster." *Time*, August 10, 1962, 34–35.

Thorp, James A., Linda O. Eckert, Matthew S. Ang, Dennis A. Johnston, Alan M. Peaceman, and Valerie M. Parisi. "Epidural Analgesia and Cesarean Section for Dystocia: Risk Factors in Nulliparas." *American Journal of Perinatology* 8 (1991): 402–410.

Thorp, James A., Daniel H. Hu, Rene M. Albin, Jay McNitt, Bruce A. Meyer, Gary R. Cohen, and John D. Yeast. "The Effect of Intrapartum Epidural Analgesia on Nulliparous Labor: A Randomized, Controlled, Prospective Trial." *American Journal of Obstetrics and Gynecology* 169 (October 1993): 851–858.

Thorp, James A., Jay D. McNitt, and Phyllis C. Leppert. "Effects of Epidural Analgesia: Some Questions and Answers." *Birth* 17 (September 1990): 157–162.

Thorpe, Kenneth E. "The Medical Malpractice 'Crisis': Recent Trends and the Impact of State Tort Reforms." *Health Affairs*, January 21, 2004.

Tollånes, Mette C., Dag Moster, Anne K. Daltveit, and Lorentz M. Irgens. "Cesarean Section and Risk of Severe Childhood Asthma: A Population-Based Cohort Study." *Journal of Pediatrics* 153 (July 2008): 112–116.e1.

"Too Posh to Push? Rising Caesarean Rates Driven by Middle Class." *Telegraph*, May 18, 2011.

Toto, Christian. "Choosing Caesarean." *Washington Times*, July 9, 2002.

Tracy, Marguerite, and Constance Leupp. "Painless Childbirth." *McClure's Magazine*, June 1914, 37–51.

Tron, Van T., et al. "Trends in Smoking Before, During, and After Pregnancy—Pregnancy Risk Assessment Monitoring System, United States, 40 Sites, 2000–2010." *Morbidity and Mortality Weekly Report* 62 (November 8, 2013): 1–19.

Tucker, Beatrice E., and Harry B. Benaron. "Maternal Mortality of the Chicago Maternity Center." *American Journal of Public Health* 27 (January 1937): 33–36.

Twist, Judy. "Story of a Home VBAC." *NAPSAC News, The National Association of Parents & Professionals for Safe Alternatives in Childbirth* 7 (Winter 1982): 7–8.

"Ultrasonography in Pregnancy." *ACOG Technical Bulletin* 187, December 1993.

"Ultrasonography in Pregnancy." *ACOG Practice Bulletin* 101, February 2009.

"The Untold Story of the Thalidomide Babies." *Saturday Evening Post*, October 1962, 19–27.

US Department of Commerce, Bureau of the Census. *Historical Statistics of the United States Colonial Times to 1970*. Washington, DC: Government Printing Office, 1975.

US Department of Health and Human Services, Public Health Service, National Institutes of Health. *Cesarean Childbirth: Report of a Consensus Development Conference Sponsored by the National Institutes of Child Health and Human Development in Conjunction with the National Center for Health Care Technology and Assisted by the Office for Medical Applications of Research, September 22–24, 1980*. NIH Publication No. 82-2067, October 1981.

US Preventive Services Task Force. "Breast Cancer Screening." December 20, 2013. www.uspreventiveservicestaskforce.org/Page/Document/RecommendationStatementFinal/breast-cancer-screening.

US Public Health Service. *Healthy People 2000: National Health Promotion and Disease Prevention Objectives.* Publication No. 93-1212-1, 1992.

"Use and Misuse of the Apgar Score." *ACOG Committee Opinion* 49, November 1986.

"Use and Abuse of the Apgar Score." *ACOG Committee Opinion* 174, July 1996.

Uygur, D., S. Kis, R. Tuncer, F. S. Özcan, and S. Erkaya. "Risk Factors and Infant Outcomes Associated with Umbilical Cord Prolapse." *International Journal of Gynecology & Obstetrics* 78 (August 2002): 127–130.

"Vaginal Delivery after a Previous Cesarean Birth." *ACOG Committee Opinion* 143 (October 1994).

"Vaginal Delivery after Previous Cesarean Birth." *ACOG Practice Patterns: Clinical Practice Guidelines for Issues in Obstetrics and Gynecology* 1 (August 1995).

"Vaginal Birth after Previous Cesarean Delivery." *ACOG Practice Bulletin: Clinical Management Guidelines for Obstetrician-Gynecologists* 2 (October 1998).

"Vaginal Birth after Previous Cesarean Delivery." *ACOG Practice Bulletin: Clinical Management Guidelines for Obstetrician-Gynecologists* 5 (July 1999).

"Vaginal Birth after Previous Cesarean Delivery." *ACOG Practice Bulletin: Clinical Management Guidelines for Obstetrician-Gynecologists* 54 (July 2004).

"Vaginal Birth after Previous Cesarean Delivery." *ACOG Practice Bulletin: Clinical Management Guidelines for Obstetrician-Gynecologists* 115 (August 2010).

Van Hoosen, Bertha. "Should Women Smoke." *Medical Woman's Journal* 34 (1927): 227.

Varner, Michael W., Dwight P. Cruikshank, and Douglas W. Laube. "X-Ray Pelvimetry in Clinical Obstetrics." *Obstetrics and Gynecology* 56 (September 1980): 296–300.

Ver Beck, Mrs. Hanna Rion. "The Painless Childbirth: Testimony of American Mothers Who Have Tried 'The Twilight Sleep.'" *Ladies' Home Journal*, September 1914, 9–10.

Ventura, S. J., J. A. Martin, S. C. Curtin, F. Menacker, and B. E. Hamilton. "Births: Final Data for 1999." *National Vital Statistics Report* 49 (2001).

Villar, Jose, et al. "Maternal and Neonatal Individual Risk and Benefits Associated with Caesarean Delivery: Multi-Center Prospective Study." *British Medical Journal* 335 (November 17, 2007): 1025–1029.

Wagner, John. "The Advocate as Politician." *Washington Post*, October 5, 2004.

Walters, D. Campbell. *Just Take It Out! The Ethics and Economics of Cesarean Section and Hysterectomy.* Mount Vernon, IL: Topiary Publishing, 1998.

Warner, Judith. *Perfect Madness: Motherhood in the Age of Anxiety.* New York: Riverhead Books, 2005.

"'Watching' the Unborn Inside the Womb." *Life*, July 25, 1969, 63–65.

Watson, B. P. "Further Experience with Pituitary Extract in the Induction of Labor." *American Journal of Obstetrics and Gynecology* 6 (December 5, 1922): 603–608.

Watson, E. M. D. "How to Have a Perfect Baby." *Cosmopolitan*, December 1959, 74–77.

Wax, J. R., A. Cartin, M. G. Pinette, et al. "Patient Choice Cesarean: An Evidence-Based Review." *Obstetric and Gynecological Survey* 59 (2004): 601–616.

Weems, M. L. "Case of Caesarian Section." *American Journal of the Medical Sciences* 18 (1836): 257–258.

"When a Cesarean Birth Is Necessary." *Good Housekeeping*, November 1963, 171.

Whitbeck, Caroline. "Fetal Imaging and Fetal Monitoring: Finding the Ethical Issues." *Women and Health* 13 (1988): 47–57.
"Why Babies Die." *Time*, May 9, 1969, 85.
"The Whys of Caesareans." *Newsweek*, August 19, 1963, 50, 53.
Williams, Gurney. "Natural Childbirth Comes of Age." *Readers' Digest*, December 1973, 153–156.
Williams, Harold. "A Comparison Between the Cesarean Section and the High Forceps Operation." *American Journal of Obstetrics and Diseases of Women and Children* 12 (1879): 23–31.
Williams, J. Whitridge. "The Abuse of Cæsarean Section." *Surgery, Gynecology, and Obstetrics* 25 (1917): 194–201.
———. "Cesarean Section at the Johns Hopkins Hospital." *Northwest Medicine* 25 (October 1926): 519–526.
———. "A Critical Analysis of Twenty-One Years' Experience with Cæsarean Section." *Bulletin of the Johns Hopkins Hospital* 32 (June 1921): 173–184.
———. "A Criticism of Certain Tendencies in American Obstetrics." *New York State Journal of Medicine* 22 (November 1922): 493–499.
———. "Medical Education and the Midwife Problem in the United States." *JAMA* 58 (1912): 1–7.
———. *Obstetrics: A Text-Book for the Use of Students and Practitioners.* New York: D. Appleton, 1909.
———. *Obstetrics: A Text-Book for the Use of Students and Practitioners.* New York: D. Appleton, 1917.
———. *Obstetrics: A Text-Book for the use of Students and Practitioners.* New York: D. Appleton, 1924.
———. "Why Is the Art of Obstetrics So Poorly Practised?" *Long Island Medical Journal* 11 (1917): 169–178.
Williams, J. Whitridge, and Ko Chi Sun. "A Statistical Study of the Incidence and Treatment of Labor Complicated by Contracted Pelvis in the Obstetric Service of the Johns Hopkins Hospital from 1896 to 1924." *American Journal of Obstetrics and Gynecology* 11 (June 1926): 735–755.
Willson, J. Robert. "Elective Induction of Labor: Is It Justifiable in Normally Pregnant Women." *American Journal of Obstetrics and Gynecology* 65 (1953): 848–858.
Withiam-Leitch, M., J. Shelton, and E. Fleming. "Central Fetal Monitoring: Effect on Perinatal Outcomes and Cesarean Section." *Birth* 33 (December 2006): 284–288.
Wong, C. A., B. M. Scavone, A. M. Peaceman, R. J. McCarthy, J. T. Sullivan, N. T. Diaz, et al. "The Risk of Cesarean Delivery with Neuraxial Analgesia Given Early versus Late in Labor." *New England Journal of Medicine* 352 (2005): 655–665.
Woodbury, Robert Morse. *Infant Mortality and Its Causes with an Appendix on the Trend of Maternal Mortality Rates in the United States.* Baltimore: Williams and Wilkins, 1926.
Woodruff, Kathryn. Letter in response to "Pay on Delivery," *New York Times Magazine*, November 21, 1999, 21.
World Health Organization. "WHO Statement on Caesarean Section Rates." Geneva: World Health Organization, 2015.

World Health Organization. *World Health Statistics 2014*. Geneva: World Health Organization, 2014.

World Health Organization, UNICEF, UNFPA, World Bank Group, and the United Nations Population Division. *Trends in Maternal Mortality 1990 to 2015*. Geneva: World Health Organization, 2015. http://apps.who.int/iris/bitstream/10665/194254/1/9789241565141_eng.pdf?ua=1.

Wright, Janet B., Alison L. Wright, Nigel A. B. Simpson, and Fiona C. Bryce. "A Survey of Trainee Obstetricians' Preferences for Childbirth." *Obstetrics & Gynecology* 97 (2001): 23–25.

Wu, Jennifer M., Andrew F. Hundley, and Anthony G. Visco. "Elective Primary Cesarean Delivery: Attitudes of Urogynecology and Maternal-Fetal Medicine Specialists." *Obstetrics & Gynecology* 105 (February 2005): 301–306.

Wu, Serena, Masha Kocherginsky, and Judith U. Hibbard. "Abnormal Placentation: Twenty-Year Analysis." *American Journal of Obstetrics and Gynecology* 192 (2005): 1458–1461.

Xu, Xiao, Aileen Gariepy, Lisbet S. Lundsberg, Sangini S. Sheth, Christian M. Pettker, Harlan M. Krumholz, and Jessica L. Illuzzi. "Wide Variation Found in Hospital Facility Costs for Maternity Stays Involving Low-Risk Childbirth." *Health Affairs* 34 (2015): 1212–1219.

Yang, Q., et al. "Association of Caesarean Delivery for First Birth with Placenta Praevia and Placental Abruption in Second Pregnancy." *British Journal of Obstetrics and Gynecology* (2007): 609–613.

Yartz, Frank C. "To the Editor." *Female Patient* 15 (March 1990): 16.

Yeh, S. Y., L. Betyar, and E. H. Hon. "Computer Diagnosis of Fetal Heart Rate Patterns." *American Journal of Obstetrics and Gynecology* 114 (December 1, 1972): 890–897.

Yunker, Barbara. "Delivery Procedures That Endanger a Baby's Life." *Good Housekeeping*, August 1975.

Zabriskie, Louise. *Nurses Handbook of Obstetrics*. Philadelphia: J. B. Lippincott, 1929.

Ziegler, C. E. "How Can We Best Solve the Midwifery Problem." *American Journal of Public Health* 12 (1922): 409.

Zinke, E. Gustav. "The Limitations of Cesarean Section." *American Journal of Obstetrics and Diseases of Women and Children* 48 (1903): 604–615.

Zlatnik, Frank J. "Elective Induction of Labor." *Clinical Obstetrics and Gynecology* 42 (1999): 757–765.

Zuckman, Jill. "Medical Bill Debate Pits Doctor vs. Lawyer." *Chicago Tribune*, June 24, 2001.

Secondary Sources

Abel, Emily. *Hearts of Wisdom: American Women Caring for Kin, 1850–1940*. Cambridge, MA: Harvard University Press, 2002.

Alexander, Diane. "Does Physician Pay Affect Procedure Choice and Patient Health? Evidence from Medicaid C-Section Use." Department of Economics, Princeton University. June 17, 2015.

Althabe, Fernando, and José M. Belizán. "Caesarean Section: The Paradox." *Lancet* 368 (2006): 1472–1473.

Altman, Lawrence K. "A Kennedy Baby's Life and Death." *New York Times*, July 29, 2013. www.nytimes.com/2013/07/30/health/a-kennedy-babys-life-and-death.html.

Anderson, Christopher. *Jack and Jackie: Portrait of an American Marriage*. New York: William Morrow, 1996.

Aronowitz, Robert A. "The Converged Experience of Risk and Disease." *Milbank Quarterly* 87 (2009): 417–442.

———. *Risky Medicine: Our Quest to Cure Fear and Uncertainty*. Chicago: The University of Chicago Press, 2015.

Baker, Jeffrey P. *The Machine in the Nursery: Incubator Technology and the Origins of Newborn Intensive Care*. Baltimore: Johns Hopkins University Press, 1996.

Becker, Gay. *The Elusive Embryo: How Women and Men Approach New Reproductive Technologies*. Berkeley: University of California Press, 2000.

Block, Jennifer. *Pushed: The Painful Truth About Childbirth and Modern Maternity Care*. Boston: DeCapo Life Long, 2007.

Blumenthal, David, and William Hsiao. "Lessons from the East—China's Rapidly Evolving Health Care System." *New England Journal of Medicine* 372 (April 2, 2015): 1281–1285.

Bodenheimer, T. S., and K. Grumbach. *Understanding Health Policy: A Clinical Approach*. New York: McGraw Hill, 2009.

Borst, Charlotte G. *Catching Babies: The Professionalization of Childbirth, 1870–1920*. Cambridge, MA: Harvard University Press, 1995.

Brandt, Allan. *The Cigarette Century: The Rise, Fall, and Deadly Persistence of the Product That Defined America*. New York: Basic Books, 2007.

Brasseaux, Carl A., and Glenn R. Conrad. *The Road to Louisiana: The Saint-Domingue Refugees 1792–1809*. Lafayette, LA: Center for Louisiana Studies, 1992.

Brody, H., and J. R. Thompson. "The Maximin Strategy in Modern Obstetrics." *Journal of Family Practice* 12 (June 1981): 977–986.

Brynner, Rock, and Trent Stephens. *Dark Remedy: The Impact of Thalidomide and Its Revival as a Vital Medicine*. Cambridge, MA: Perseus, 2001.

Casper, Monica J. *The Making of the Unborn Patient: A Social Anatomy of Fetal Surgery*. New Brunswick, NJ: Rutgers University Press, 1998.

Caton, Donald. *What a Blessing She Had Chloroform: The Medical and Social Response to the Pain of Childbirth from 1800 to the Present*. New Haven, CT: Yale University Press, 1999.

Cie, Kedarnath Das. *Obstetric Forceps: Its History and Evolution*. Leeds: Medical Museum Publishing, 1993 [1929].

Clarke, Thurston. "A Death in the First Family." *Vanity Fair*, July 2013. www.vanityfair.com/news/politics/2013/07/icebergs-jfk-jackie-death-patrick.

Coontz, Stephanie. *The Way We Never Were: American Families and the Nostalgia Trap*. New York: Basic Books, 1992.

Dally, Ann. *Women Under the Knife: A History of Surgery*. New Jersey: Castle Books, 2006.

Davis-Floyd, Robbie E. *Birth as an American Rite of Passage*. Berkeley: University of California Press, 1992.

Demleitner, Nora V. "Maternity Leave Policies of the United States and Germany: A Comparative Study." *New York Law School Journal of International and Comparative Law* 13 (1992): 229–255.

Douglas, Mary. "Risk as a Forensic Resource." *Daedalus* 119 (Fall 1990): 1–16.

Drachman, Virginia G. *Hospital with a Heart: Women Doctors and the Paradox of Separatism at the New England Hospital, 1862–1969*. Ithaca, NY: Cornell University Press, 1984.

Dubay, Lisa, Robert Kaestner, and Timothy Waidman. "The Impact of Malpractice Fears on Cesarean Section Rates." *Journal of Health Economics* 18 (1999): 491–522.

Dunn, Peter M. "Dr. Francis Ramsbotham (1801–1868) and Obstetric Practice in London." *Archives of Disease in Childhood* 73 (1995): F118–F120.

Fenster, Julie M. *Ether Day: The Strange Tale of America's Greatest Medical Discovery and the Haunted Men Who Made It*. New York: HarperCollins, 2001.

Freeman, Andrew D., and John M. Freeman. "No-Fault Cerebral Palsy Insurance: An Alternative to the Obstetrical Malpractice Lottery." *Journal of Health Politics, Policy and Law* 14 (Winter 1989): 708–718.

Gabe, Jonathan. "Health, Medicine and Risk: The Need for a Sociological Approach." In *Medicine, Health and Risk: Sociological Approaches*, edited by Jonathan Gabe. Blackwell, 1995.

Garrett, Eilidh, Chris Galley, Nicola Shelton, and Robert Woods, eds. *Infant Mortality: A Continuing Social Problem*. Hampshire, UK: Ashgate, 2006.

Gerl, Ellen. "Out of the Back Rooms." *Journalism History* (Fall 2016): 122–129.

Gilfix, Myra Gerson. "Electronic Fetal Monitoring: Physician Liability and Informed Consent." *American Journal of Law and Medicine* 10 (Spring 1984): 31–90.

Gold, Rachel Benson, Asta M. Kenney, and Susheela Singh. "Paying for Maternity Care in the United States." *Family Planning Perspectives* 19 (September/October 1987): 190–193, 195–206.

Gordon, Linda. *Woman's Body, Woman's Right: Birth Control in America*. New York: Penguin, 1990.

Gould, Lewis L. *America in the Progressive Era, 1890–1914*. New York: Longman, 2001.

Greene, Jeremy A. *Prescribing by Numbers: Drugs and the Definition of Disease*. Baltimore: Johns Hopkins University Press, 2007.

Haliday, H. L. "Surfactants: Past, Present, and Future." *Journal of Perinatology* 28 (2008): S47–S56.

Halpern, Sydney A. *American Pediatrics: The Social Dynamics of Professionalism, 1880–1980*. Berkeley: University of California Press, 1998.

Hibbard, Bryan. *The Obstetrician's Armamentarium: Historical Obstetric Instruments and Their Inventors*. San Anselmo, CA: Norman, 2000.

Hoffman, Beatrix. *Health Care for Some: Rights and Rationing in the United States since 1930*. Chicago: University of Chicago Press, 2012.

Howell, Joel D. *Technology in the Hospital: Transforming Patient Care in the Early Twentieth Century*. Baltimore: Johns Hopkins University Press, 1995.

Huston, Perdita. *Motherhood by Choice: Pioneers in Women's Health and Family Planning*. New York: The Feminist Press at CUNY, 1993.

Issacharoff, Samuel, and Elyse Rosenblum. "Women and the Workplace: Accommodating the Demands of Pregnancy." *Columbia Law Review* (1994): 2154–2221.

Jellison, Katherine. *It's Our Day: America's Love Affair with the White Wedding, 1945–2005.* Lawrence: University Press of Kansas, 2008.

Joffe, Carole. *Dispatches from the Abortion Wars. The Costs of Fanaticism to Doctors, Patients, and the Rest of Us.* Boston: Beacon, 2011.

———. *Doctors of Conscience: The Struggle to Provide Abortion before and after Roe v. Wade.* Boston: Beacon, 1996.

Johnson, Timothy R. B. "John Whitridge Williams, MD." In *Department of Gynecology and Obstetrics, The Johns Hopkins University School of Medicine, The Johns Hopkins Hospital: The First 100 Years,* edited by John A. Rock, Timothy R. B. Johnson, and J. Donald Woodruff. Baltimore: Johns Hopkins University, 1991.

Kachlik, David, Ingrid Kästner, and Vaclav Baca. "Christian Gerhard Leopold: Fascinating History of a Productive Obstetrician Gynecologist." *Obstetrical and Gynecological Survey* 67 (2012): 1–5.

Kass, Amalie M. *Midwifery and Medicine in Boston: Walter Channing, MD 1786–1876.* Boston: Northeastern University Press, 2002.

King, J. C. "Maternal Mortality in the United States—Why Is It Important and What Are We Doing about It?" *Seminars in Perinatology* 36 (February 2012): 14–18.

Klimpel, Jill M. "Performing Modernity through Birth: Exploring the High Rates of C-Sections in São Paulo, Brazil." MA thesis, Ohio University, 2011.

Kline, Wendy. *Building a Better Race: Gender, Sexuality, and Eugenics from the Turn of the Century to the Baby Boom.* Berkeley: University of California Press, 2005.

Kolker, Aliza, and B. Meredith Burke. *Prenatal Testing: A Sociological Perspective.* Westport, CT: Bergin & Garvey, 1998.

Korenstein, Deborah, Raphael Falk, Elizabeth A. Howell, Tara Bishop, and Salomeh Keyhani. "Overuse of Health Care Services in the United States: An Understudied Problem." *Archives of Internal Medicine* 177 (January 23, 2012): 171–178.

Ladd-Taylor, Molly. "'Grannies' and 'Spinsters': Midwife Education under the Sheppard-Towner Act." *Journal of Social History* 22 (Winter 1988): 255–275.

———. "'My Work Came Out of My Agony and Grief': Mothers and the Making of the Sheppard-Towner Act." In *Mothers of a New World: Maternalist Politics and the Origins of Welfare States,* edited by Seth Koven and Sonya Michel, 321–342. London: Routledge, 1993.

Lane, Karen. "The Medical Model of the Body as a Site of Risk: A Case Study of Childbirth." In *Medicine, Health and Risk: Sociological Approaches,* edited by Jonathan Gabe, 53–69. Oxford, UK: Blackwell, 1995.

Lax, Eric. *The Mold in Dr. Florey's Coat: The Story of the Penicillin Miracle.* New York: Henry Holt, 2004.

Leaming, Barbara. *Mrs. Kennedy: The Missing History of the Kennedy Years.* New York: Free Press, 2002.

Leavitt, Judith Walzer. *Brought to Bed: Childbearing in America, 1750–1950.* New York: Oxford University Press, 1986.

———. "Joseph B. DeLee and the Practice of Preventive Obstetrics." *American Journal of Public Health* 78 (October 1988): 1353–1361.

———. *Make Room for Daddy: The Journey from Waiting Room to Birthing Room.* Chapel Hill: University of North Carolina Press, 2009.

Lent, Margaret. "The Medical and Legal Risks of the Electronic Fetal Monitor." *Stanford Law Review* 51 (April 1999): 807–837.

Leopold, Ellen. *A Darker Ribbon: Breast Cancer, Women, and Their Doctors in the Twentieth Century.* Boston: Beacon Press, 1999.

Lerner, Barron H. *The Breast Cancer Wars: Hope, Fear, and the Pursuit of a Cure in Twentieth-Century America.* New York: Oxford University Press, 2001.

Levingston, Steven. "For John and Jackie Kennedy, the Death of a Son May Have Brought Them Closer." *Washington Post*, October 24, 2013.

Lewis, Carolyn Herbst. "The Gospel of Good Obstetrics: Joseph Bolivar DeLee's Vision for Childbirth in the United States." *Social History of Medicine* 29 (2016): 112–130.

Lindenmeyer, Kriste. *"A Right to Childhood": The US Children's Bureau and Child Welfare, 1912–46.* Champaign: University of Illinois Press, 1997.

Lombardo, Paul A. *Three Generations, No Imbeciles: Eugenics, the Supreme Court, and* Buck v. Bell. Baltimore: Johns Hopkins University Press, 2008.

Loudon, Irvine. *Death in Childbirth: An International Study of Maternal Care and Maternal Mortality 1800–1950.* Oxford: Oxford University Press, 1992.

———. *The Tragedy of Childbed Fever.* Oxford: Oxford University Press, 2000.

Lyerly, Anne Drapkin, et al. "Risk and the Pregnant Body." *Hastings Center Report* 39 (November–December 2009): 34–42.

May, Elaine Tyler. *Homeward Bound: American Families in the Cold War Era.* New York: Basic Books, 1999.

McGregor, Deborah Kuhn. *From Midwives to Medicine: The Birth of American Gynecology.* New Brunswick, NJ: Rutgers University Press, 1998.

Meckel, Richard A. *Save the Babies: American Public Health Reform and the Prevention of Infant Mortality, 1850–1929.* Baltimore: Johns Hopkins University Press, 1990.

Mennill, Sally Elizabeth. "Prepping the Cut: Caesarean Section Scenarios in English Canada, 1945–1970." PhD diss., University of British Columbia, 2012.

Metzel, Jonathon Michel. "'Mother's Little Helper': The Crisis of Psychoanalysis and the Miltown Resolution." *Gender and History* 15 (August 2003): 228–255.

Mitchinson, Wendy. *Giving Birth in Canada, 1900–1950.* Toronto: University of Toronto Press, 2002.

Morris, Theresa. *Cut It Out: The C-Section Epidemic in America.* New York: New York University Press, 2013.

Nicolson, Malcolm, and John E. E. Fleming. *Imaging and Imagining the Fetus.* Baltimore: Johns Hopkins University Press, 2013.

Noble, Charles P. "Memoir of Dr. Robert P. Harris Born 1822 Died 1899." *The American Gynaecological and Obstetrical Journal* 15, 227–230. https://books.google.com/books?id=6-IhAQAAMAAJ.

Nuland, Sherwin B. *The Doctors' Plague: Germs, Childbed Fever, and the Strange Story of Ignác Semmelweis.* New York: W. W. Norton, 2003.

Office of NIH History. "A Thin Blue Line: A History of the Pregnancy Test Kit." http://history.nih.gov/exhibits/thinblueline/timeline.html.

Oshinsky, David M. *Polio: An American Story.* New York: Oxford University Press, 2005.

Paim, Jairnilson, Claudia Travassos, Celia Almeida, Ligia Bahia, and James Macinko. "The Brazilian Health System: History, Advances, and Challenges." *Lancet* 377 (May 21, 2011): 1778–1797.

Pernick, Martin S. *The Black Stork: Eugenics and the Death of 'Defective' Babies in American Medicine and Motion Pictures Since 1915*. New York: Oxford University Press, 1996.

———. *A Calculus of Suffering: Pain, Professionalism, and Anesthesia in Nineteenth-Century America*. New York: Columbia University Press, 1985.

Perry, Barbara. *Jacqueline Kennedy: First Lady of the New Frontier*. Lawrence, KS: University of Kansas Press, 2004.

Preston, Samuel H., and Michael R. Haines. *Fatal Years: Child Mortality in Late Nineteenth-Century America*. Princeton, NJ: Princeton University Press, 1991.

Randall, Clyde L. *Developments in the Certification of Obstetricians and Gynecologists in the United States, 1930–1980: The American Board of Obstetrics and Gynecology*. American Board of Obstetrics and Gynecology, 1989.

Rapp, Rayna. *Testing Women, Testing the Fetus: The Social Impact of Amniocentesis in America*. London: Routledge, 2000.

Reagan, Leslie J. *Dangerous Pregnancies: Mothers, Disabilities, and Abortion in Modern America*. Berkeley: University of California Press, 2010.

———. *When Abortion Was a Crime: Women, Medicine, and Law in the United States, 1867–1973*. Berkeley: University of California Press, 1997.

Rothman, Barbara Katz. *In Labor: Women and Power in the Birthplace*. New York: Norton, 1991.

———. *The Tentative Pregnancy: How Amniocentesis Changes the Experience of Motherhood*. New York: W. W. Norton, 1986.

Rosenberg, Charles E. *The Care of Strangers: The Rise of America's Hospital System*. New York: Basic Books, 1987.

Rosner, David. *A Once Charitable Enterprise: Hospitals & Health Care in Brooklyn & New York 1885–1915*. Cambridge, UK: Cambridge University Press, 1982.

Rhoden, Nancy Y. "Informed Consent in Obstetrics: Some Special Problems." *Western New England Law Review* 9 (1987): 67–88.

Sachs, Benjamin P. "Is the Rising Rate of Cesarean Sections a Result of More Defensive Medicine?" In *Medical Professional Liability and the Delivery of Obstetrical Care*. Vol. 2, *An Interdisciplinary Review*, edited by Victoria P. Rostow and Roger J. Bulger, 27–40. Washington, DC: Institute of Medicine, National Academy Press, 1989.

Sartwelle, Thomas P. "Electronic Fetal Monitoring: A Bridge Too Far." *Journal of Legal Medicine* 33 (2012): 313–379.

Sartwelle, Thomas P., and James C. Johnston. "Cerebral Palsy Litigation: Change Course or Abandon Ship." *Journal of Child Neurology* (2014): 1–14.

Sartwelle, Thomas P., James C. Johnston, and Berna Arda. "Perpetuating Myths, Fables, and Fairy Tales: A Half Century of Electronic Fetal Monitoring." *The Surgery Journal* 1 (November 2015).

Schwartz, Marie Jenkins. *Birthing a Slave: Motherhood and Medicine in the Antebellum South*. Cambridge, MA: Harvard University Press, 2006.

Slovic, P. "Perception of Risk: Reflections on the Psychometric Paradigm." In *Social Theories of Risk*, edited by S. Krimsky and D. Golding. Westport, CT: Praeger, 1992.

Smith, Sally Bedell. *Grace and Power: The Private World of the Kennedy White House.* New York: Random House, 2004.
Speert, Harold. *Essays in Eponymy: Obstetric and Gynecologic Milestones.* New York: Macmillan, 1958.
Starr, Chauncey. "Social Benefit versus Technological Risk." *Science* 165 (September 19, 1969): 1232–1238.
Starr, Douglas. *Blood: An Epic History of Medicine and Commerce.* London: Little, Brown, 1999.
Starr, Paul. *The Social Transformation of American Medicine: The Rise of a Sovereign Profession and the Making of a Vast Industry.* New York: Basic Books, 1982.
Stern, Alexandra Minna. *Eugenic Nation: Faults and Frontiers of Better Breeding in Modern America.* Berkeley: University of California Press, 2005.
Stevens, Rosemary. *American Medicine and the Public Interest: A History of Specialization.* Berkeley: University of California Press, 1998.
Stratmann, Linda. *Chloroform: The Quest for Oblivion.* United Kingdom: Sutton, 2003.
Strong, Thomas H. *Expecting Trouble: The Myth of Prenatal Care in America.* New York: New York University Press, 2000.
Taylor, Janelle S. "The Public Fetus and the Family Car: From Abortion Politics to a Volvo Advertisement." *Public Culture* 4 (1992): 167–183.
———. *Public Life of the Fetal Sonogram: Technology, Consumption, and the Politics of Reproduction.* New Brunswick, NJ: Rutgers University Press, 2008.
"Ten Great Public Health Achievements in the 20th Century." www.cdc.gov/about/history/tengpha.htm.
Tomes, Nancy. *The Gospel of Germs: Men, Women, and the Microbe in American Life.* Cambridge, MA: Harvard University Press, 1998.
Ulrich, Laurel Thatcher. "'The Living Mother of a Living Child': Midwifery and Mortality in Post-Revolutionary New England." *William and Mary Quarterly* 46 (1989): 27–48.
———. *A Midwife's Tale: The Life of Martha Ballard, Based on Her Diary, 1785–1812.* New York: Vintage Books, 1991.
Walker, Nancy A. *Shaping Our Mothers' World: American Women's Magazines.* Jackson: University Press of Mississippi, 2000.
Watkins, Elizabeth Siegel. *On the Pill: A Social History of Oral Contraceptives, 1950–1970.* Baltimore: Johns Hopkins University Press, 2001.
Wolf, Jacqueline H. *Deliver Me from Pain: Anesthesia and Birth in America.* Baltimore: Johns Hopkins University Press, 2009.
———. *Don't Kill Your Baby: Public Health and the Decline of Breastfeeding in the 19th and 20th Centuries.* Columbus: Ohio State University Press, 2001.
———. "Saving Mothers and Babies: Pioneering Efforts to Decrease Infant and Maternal Mortality." In *Silent Victories: The History and Practice of Public Health in Twentieth-Century America,* edited by John W. Ward and Christian Warren, 135–160. New York: Oxford University Press, 2007.

Index